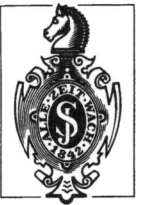

Gottfried Lemperle   Jürg Nievergelt

Plastic and Reconstructive Breast Surgery

An Atlas

Foreword by J. O. Strömbeck

With 538 Figures

Springer-Verlag Berlin Heidelberg GmbH

Professor Dr. med. G. Lemperle

Klinik für Plastische- und
Wiederherstellungschirurgie
St. Markus Krankenhaus
Wilhelm-Epstein-Str. 2
D-6000 Frankfurt/Main 50

Dr. med. J. Nievergelt

Service de chirurgie
plastique et reconstructive
Centre des Brûlés
Centre Hospitalier Universitaire Vaudois
CH-1011 Lausanne

Title of German Edition:
G. Lemperle, J. Nievergelt/Plastische Mammachirurgie
ISBN 978-3-662-01575-9

ISBN 978-3-662-01575-9

Library of Congress Cataloging-in-Publication Data
Lemperle, G. (Gottfried) [Plastische Mammachirurgie. English] Plastic and reconstructive breast surgery / Gottfried Lemperle, Jürg Nievergelt : foreword by J. O. Strombeck. p. cm. Translation of: Plastische Mammachirurgie. Includes bibliographical references and index.
ISBN 978-3-662-01575-9   ISBN 978-3-662-01573-5 (eBook)
DOI 10.1007/978-3-662-01573-5
1. Breast-Surgery. 2. Surgery, Plastic. I. Nievergelt. Jürg, 1943-   . II. Title. [DNLM: 1. Breast-surgery-atlases.
2. Surgery, Plastic-atlases.

© Springer-Verlag Berlin Heidelberg 1991
Originally published by Springer-Verlag Berlin Heidelberg New York in 1991
Softcover reprint of the hardcover 1st edition 1991

The use of general descriptive names, registered names, trademarks, etc. in this publication does not imply, even in the absence of a specific statement, that such names are exempt from the relevant protective laws and regulations and therefore free for general use.

Product Liability: The publisher can give no guarantee for information about drug dosage and application thereof contained in this book. In every individual case the respective user must check its accuracy by consulting other pharmaceutical literature.

24/3145-543210 - Printed on acid-free paper

Foreword

Plastic surgery of the breast has made tremendous progress in recent decades and today accounts for much of the work done in plastic surgical departments. The development of silicone prostheses and musculocutaneous flaps, for example, has made possible augmentation and reconstruction of the female breast as we know it today.

A mastery of the many problems in plastic and reconstructive surgery demands a high degree of training and experience. Because every surgeon cannot be expected to have the latter, he must take full advantage of the knowledge and experience of his colleagues. In response to this need, Gottfried Lemperle and Jürg Nievergelt have compiled a book which covers all major aspects of breast surgery. I am impressed by the wealth of experience that is reflected in the case selections and operative recommendations, and I am convinced that every surgeon can learn something from this book. Of particular value are the detailed discussions of complications and problems that every surgeon must eventually confront.

This atlas covers the complete range of plastic breast surgery in chapters that are clearly organized and logically arranged. The book is copiously illustrated and very easy to read.

I wish this work the great success that it deserves.

Stockholm, January, 1991   Jan Olof Strömbeck

Preface

A busy surgeon generally has little time for reading. His work requires him to look, evaluate, and act. We therefore conceived this book as a reference work in which the surgeon could look up a case that parallels his own problem and find a direct answer in the form of a series of pictures with accompanying text.

This book is not an introduction to breast surgery but is written for the experienced breast surgeon. It is intended to help the experienced surgeon with case-by-case decision making while directing his attention to specific details and complications. We have included many less common types of cases to provide the broadest possible coverage.

The advantage of this book over a multi-author text is that it originates from a single hospital and thus provides up-to-date information based on techniques and publications available as of early 1990. To keep the book concise, we describe only the methods and techniques that have proved most successful at our hospital over the past 20 years. To get the most from the book, the reader should have a solid foundation in plastic surgery and should be familiar with the various operative methods. The stimulating aspect of our field, after all, lies in the flexibility of its methods and techniques.

We are grateful to our senior staff members Dr. Dorin Radu, Dr. Klaus Exner, and Dr. Hermann Lampe and to all of our colleagues whose many ideas contributed to the refinement of techniques. We also express thanks to Mrs. Margarete Markert for performing the typing and bibliographic searches connected with this book, to Karl Weil of the Frankfurt University Pathology Department for his lucid drawings, and to the staff at Springer Verlag for their outstanding production work.

Frankfurt and Lausanne, January 1991
Gottfried Lemperle
Jürg Nievergelt

Table of Contents

Part A

Hypoplasias

1 Augmentation Mammoplasty

In a time when increasing emphasis is placed upon the female breast in fashion, movies, advertising, and personal affairs, it is not surprising that many women are unhappy with small or flabby breasts and become interested in augmentation. The development of the silicone gel prosthesis, introduced by Cronin in 1962, and the simplification of surgical technique have caused breast augmentation to become one of the most requested plastic surgical operations (Cronin and Gerow 1964).

The best candidates for augmentation mammoplasty are small-breasted women with an adequate distance between the nipple and inframammary line (more than 4 cm) or women with involuted, atrophic breasts that overhang the inframammary crease by no more than 2 cm.

Augmentation is not indicated for flabby, moderately ptotic breasts that would require simultaneous nipple elevation or skin reduction. When the patient is counseled, it should be emphasized that the implant will be placed within a natural space between the chest muscles and mammary gland, so that lactation will be unaffected and the glandular tissue will still be accessible for manual examination and radiography. The operation does not increase the risk of breast cancer, nor will it mask the presence of incipient cancer for the experienced examiner. Indeed, the implant so flattens the overlying breast tissue that the patient herself can palpate and detect even the smallest nodule.

The only risk to the patient is that of fibrous capsular contracture, whose pathogenesis is not yet fully understood.

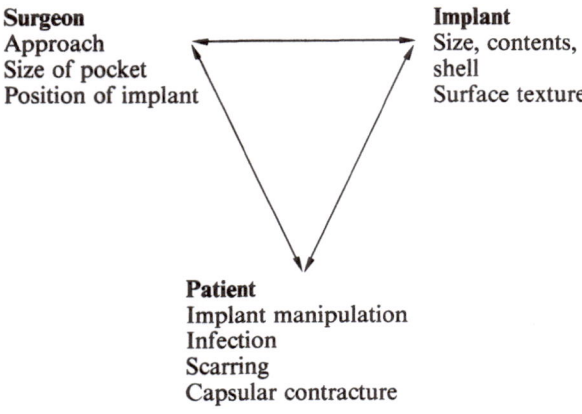

Surgeon
Approach
Size of pocket
Position of implant

Implant
Size, contents, shell
Surface texture

Patient
Implant manipulation
Infection
Scarring
Capsular contracture

Fig. 1.1. Factors that influence the result of augmentation mammoplasty

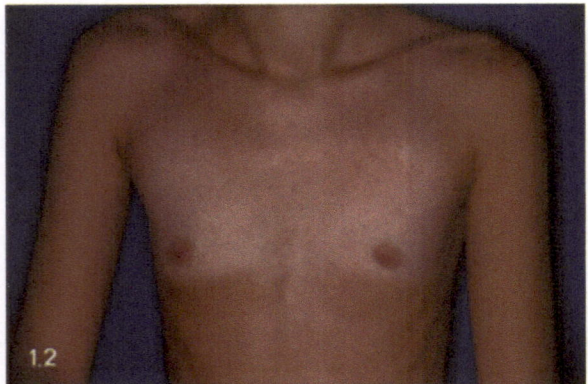

Fig. 1.2. Young woman with extreme mammary hypoplasia

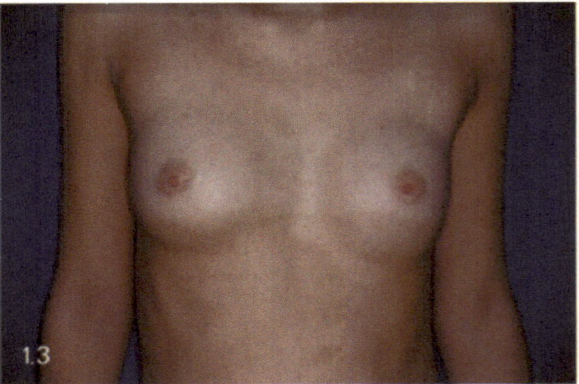

Fig. 1.3. With silicone implant augmentation, care must be taken that the center of the dissected pocket is directly beneath the areola

Technique: Transaxillary Approach

The operation should be performed under general anesthesia, as considerable force may be needed to separate the breast tissue from the pectoralis fascia. The upper arms are abducted about 70° from the body to create sufficient space in the axilla for insertion of the implant. Before draping, we inject 50 ml of a 0.5% local anesthetic containing 1 ml of POR 8 (Sandoz) or 1:400,000 epinephrine circumferentially around both breasts.

For development of the prepectoral space, we use a No. 14 Hegar dilator (Aesculap) that has been lengthened by 8 cm (Fig. 1.5). The dissection must be carried 2 cm past the border of the pectoralis muscle medially and inferiorly, as a smaller pocket would compress the implant into a spherical shape.

Tube drainage is almost never required, because blunt dissection of the pocket rarely provokes bleeding. In vessels that are bluntly disrupted, the media will retract in the adventitia and provide a physical hemostasis.

When the pocket is developed laterally, attention must be given to the "mammillary nerve" (Jäger and Schneider 1982), which emerges from the fourth intercostal space at the level of the midaxillary line. Division of this nerve will cause loss of deep sensation in the nipple area!

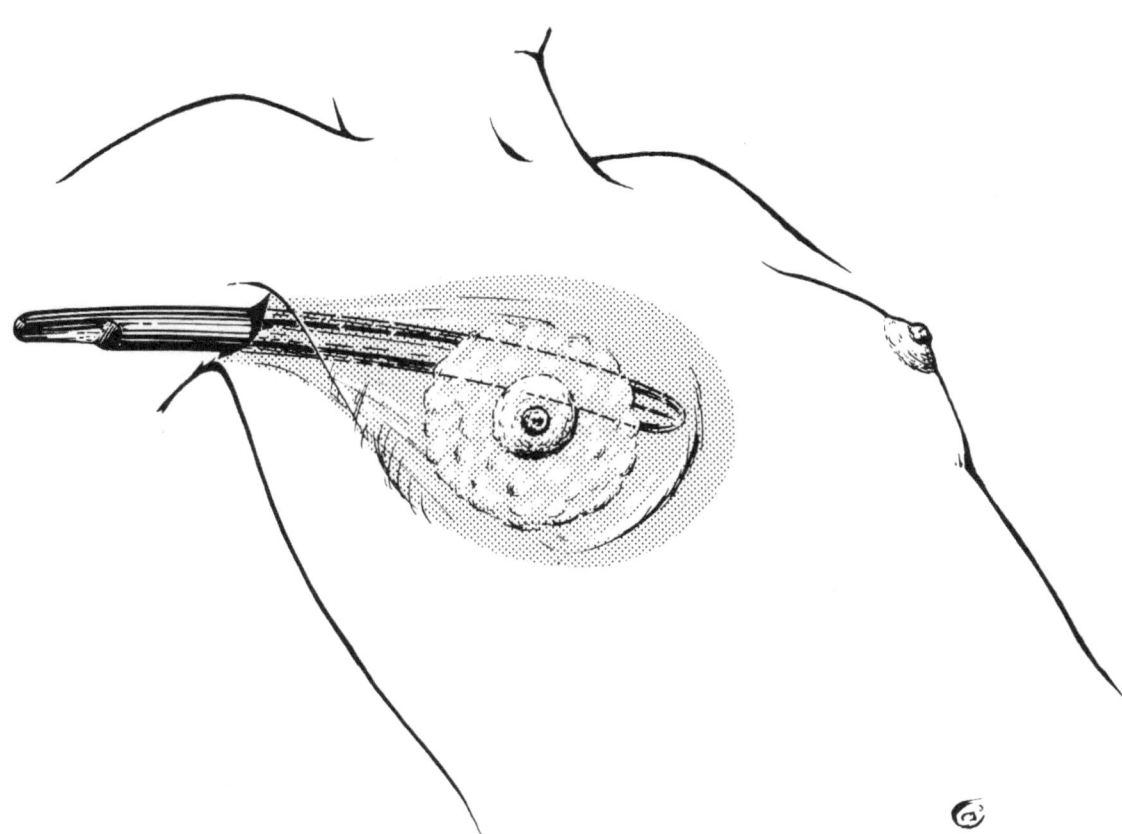

Fig. 1.4. The transaxillary approach to the retromammary space is made through a 4-cm sagittal incision in the dome of the axilla. The incision may be extended 1–3 cm posteriorly if required, but it should not be visible from the front. The first 2 cm of the pocket is developed by sharp scissors dissection until the anterior border of the pectoralis muscle is reached. From there the surgeon dissects bluntly with the middle finger toward the clavicle and manubrium sterni and then clockwise along the sternum to the inframammary crease. If the middle finger is not long enough (this is often the case in the lower medial quadrant), a dissecting instrument must be used

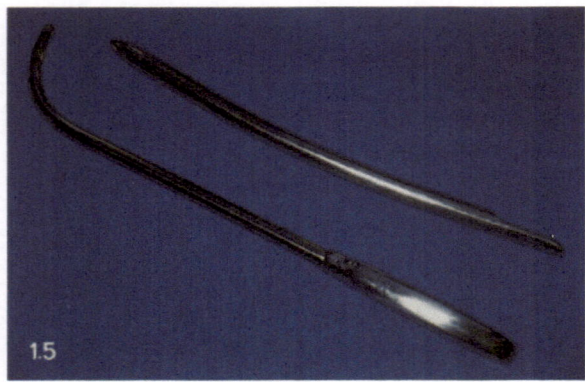

Fig. 1.5. Agris dissector (Padgett) and extended Hegar dilator (Aesculap)

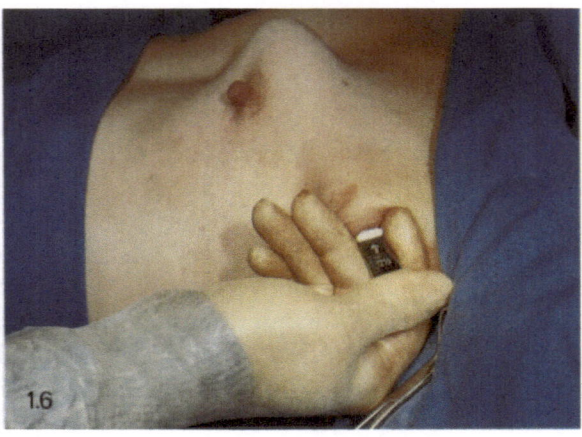

Fig. 1.6. The tip of the instrument must rupture the suspensory ligaments between the breast tissue and skin in the area of the inframammary crease. The tip is directed toward the skin, therefore

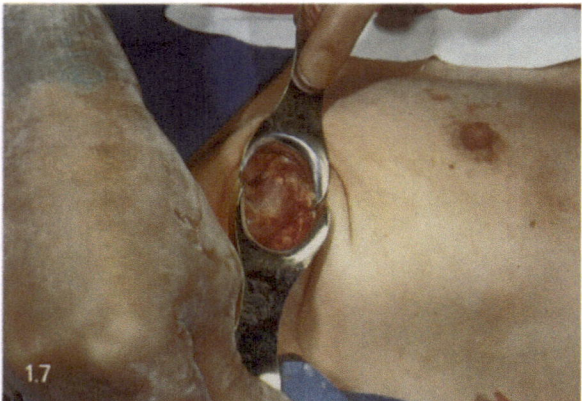

Fig. 1.7. Holding the incision open with Langenbeck retractors may tear the wound anteriorly. This is avoided by using buccal retractors to hold the incision open and direct the plane of the opening toward the surgeon's face. During insertion of the implant, the right index finger first pushes the valve in the direction of the pectoralis major muscle. The five fingers of the left hand exert a concentric pressure on the implant to keep it within the pocket. The surgeon confirms that the valve is placed posteriorly before closing the skin

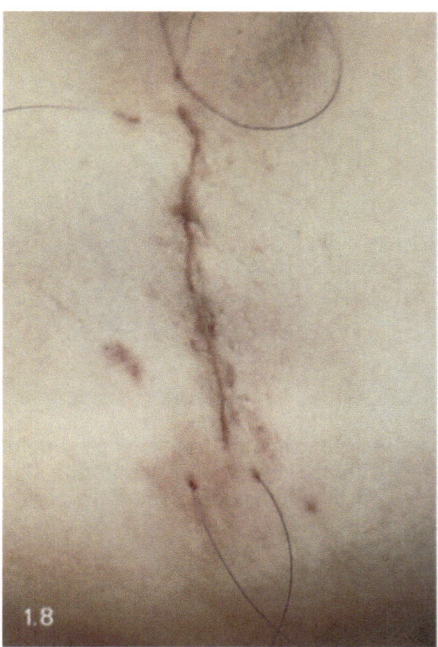

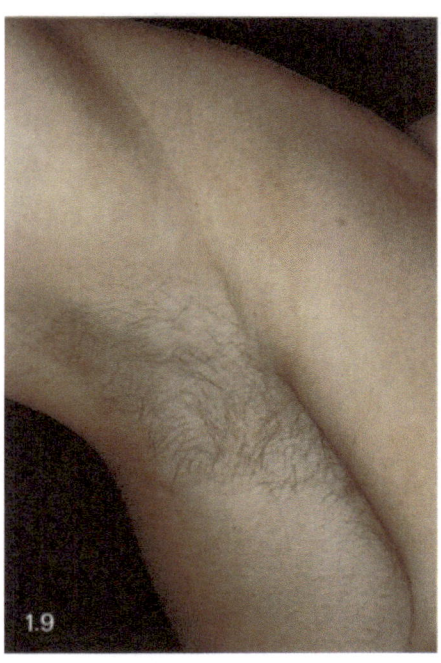

Fig. 1.8. Double intracutaneous closure of the axillary incision after the instillation of 40 mg gentamycin or 1 g Cephalothin in 20 ml of saline. On completion of the operation, the implant should be moved about to ensure that all surfaces of the pocket are wetted with the antibiotic solution

Fig. 1.9. Even light axillary hair growth at several weeks postoperatively is sufficient to hide the scar, especially since the skin in the hair-bearing portion of the axilla is not prone to hypertrophic scarring

Fig. 1.10. Scar hypertrophy is a danger in the inframammary approach. Up to 30% of European women and up to 50% of young Asian and black women tend to develop this complication. We see no advantages in the inframammary route, as bleeding is extremely rare when the submammary space is bluntly dissected and can be managed in any case with a suction drain. If scar hypertrophy is feared, the incision can be made *vertically* between the areola and inframammary crease, or it can even be *angled* (Planas) so that part is vertical and part is on the inframammary line

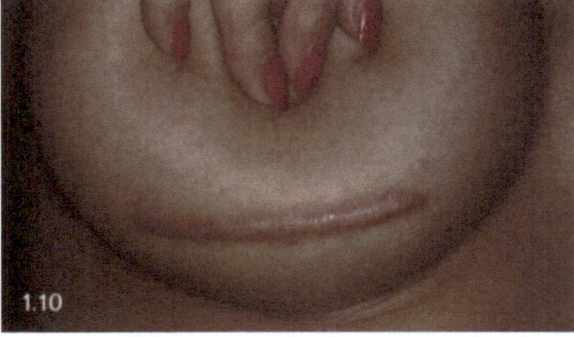

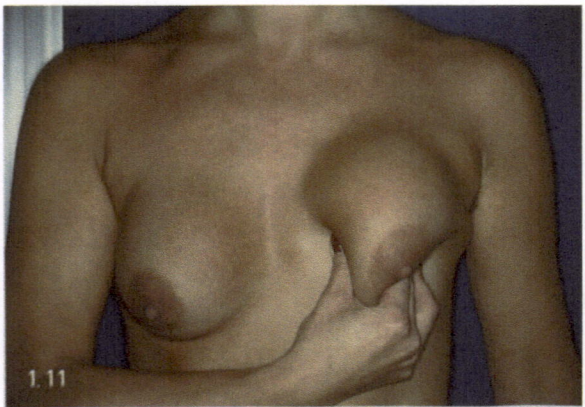

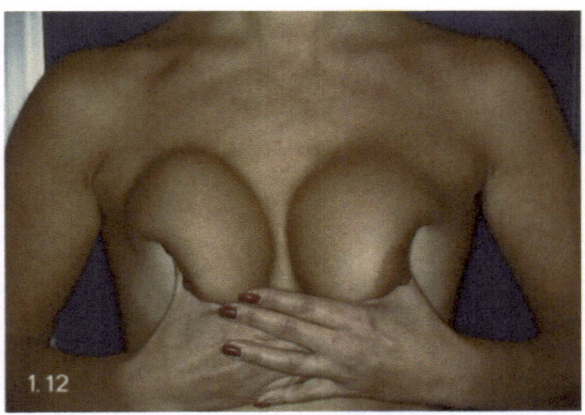

Fig. 1.11. Starting on the first postoperative day, the implant is moved about in all directions to ensure that the pocket maintains its full size and acquires a good fibroblast lining. The patient should understand this and should massage her breasts twice daily for the first six months, forcibly pressing the implant toward the pocket periphery to disrupt any adhesive bands that have formed there. Special care is taken to push the implant upward and medially, where there may still be soreness during the first week. If necessary this maneuver can be assisted with the free hand

Fig. 1.12. For the first few months the patient should sleep on her side with the lower arm supporting the breast. This helps to push both implants toward the center so that cleavage is maintained

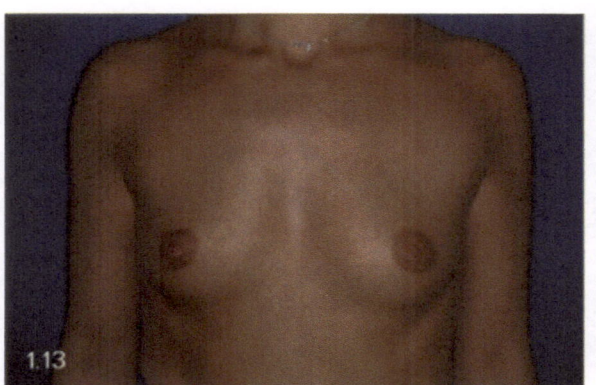

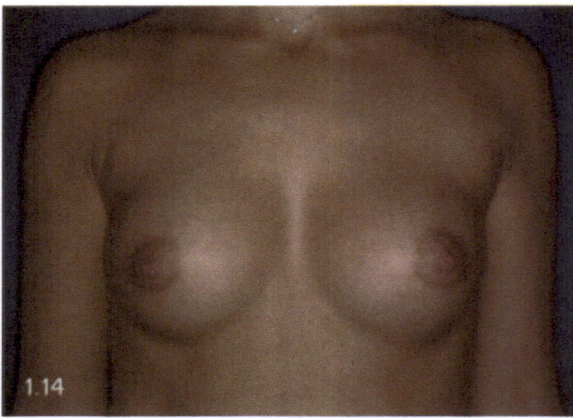

Fig. 1.13. Postpartum involutional atrophy of both breasts

Fig. 1.14. Breast volume restored bilaterally with 180-ml silicone implants

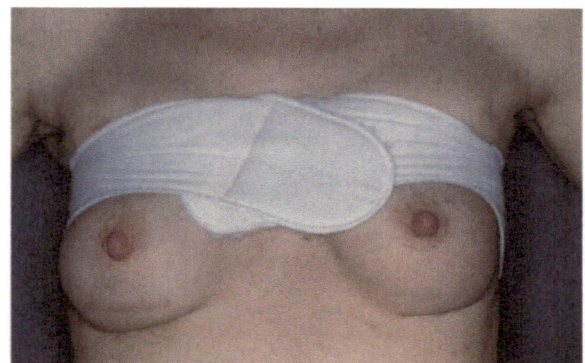

Fig. 1.15. If textured implants are used (Hester 1988), it is wise to apply an elastic girdle day and night for about 4 weeks to keep the implant down at the level of the inframammary fold

Implants

There are about ten manufacturers of implantable breast prostheses, mostly in the U.S., which offer four basic types of silicone implant for breast augmentation:

1. Saline-filled silicone shells have the advantage of being radiolucent on mammograms, and they eliminate the danger of "siliconomas" in case of rupture. However, saline-filled implants are subject to perforation as a result of material fatigue and abrasion at small ridges. Such an implant can deflate overnight, necessitating replacement. Saline-filled shells still have a greater than 20% rate of spontaneous perforation!

2. Older types of simple silicone gel prosthesis had a serious problem with "bleeding" (Fig. 2.3), and very thin-shelled implants (manufactured from 1974 to 1977) were prone to spontaneous rupture leading to siliconoma formation. The gel implants available today have a protective layer that largely prevents bleeding between the semipermeable silicone membranes. Additionally, the silicone shells are made from a far more tear-resistant material than was previously used.

3. Bilumen implants (after Hartley 1976) (Fig. 2.1) have been available since 1975. Their great advantages are negligible bleeding and the ability to add diffusible agents such as cortisones or antibiotics for prophylaxis of capsular contracture and infection. Because of this, we use these implants almost exclusively for simple augmentations. We routinely instill 12.5 mg of prednisolone in 30–50 ml of saline solution.

4. Implants with a polyurethane foam coating (Meme, Replicon) are associated with a significantly lower rate of capsular contracture. However, because the polyurethane coating separates from the silicone shell over time and is broken down by macrophages and foreign-body giant cells (i.e., incites an intense foreign-body reaction), we currently use these implants only after subcutaneous mastectomies. Another problem is the necessity of removing all surrounding granulation and capsular tissue in case the implant must be changed. (Fig. 2.19)

5. Since 1988, silicone implants with a textured surface (Fig. 1.16) have been introduced in the U.S. with claims of good results. These "textured" implants are said to have a less than 2% incidence of capsular contracture. These implants (Biocell by McGhan, Siltex by Mentor, Misti by Bioplasty, Silastic MSI by Dow Corning) may well replace implants with smooth surfaces. Siltex has a pore size of 30–50 μm, Misti, a particle size of 80–400 μm, Biocell - a pore size of 300–800 μm, and Silastic MSI - interstices of 200–300 μm between cones 750 μm in length. Instead of a constricting fibrous capsule, the textured implants incite the formation of a granulation layer with an irregular fiber network.

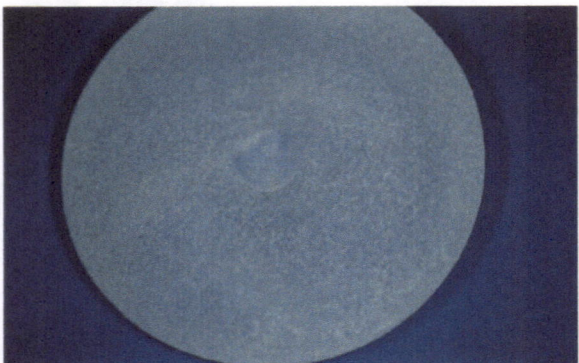

Fig. 1.16. "Textured" implants (here a Biocell implant, McGhan) still have to prove the reduced capsule rate claimed by the manufacturers. In our first series of 142 textured implants of different origin, we had a 23% rate of Baker III and IV capsule formation in subcutaneous mastectomy patients (see Caffee 1990)

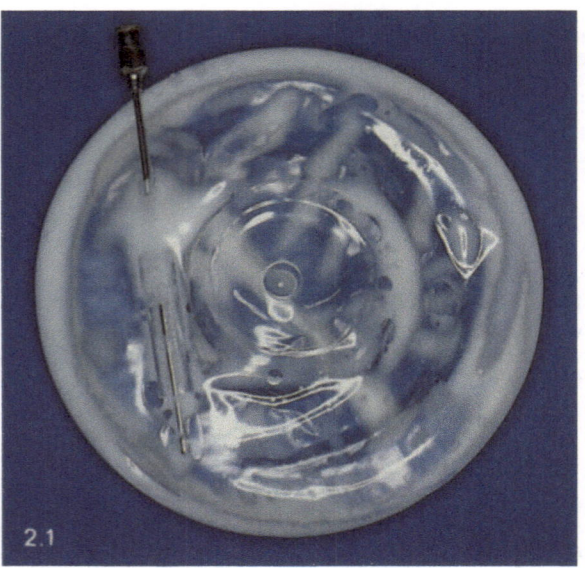

Fig. 2.1. Double-lumen silicone implant with 12.5 mg of prednisolone instilled into the outer shell

2 Complications

While great strides have been made in the prevention of fibrous capsular contracture during the last decade (addition of cortisone, implant massage, closed capsulotomy), there is still a certain percentage of women who will develop unilateral or bilateral capsular contracture within a period of weeks, or in some cases, years following augmentation mammoplasty.*

Among our own patients, the incidence of capsular contracture has declined from 18% before 1976 to 4.9% owing to the three manipulations listed above. It has been found that hematomas and seromas have as little etiologic significance

in capsular contracture as the "silicone bleed" implicated by so many authors. On the other hand, there is compelling evidence (Burkhardt et al. 1986, Lemperle and Exner 1990) that infection with nonpathogenic cutaneous organisms, most notably *Staphylococcus epidermidis,* constitutes the major cause of capsular contracture. These subclinical infections are very difficult to detect in their early stage, for the risk of implant perforation makes bacterial smears difficult to obtain.

For prophylaxis, then, we routinely instill 40 mg of gentamycin or 1 g cephalothin in 20 ml of saline solution into the implant pocket at the end of the operation.

Thinning of the skin overlying the implant has been described in the literature (Ellenberg 1977, Eder et al. 1981) and observed by us in patients treated with cortisone. So far it has affected only augmentations in which triamcinolone (Volon-A) had been instilled into double-lumen implants. Currently we use bilumen implants with 20 mg of triamcinolone added only when there is an extreme tendency toward recurrent capsule formation, and we carefully counsel the patient about the risk of cutaneous thinning.

---

* The Baker classification (Baker 1976) is used to grade the severity of capsular contractures:
Baker 1: The prosthesis cannot be felt or seen.
Baker 2: The prosthesis can be felt but not seen.
Baker 3: The prosthesis can be felt and seen.
Baker 4: The breast is hard, painful, and cold. Distortion is often marked.

In the course of physiologic aging, the breast undergoes a gradual ptosis with a corresponding descent of the nipple. But a silicone prosthesis, once implanted, becomes fixed to the chest wall by the fibrous capsule and will remain at that level for the patient's lifetime. The result is a gradual sagging of the breast over the fixed implant until the nipple points downward. The crescent-shaped periareolar skin excision offers a relatively simple technique for returning the nipple to the most prominent part of the breast (Figs. 3.12–3.14).

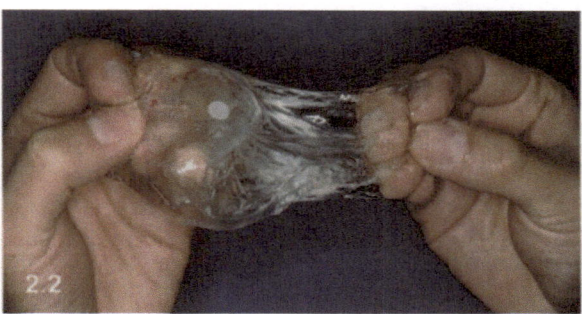

Fig. 2.2. Ruptured silicone implant, showing its gelatinous filling

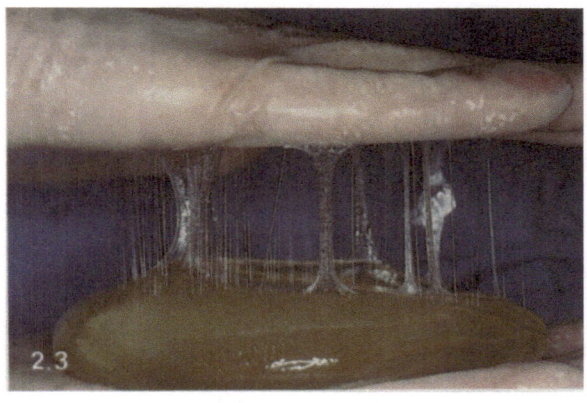

Fig. 2.3. Extreme "gel bleed" from a prosthesis removed 10 years after implantation

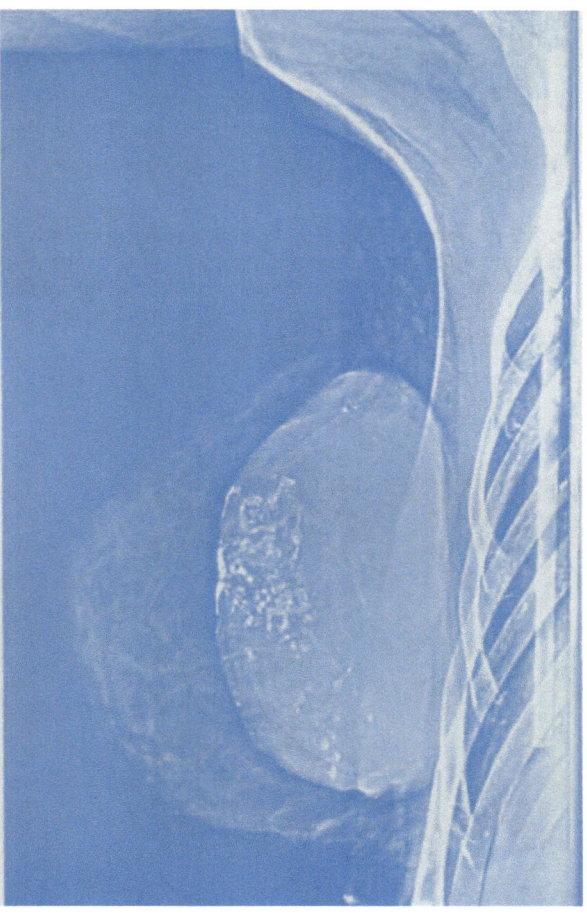

Fig. 2.4. Xeroradiograph showing marked calcification of the capsule and "siliconomas" in the axillary lymphatics four years after the implant was replaced due to rupture

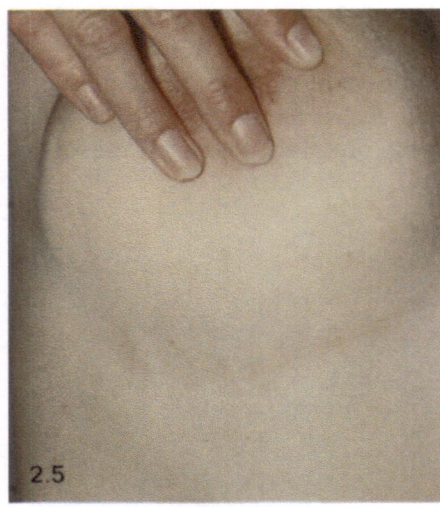

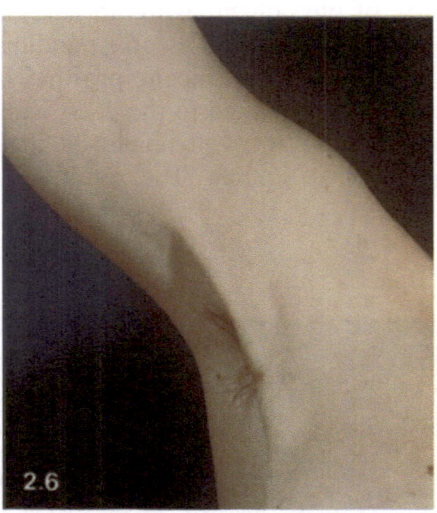

Fig. 2.5. Mondor's sign. For several weeks, thrombosed cutaneous veins can form palpable and visible bands that may extend from the inframammary crease as far as the lower abdomen. Though sometimes quite painful, they resolve spontaneously within three months

Fig. 2.6. Mondor's bands can develop in all operations on the breast. Occurring in the axilla, they can cause discomfort when the arm is raised. Treatment is not required

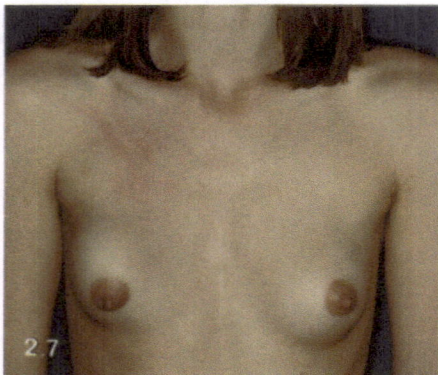

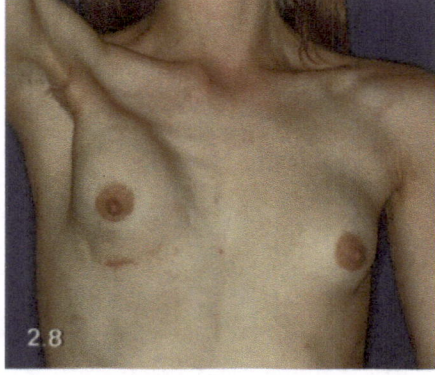

Fig. 2.7. Unilateral capsular contracture of the right breast, probably secondary to infection by *Staphylococcus epidermidis*

Fig. 2.8. In the same patient, a very prominent band is seen extending between the axilla and inframammary crease when the right arm is raised. Extreme cases of this kind can be managed by injecting triamcinolone (Volon-A) into the band at intervals of four weeks

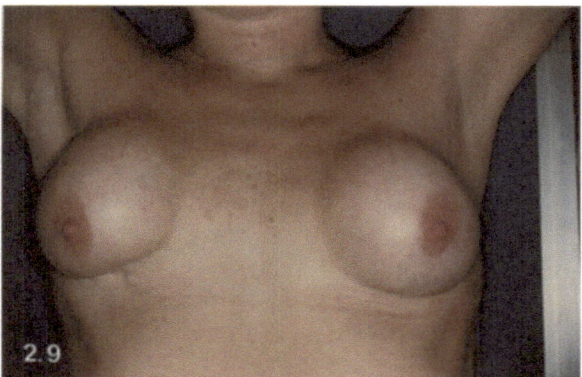

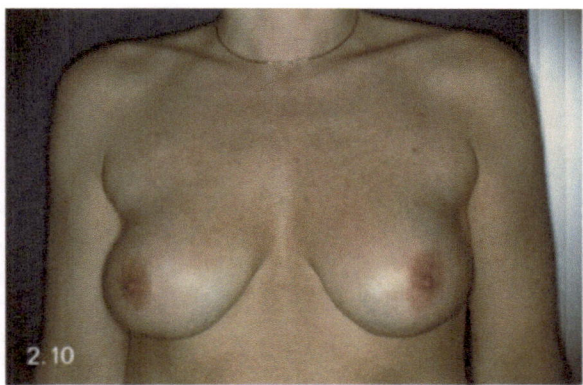

Fig. 2.9. Even an implant with minimal capsule formation becomes conspicuous when the arms are raised. In this patient the capsular contracture is associated with superolateral displacement (Baker III) not correctible by squeeze capsulotomy, necessitating replacement of the implants

Fig. 2.10. If the patient responds well to the small dose of 12.5 mg prednisolone, the constriction may loosen during the first postoperative year with a corresponding descent of the inframammary crease. In this patient (the same as in Fig. 2.9) the prostheses had to be changed for bilumen implants with 50 mg prednisolone due to severe capsular contracture. Five months later the revisionary prostheses had to be changed for prednisolone-free implants

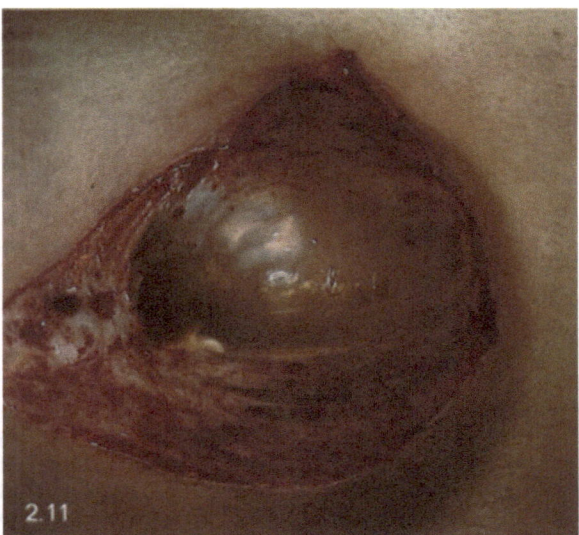

Fig. 2.11. In patients treated with cortisone, the capsule can become greatly thinned, and there may be simultaneous thinning of the overlying skin. The patient must be informed of this possibility. In all cases the cortisone effect is reversible after replacement of the implant

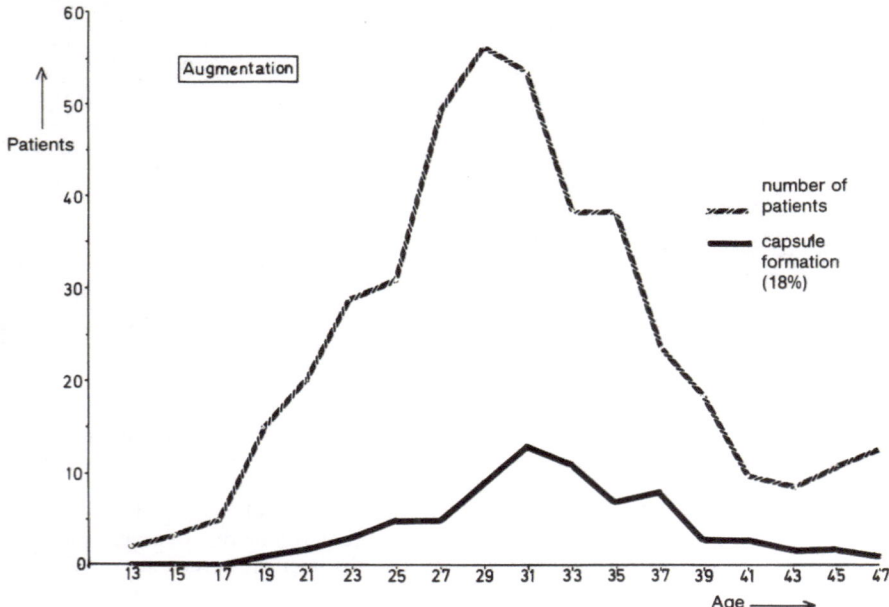

Fig. 2.12. The incidence of capsular contracture is similar for all age groups. (Patients with simple silicone prostheses, 1971–1978)

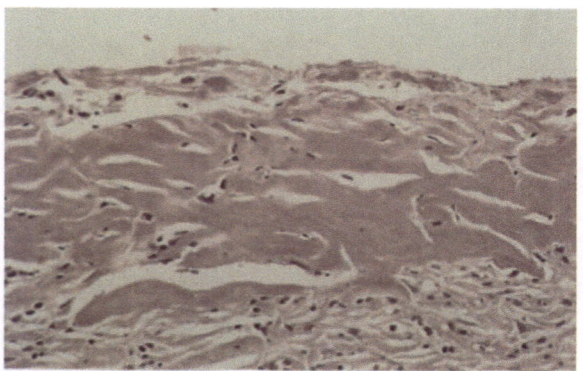

Fig. 2.13. Histologic appearance of a constrictive fibrous capsule 6 weeks after implantation of a smooth-walled prosthesis. The paucity of cell nuclei and the absence of blood vessels are noteworthy features. The clinical and histologic thickness of a fibrous capsule do not relate to the clinical prominence of the contracture. A successful capsulotomy requires only that the capsule (=scar) is mature; this "ripening" generally takes at least 6 months

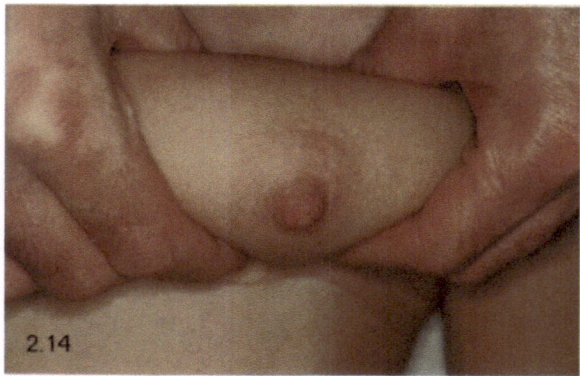

Fig. 2.14. Compression capsulotomy: To achieve a cruciate capsulotomy, the fibrous capsule is first broken horizontally by exerting a strong squeezing force toward the base. The surgeon can do this most easily by standing at the patient's head

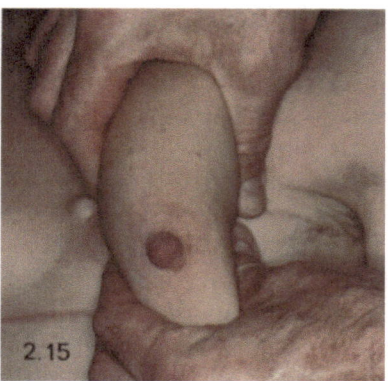

Fig. 2.15. After pausing a few seconds to let the pain from the initial rupture subside, the surgeon applies an equally strong squeezing force in the vertical direction. Note: If the implant is too high, it cannot be lowered by external manipulation

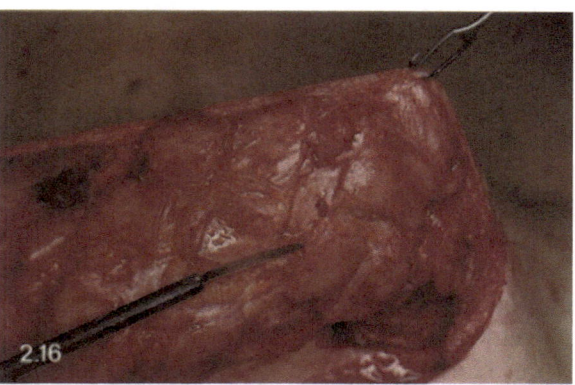

Fig. 2.16. If closed capsulotomy is unsuccessful even after one year, an open capsulotomy is performed in which the contracture is released by "cross-hatching" the capsule with an electrocautery. Some authors recommend complete excision of the capsule

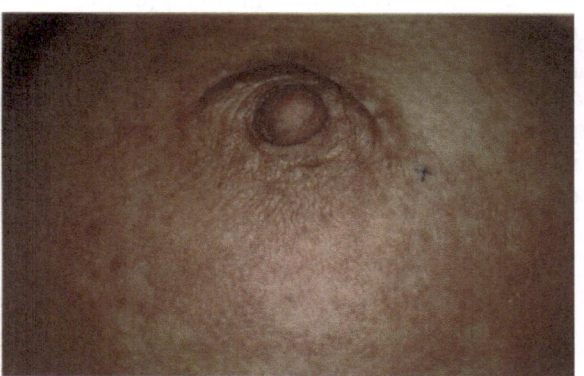

Fig. 2.17. Typical nonitching rash occurring in about 50% of patients with polyurethane foam coated implants 3-6 weeks after operation. Extent, duration, and severity of the rash can be reduced by administration of 40 mg triamcinolone acetonide (Kenalog, Squibb)

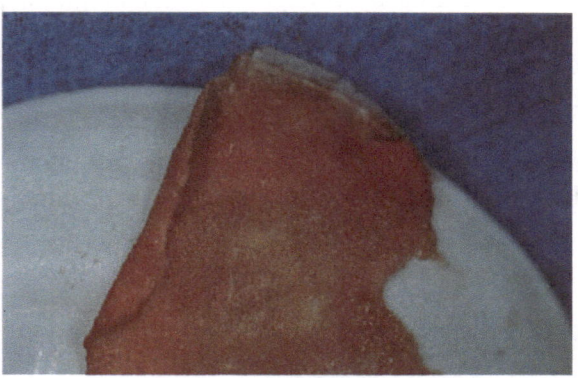

Fig. 2.18. Polyurethane foam coating separates as early as 1 week after implantation from the silicone shell of a "même" implant

Fig. 2.19. Polyurethane foam coating of a natural Y prosthesis (Ashley) still present in the capsule 18 years after implantation

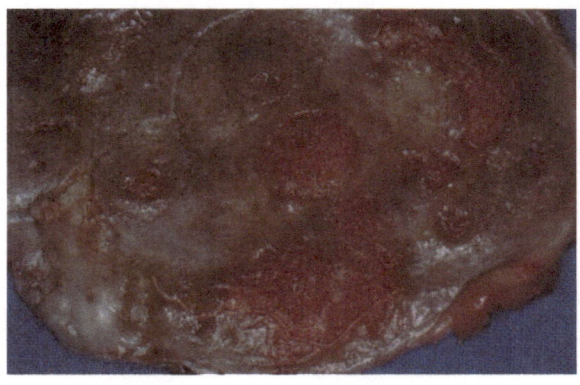

3 Siliconomas

The formation of silicone masses ("siliconomas") following the rupture of a breast implant was most commonly seen in the early days of the compression capsulotomy, i.e., in the period from 1976 to 1980. From 1974 to 1977, various manufacturers offered very thin-walled prostheses with thin gel that could easily be ruptured by a closed capsulotomy. An extremely soft breast in which an implant is no longer palpable should raise suspicion of an implant rupture. A simple clinical test is to push the gel upward with the patient seated and then release it. With a ruptured implant, the gel will adhere strongly to the surrounding capsule and will be very slow in settling back to its original position. The rupture can be verified by sonography, mammography, or preferably by xeroradiography, which will demonstrate the uneven surface of the ruptured prosthesis.

In theory, a ruptured implant surrounded by an intact capsule could simply be left alone. However, the persistent gel bleed might eventually lead to calcifications of the capsule (Fig. 3.9) with thickening and further constriction, so a change of implants is always advised.

In cases where a closed capsulotomy has breached the capsule but has also caused a rupture of the prosthesis, the latter should be removed at once before the extracapsular gel can disseminate into the chest muscles, migrate to axillary nodes, or even travel to the elbow through the neurovascular sheath of the upper arm (Fig. 3.7). All palpable siliconomas that develop within a period of weeks to years after the rupture must be surgically removed. A suction cannula is used to remove free gel from muscle and axillary tissue. Six-month follow-up visits with sonography (Herzog 1989) are mandatory for the next five years.

There is much speculation about a possible link between silicone implants and "human adjuvant disease" (Weisman et al. 1988) (certain rheumatoid symptoms without typical laboratory proof) as well as systemic sclerosis (Varga et al. 1989). So far, however, there is no statistical proof that these two syndromes occur more often in patients with silicone implants than in the general population.

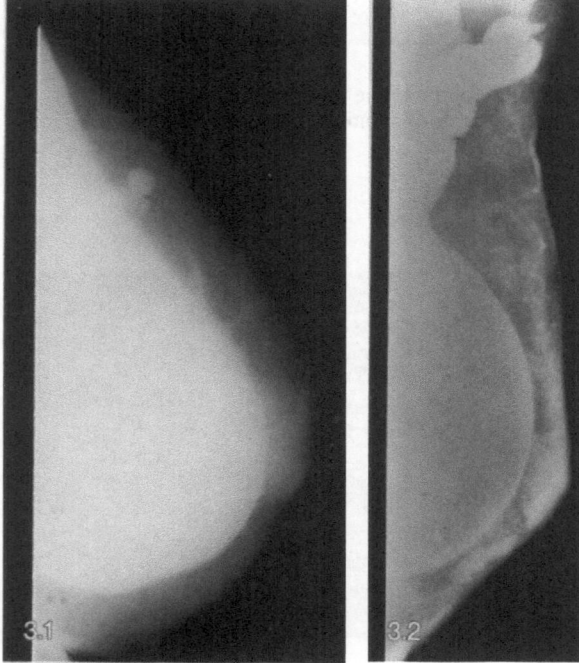

Fig. 3.1. Palpable nodes developing after breast augmentation should raise suspicion of a siliconoma. These masses are best documented by xeroradiography (see Fig. 2.4)

Fig. 3.2. The path to the axilla should be palpated with particular care, since extravasated gel is transported there by the pumping action of the pectoralis major muscle and by lymphatic drainage

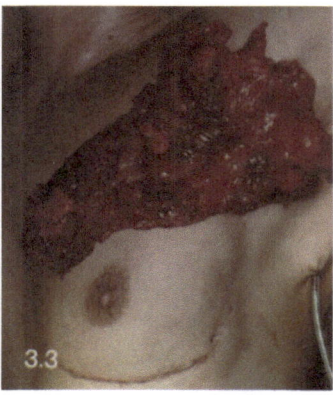

Fig. 3.3. Here the whole pectoral muscle is permeated by siliconomas, necessitating its complete removal

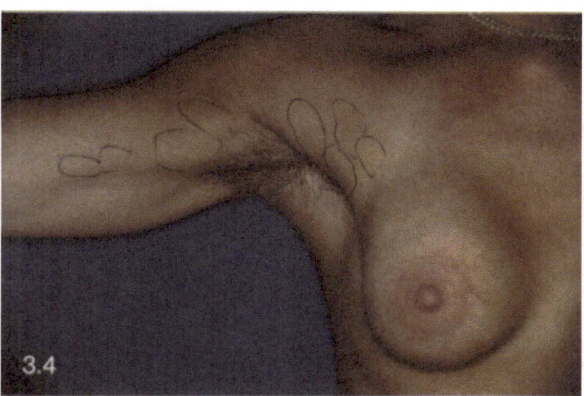

Fig. 3.4. Multiple siliconomas detected three years after a compression capsulotomy. By this time the gel has migrated along the arm muscles and into the septa. The breast was augmented with a thin-shell, soft-gel implant manufactured betwen 1974 and 1976

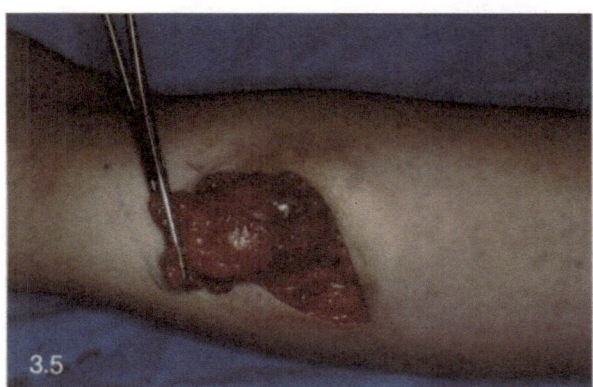

Fig. 3.5. All palpable silicone masses are excised, even though these giant-cell granulomas have not been known to undergo malignant change. Siliconomas are an indication for total capsulectomy, at which time the muscles are carefully inspected and palpated. Here, heavily infiltrated fascia is being excised from the ventral side of the upper arm

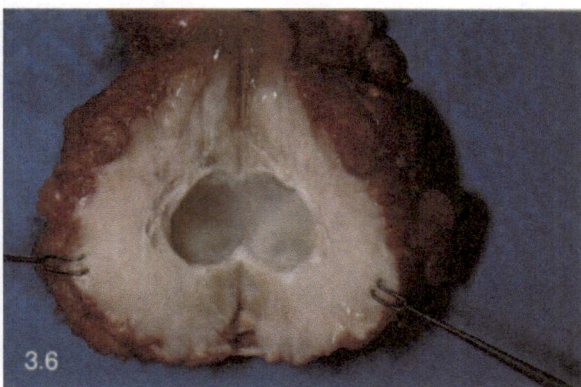

Fig. 3.6. Siliconoma found in a Korean woman 18 years after breast augmentation by liquid silicone injection

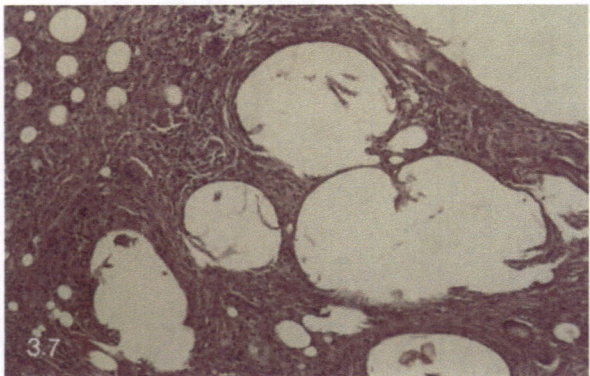

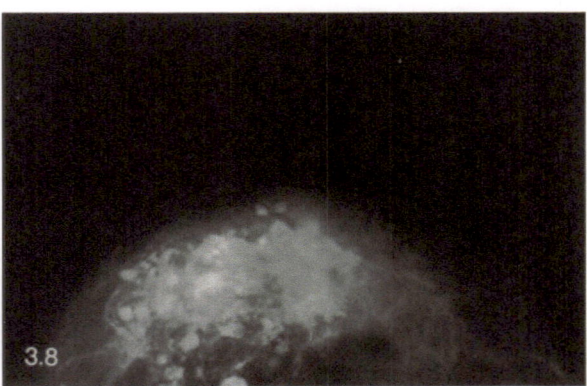

Fig. 3.7. Histologic section from a siliconoma shows multiple vacuoles of varying size and prominent giant cells with up to 50 nuclei. In theory, masses of this kind should resolve spontaneously through gradual absorption of all the silicone

Fig. 3.8. Mammogram showing silicone drops 22 years after the injection of silicone oil

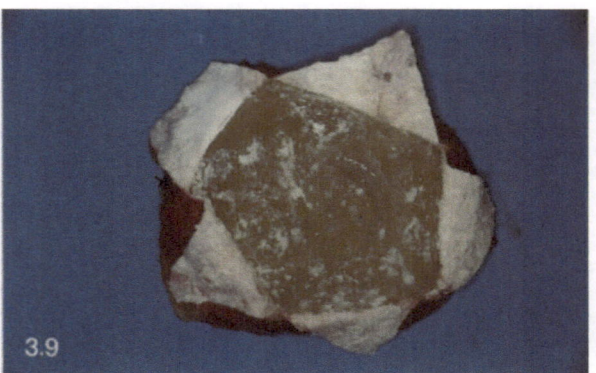

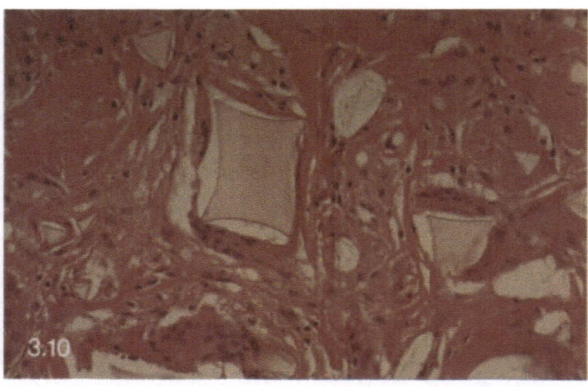

Fig. 3.9. Heavily calcified capsule 21 years after the insertion of a prosthesis that bled a large amount of gel (see Fig. 2.4). This problem should not occur with the reinforced shells (HP material, interposed teflon layer) available today

Fig. 3.10. Histologic appearance of the cellular reaction to the polyurethane coating on the Ashley prosthesis. The trabecular structure of the polyurethane is gradually broken down by giant cells. Polyurethane-coated prostheses (Replicon) are currently undergoing a renaissance (Hester) owing to their tendency to incite the formation of nonconstricting granulation tissue rather than a fibrous capsule

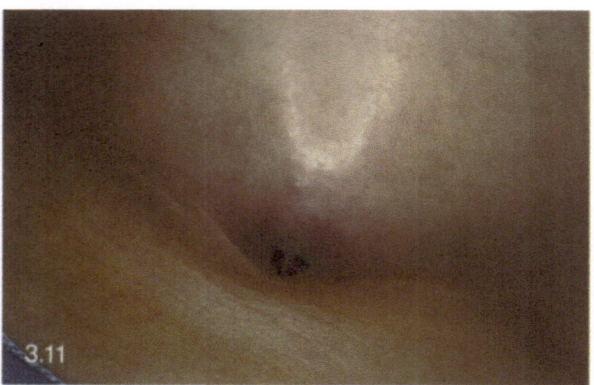

Fig. 3.11. Perforation of the skin over a fold in the implant, which eroded through the skin during respiratory movements. This complication is managed by open capsulotomy, suction drainage for six days (see Fig. 15.28), and closure of the perforation site in layers

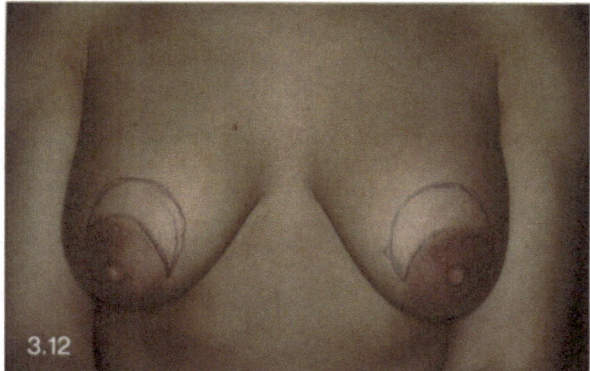

Fig. 3.12. Over the years, the nipple descends due to physiologic stretching of the skin over the implant and eventually points downward

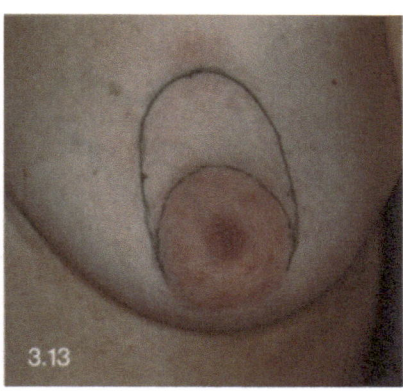

Fig. 3.13. The nipple can be raised to a more prominent site on the breast by making a simple crescent-shaped skin excision above the areola

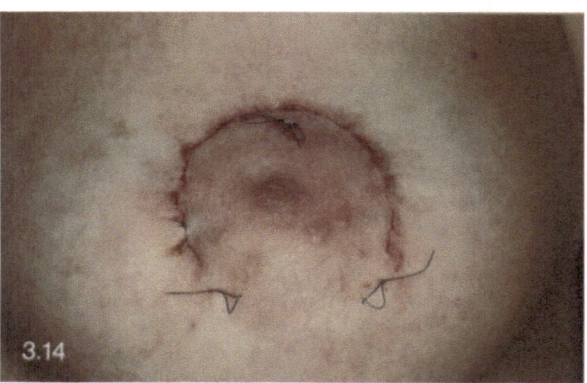

Fig. 3.14. Completion of the outpatient procedure. The corium of the nipple-areola complex has been sutured to the corium of the skin with buried monofilament absorbable threads. A silicone implant does not follow the ptotic descent of the aging breast, but remains fixed at the level of the inframammary crease

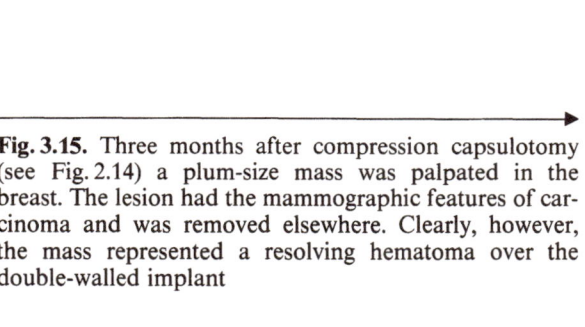

Fig. 3.15. Three months after compression capsulotomy (see Fig. 2.14) a plum-size mass was palpated in the breast. The lesion had the mammographic features of carcinoma and was removed elsewhere. Clearly, however, the mass represented a resolving hematoma over the double-walled implant

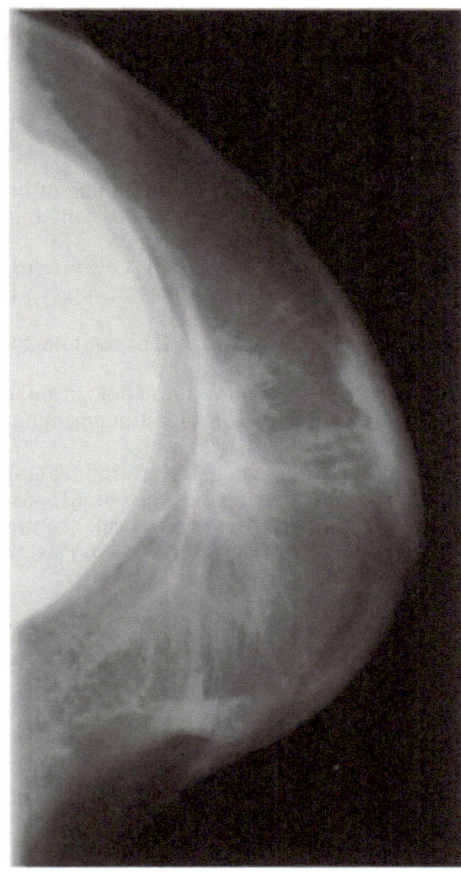

References

Agris JR, Ding O, Wilensky RJ (1976) A dissector for the transaxillary approach in augmentation mammaplasty. Plast Reconstr Surg 57: 10

Baker JL, Bartels RJ, Douglas WM (1976) Closed compression technique for rupturing a contracted capsule around a breast implant. Plast Reconstr Surg 58: 137–141

Becker H (1987) Breast augmentation using the expander mammary prosthesis. Plast Reconstr Surg 79: 192–199

Brand KG (1988) Foam-covered mammary implants. Clin Plast Surg 15: 533

Burkhardt BR, Dempsey PD, Schnur PL, Tofield JJ (1986) Capsular contracture: a prospective study of the effect of local antibacterial agents. Plast Reconstr Surg 77: 919–930

Caffee H (1990) Textured silicone and capsule contracture Ann Plast Surg (in press)

Cronin TD, Gerow FJ (1964) Augmentation mammaplasty: a new „natural feel" prosthesis. In: Transact. III. Int Congr Plast Surg, I. P. R. S. Excerpta Medica, Amsterdam (Int Congr Series 66, pp 41–49)

De Cholnoky T (1970) Augmentation mammaplasty: Surgery of complications in 10941 patients by 265 surgeons. Plast Reconstr Surg 45: 573

Eder H, Lejour M, Smahel J (1981) Steroid related complications of double-lumen prostheses with cortisone. Chir Plast 6: 95–103

Ellenberg AH (1977) Marked thinning of breast skin flap after the insertion of implants containing triamcinolone. Plast Reconstr Surg 60: 755–758

Ellenberg AH, Braun H (1980) A 3½ year experience with double lumen implants in breast surgery. Plast Reconstr Surg 65: 307–313

Ersek RA (1989) Prostheses for breast augmentation. Travis County Med Soc J, May

Ferreira JA (1984) The various etiological factors of „hard capsule" formation in breast augmentations. Aesthetic Plast Surg 8: 109–117

Gassel WD, Eisenmann A, Kaffarnik H (1982) Die Mondor'sche Krankheit. Chir Prax 30: 635–637

Gayou R, Rudolph R (1979) Capsular contraction around silicone mammary prostheses. Ann Plast Surg 2: 62–71

Hartley JH (1976) Specific applications of the double lumen prosthesis. Clin Plast Surg 3: 247–263

Herzog P (1989) Silicone granulomas: detection by ultrasonography. Plast Reconstr Surg 84: 856–857

Hester TR, Nahai F, Bostwick J, Cukic J (1988) A 5-year experience with polyurethane-covered mammary prostheses for treatment of capsular contracture, primary augmentation mammoplasty, and breast reconstruction. Clin Plast Surg 15: 569

Höhler H (1973) Breast augmentation: the axillary approach. Br J Plast Surg 26: 373–376

Höhler H (1977) Further progress in the axillary approach in augmentation mammaplasty: Prevention of incapsulation. Aesthetic Plast Surg 1: 107–113

Lemperle G (1979) Die Behandlung von Silikonprothesen für den Wiederaufbau und die Vergrößerung der weiblichen Brust. Schwester/Pfleger 18: 82–84

Lemperle G (1980) Unfavourable results after breast reconstruction with silicone implants. Acta Chir Belg 79: 159

Lemperle G, Exner K (1990) The effect of cortisone on capsule contracture in double lumen breast implants. (to be published)

Little G, Baker JL (1980) Results of closed compression capsulotomy for treatment of contracted breast implant capsules. Plast Reconstr Surg 65: 30–33

Perrin ER (1976) The use of soluble steroids within inflatable breast prothesis. Plast Reconstr Surg 57: 163–166

Peterson HE, Burt GB (1974) The role of steroids in the prevention of circumferential scaring in augmentation mammaplasty. Plast Reconstr Surg 54: 28

Shapiro MA (1989) Smooth versus rough: an 8-year survey of mammary prostheses. Plast Reconstr Surg 84: 44

Varga J, Schumacher R, Jimenez SA (1989) Systemic sclerosis after augmentation mammoplasty with silicone implants. Ann Int Med 111: 377–383

Vasquez B, Given KS, Houston GC (1987) Breast augmentation: a review of subglandular and submuscular implantation. Aesthetic Plast Surg 11: 101–105

Viñas JC (1966) Protesis mamarias por via axilar. Rev Actual Med 1: 1

Weisman MH, Vecchione TR, Albert D, Moore LT, Mueller MR (1988) Connective tissue disease following breast augmentation: a preliminary test of the human adjuvant disease hypothesis. Plast Reconstr Surg 82: 626–630

Part B

Hyperplasias

4 Reduction Mammoplasty

Indications

True instances of mammary hyperplasia and macromastia become apparent during adolescence and should be operatively treated at that time. Erosion of self-confidence, social isolation, and deterioration of self-image are some of the early psychological effects associated with this deformity. In addition, the weight of the enlarged breasts can lead to physical problems such as postural defects and myogeloses in the area of the cervical and upper thoracic spine, shoulder pain and furrowing from brassiere straps, and intertriginous eczema in the inframammary creases. The patient may be handicapped in her ability to engage in sports and other recreational activities, leading to problems in social adjustment and sometimes to neurotic postural attitudes.

If the hypertrophy is already extreme by 13 years of age, the importance of breast reduction justifies the residual – often hypertrophic – scarring, and early mammoplasty will spare the patient considerable anguish. If further breast growth takes place after the procedure, a second reduction mammoplasty may be considered at the age of 18.

The question of whether surgery is indicated on medical or aesthetic grounds should be decided case by case. A resected tissue volume greater than 400 g usually constitutes a medical indication, while a lesser resection is regarded as aesthetic. Exceptions where the reduction is done for psychologic need would include extreme ptosis in a young woman, asymmetry, and any type of malformation.

The goal of the reduction is to produce a breast shape and size that conform to the patient's body proportions. Thus, it is well for the surgeon to master various techniques that he can apply in accordance with the patient's age, skin characteristics, and anatomy. Of the many operations that have been devised for mammary reduction, we shall demonstrate the one that has given us the best results. It is based on the skin pattern of Wise (1956) (Fig. 4.8) and Strömbeck (1960) and involves resection of the lower quadrants. To decrease the length of the inframammary scar, we have modified the pattern markings by rounding the medial and lateral corners (Fig. 4.10).

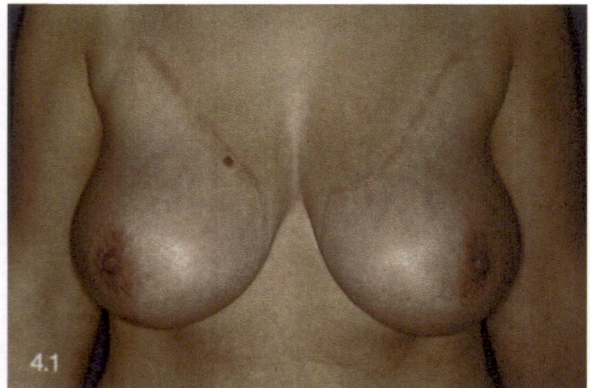

Fig. 4.1. Woman 40 years of age showing typical age-related ptosis of a formerly large and well-shaped breast

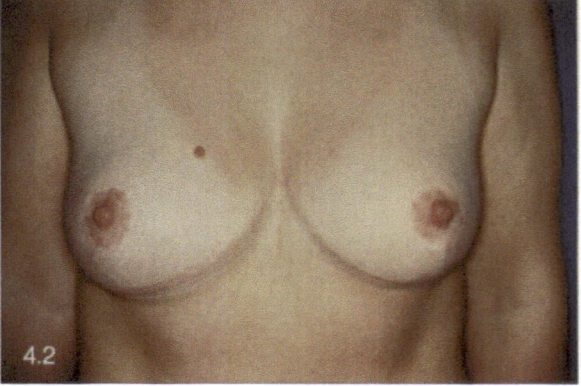

Fig. 4.2. Appearance one year after reduction mammoplasty, showing scar formation of average conspicuity

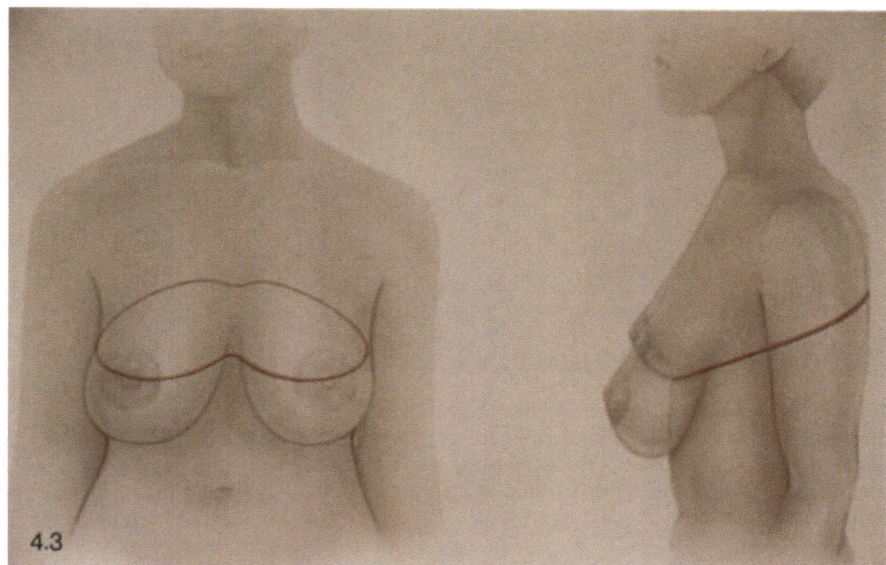

Fig. 4.3. The inframammary line encircles the chest like a belt. As its height is determined by the shape of the thoracic cage and not by the elasticity of the skin, its position is constant

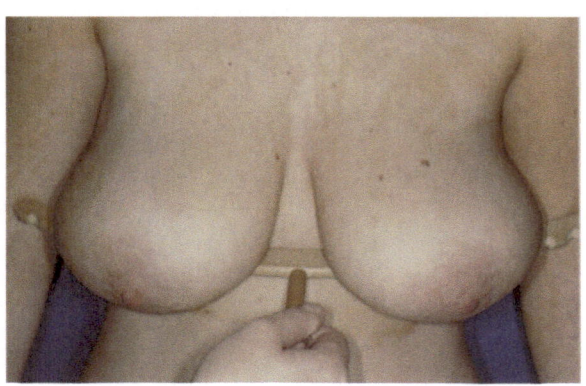

Fig. 4.4. The new nipple site should not be determined from a predefined set of measurements. It is located by pressing the index or index finger forward from the inframammary line

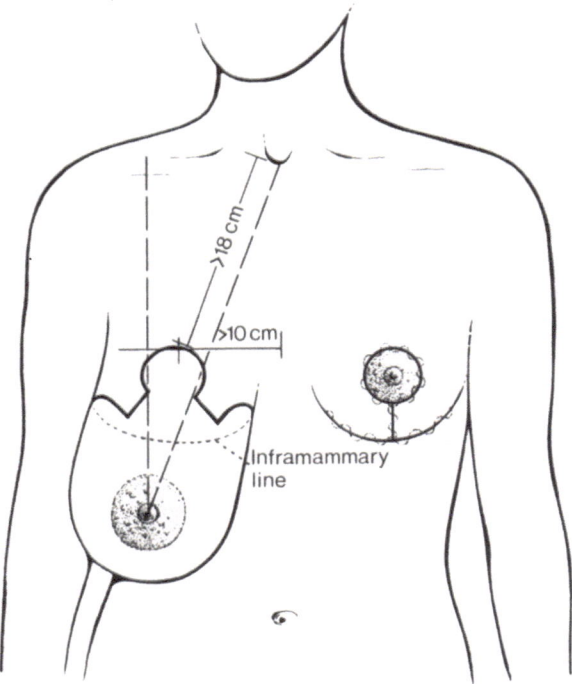

Fig. 4.5. The superior border of the new areola should be at least 18 cm from the sternal notch and 10 cm from the midsternal line

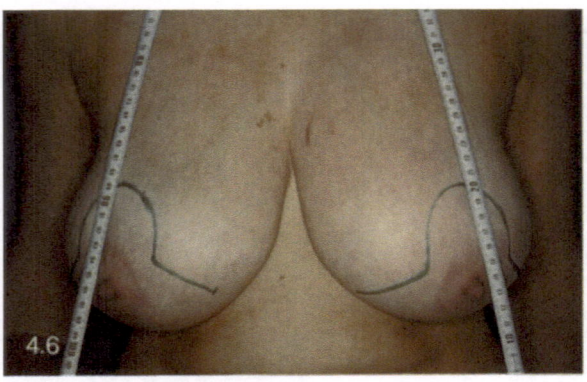

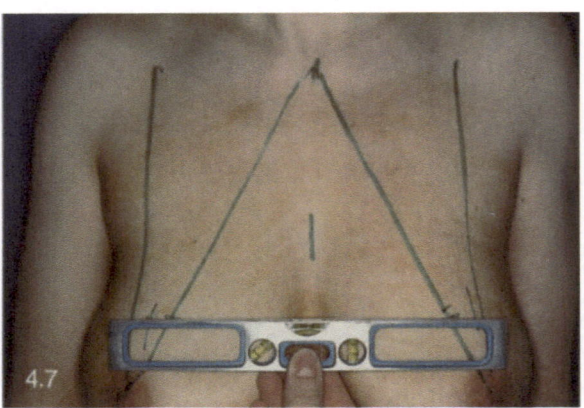

Fig. 4.6. The nipple level on one side is transferred to the opposite side by draping a measuring tape around the patient's neck so that it extends from the tip of one nipple to the other. The new nipple site is found by moving medially upward along the tape

Fig. 4.7. In large breasts, a line is drawn from the sternal notch to the nipple, and from there a second line is drawn vertically upward. The upper border of the nipple-areola is located by halving the horizontal distance between the two lines. A spirit level can be used to transfer the markings to the opposite side

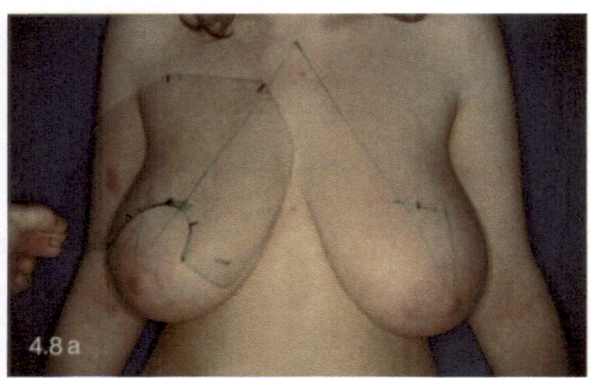

Fig. 4.8. a, b The breasts are now marked for resection using the skin pattern of Wise (1956) and Strömbeck (1964) (**a**). We have developed two additional patterns for use on large breasts (**b**)

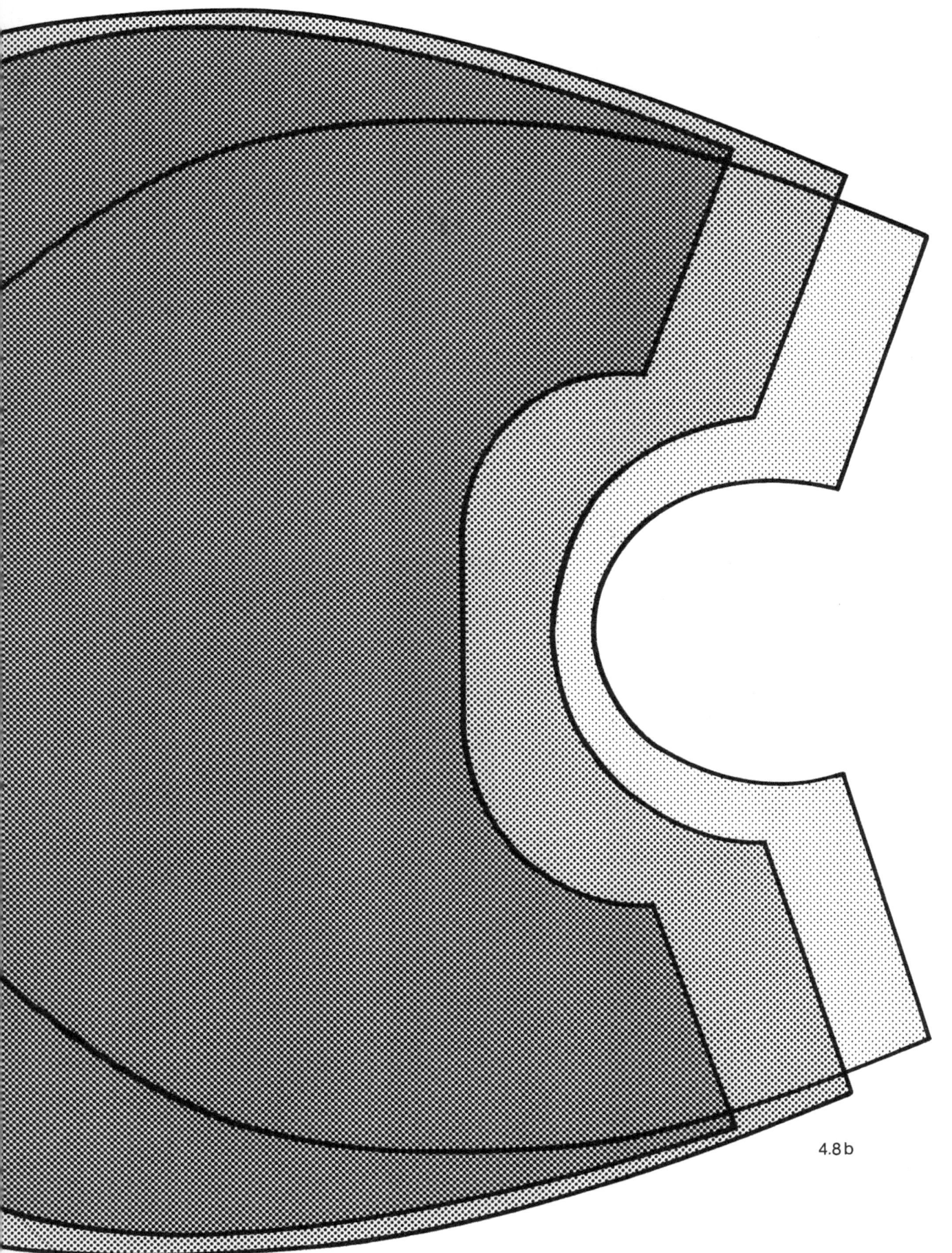

4.8 b

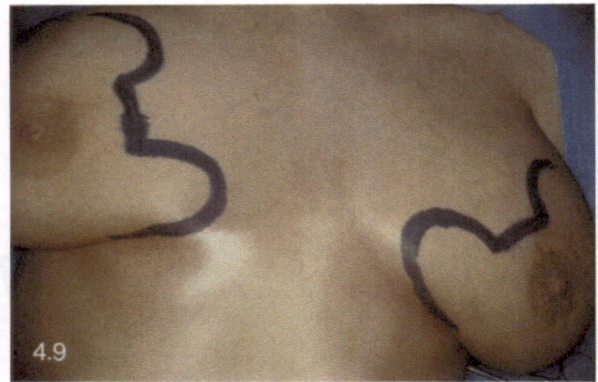

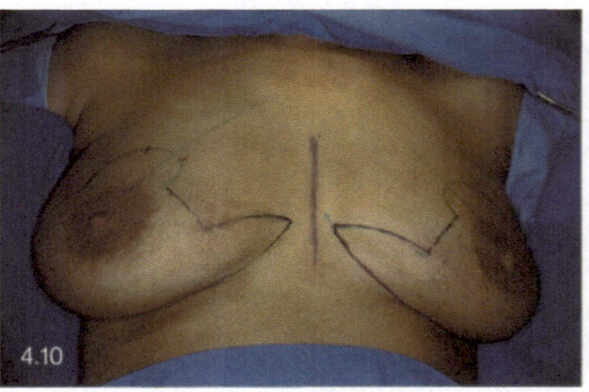

Fig. 4.9. The first step on the operating table is to incise the pattern marks with a scalpel. To reduce the length of the inframammary scar, which is very often hypertrophic and conspicuous in its medial portion, we have rounded the traditionally sharp medial and lateral corners of the pattern. The rounded edge will serve as the upper wound margin during reshaping of the breast

Fig. 4.10. In older women with hypotrophic scarring, sharp medial and lateral pattern corners may be drawn

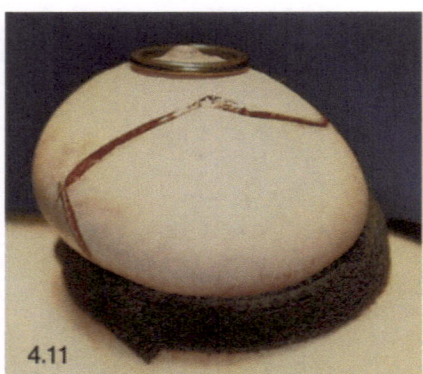

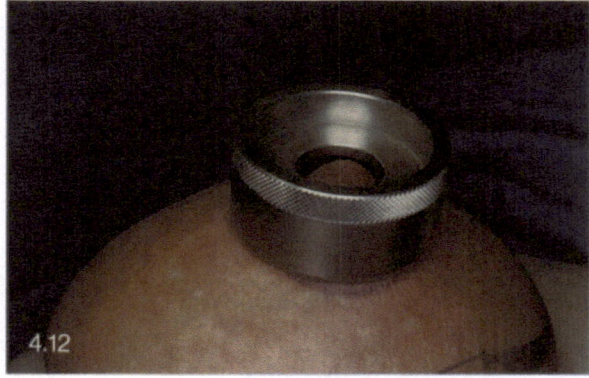

Fig. 4.11. Prior to deepithelialization of the periareolar area, a velcro tape is wrapped tightly around the base of the breast

Fig. 4.12. The areolar circle that is to be transposed can be outlined by drawing around a curtain ring (Fig. 4.11), or it can be circumcised with a "cookie cutter" (Padgett)

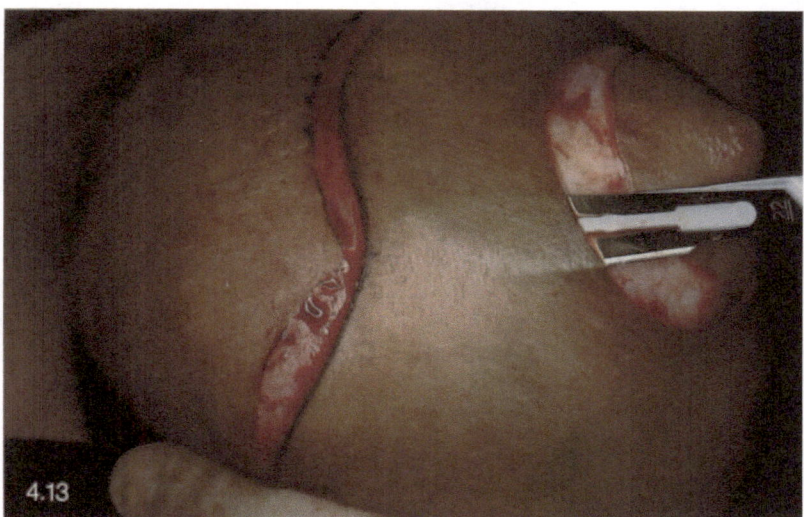

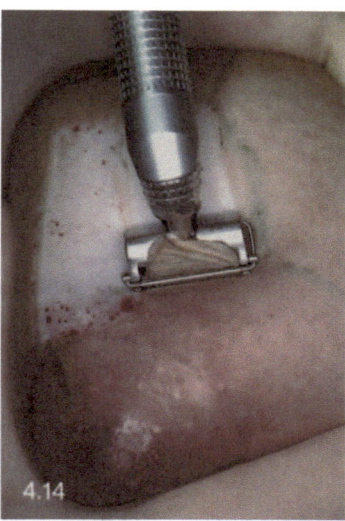

Fig. 4.13. Deepithelization in the corium

Fig. 4.14. In large breasts, deepithelialization can be accomplished more quickly with a minidermatome (Aesculap). Unfortunately the blades dull quickly, and as many as three blades may be needed for each side (!)

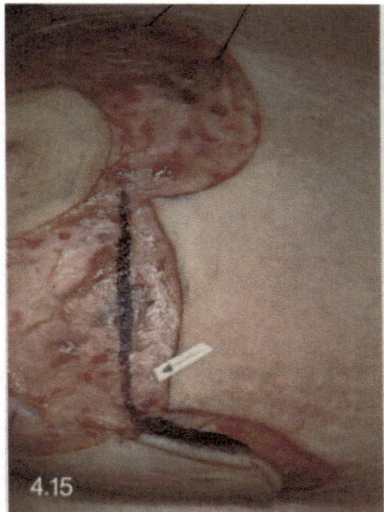

Fig. 4.15. During the resection, a border of corium should be left along the vertical limbs to facilitate later approximation of the tight skin margins with buried interrupted sutures

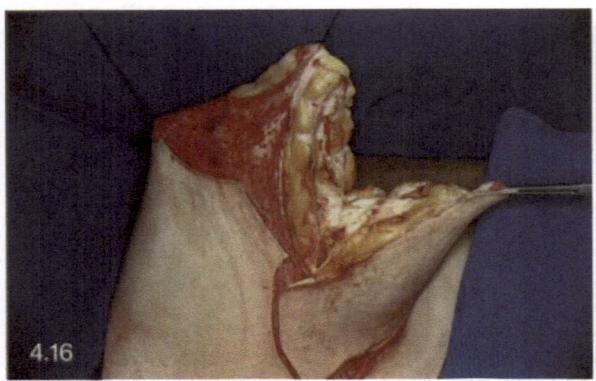

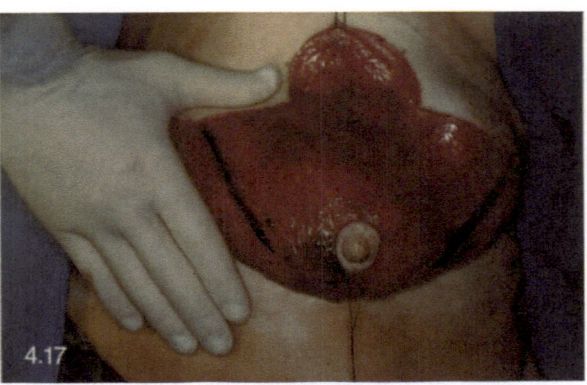

Fig. 4.16. With upward traction on the nipple-aerola, the resection proceeds horizontally toward the center of the mammary gland

Fig. 4.17. The thickness of the pedicle supplying the nipple-areola complex is critical. In large resections, we have found it helpful to relate the pedicle to the shape and size of the surgeon's hand, picturing the nipple-areola complex as overlying the fingernails. When the pedicle is fashioned in this way, the nipple-areola complex can easily be transposed up to 25 cm superiorly

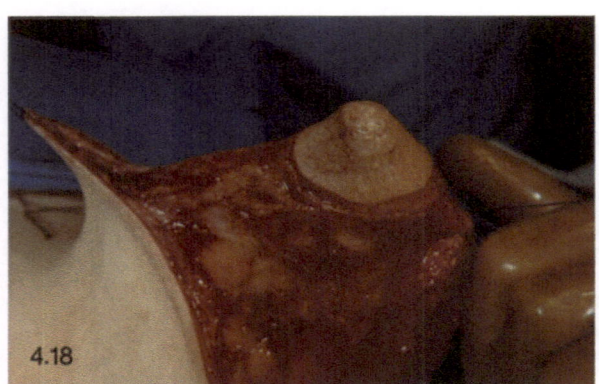

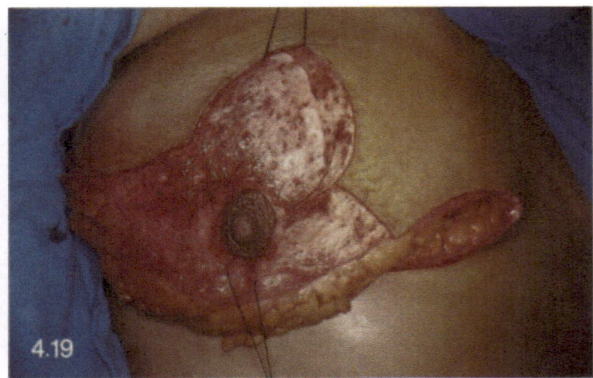

Fig. 4.18. In large resections all the tissue below and around the nipple-areola complex should be removed so that the pedicular vessels will not have to supply it in addition to the complex. A 1-cm thickness of retroareolar tissue is sufficient. When the resection is completed, additional subcutaneous fat should be removed from the medial and lateral ends to eliminate "dog ears" upon closure

Fig. 4.19. The wound edges along the Wise pattern are undermined for a distance of 1–2 cm (see Fig. 4.18), and the nipple-areola is transposed into the "keyhole." Next the vertical edges are approximated and fixed with buried simple interrupted sutures and a row of intracutaneous sutures

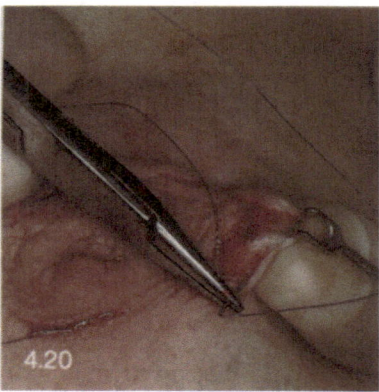

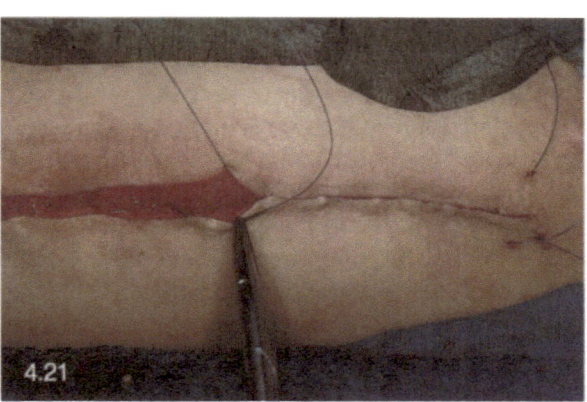

Fig. 4.20. The nipple-aerolar complex is initially fixed in its new position with four simple interrupted sutures, then the wound margins are coapted with intracutaneous threads. The needle should enter and exit within the areola so that the needle tracks will not be visible later

Fig. 4.21. The horizontal suture should also be placed intracutaneously to allow for the hypertrophic scarring that frequently occurs in young women

Fig. 4.22. To minimize the length of the horizontal scar (see Fig. 4.9), the lower wound margin should be well pleated and any "dog ears" resected. At the end of the operation, a rubber Penrose drain is brought out through the lateral end of the wound (a suction drain is likely to become blocked). The simple interrupted sutures should be removed no later than day four, the periareolar intracutaneous sutures at two weeks, and the inframammary sutures at four weeks

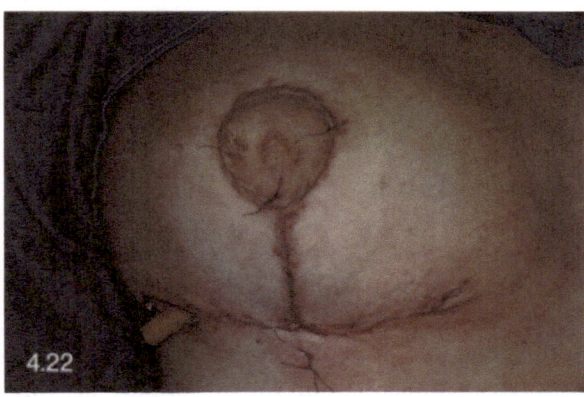

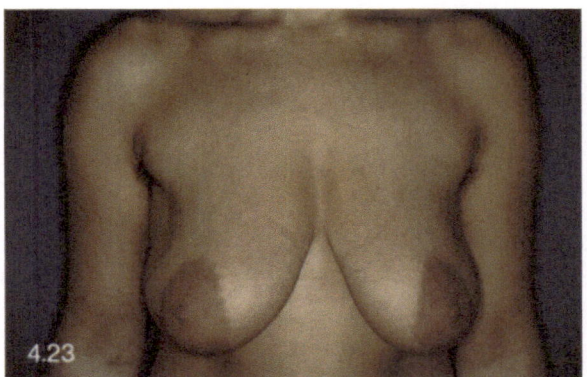

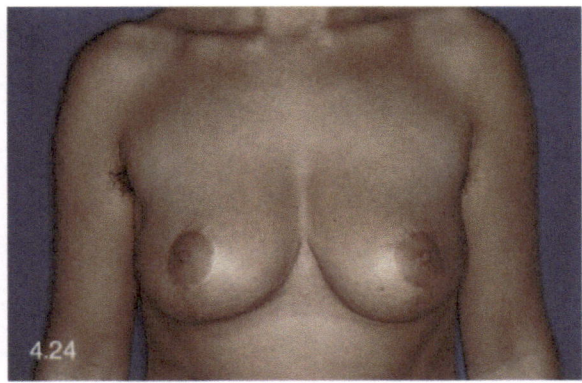

Fig. 4.23. Severely ptotic breasts in a 45-year-old woman

Fig. 4.24. Good postoperative result one year later

5 Other Methods

During the past 17 years, we have performed more than 3000 reduction mammoplasties using a variety of methods. In 1978 we abandoned the reduction devised by Pitanguy in 1960 (Pitanguy 1967), in which the nipple location is determined at the end of the operation, because the nipple sites were never completely symmetrical. The vertical nipple pedicle described by McKissock in 1972 is subject to blood-flow problems in inexperienced hands. Additionally, this procedure invariably disrupts the nerve supply to the nipple (Jaeger and Schneider 1982). The L-shaped suture line eliminates a scar in the medial inframammary crease, but at the cost of a longer lateral scar. Meyer (1979) himself writes that it is sometimes necessary to extend the excision medially to avoid coning or bulging of the breast in the lower medial quadrant (Meyer and Kesselring 1979). We have also abandoned the L-shaped incision and believe that the inverted T shape left by skin resection in the vertical and horizontal directions is necessary for an optimum breast shape.

Today only innovation among breast reduction techniques is that greater emphasis is placed on minimizing the length of the inframammary scar, as described by Marchac (Marchac and De-Olarte 1982; Maillard 1986; Lejour et al. 1987).

Scars on the reduced breast itself are generally less conspicuous than on the inframammary line.

This led Maillard (1986) to devise a method in which the skin surrounding the areola is tightened like the diaphragm of a camera. This technique results in a Z-shaped scar on the lower half of the breast. We can recommend this procedure (Figs. 15.7–15.15) only for adolescent breasts, because the Z-plasty often creates "dog ears" that necessitate medial and lateral extension of the incisions (Fig. 15.14).

For the past ten years we have found it unnecessary to perform free nipple transplantations in our practice. We have found that up to 1500 g of tissue can be resected per breast without jeopardizing the nipple-areolar blood supply. The Strömbeck modification is good for relatively flaccid breasts, and in firm adolescent breasts we have had better results with the method of Robbins (1977) using an inferiorly based nipple pedicle (Fig. 5.2). Nevertheless, we would recommend that surgeons less experienced in glandular resections apply the more reliable method of free nipple grafting beyond a resection volume of approximately 1000 g. The great advantage of this method is that it avoids nipple retraction in the first postoperative weeks ("kangaroo nipple"), which frequently occurs after Strömbeck's operation on large breasts in which a supramamillary disc has not been excised. On the other hand, free nipple grafting is more time-consuming than transfer on a pedicle, since it is a basic rule that *one* operator should perform the pyramid-shaped resections successively on both sides.

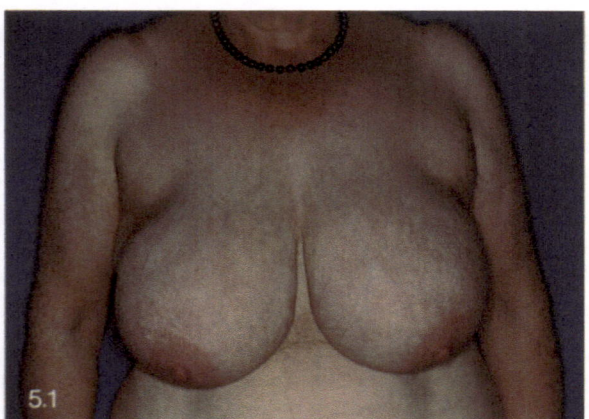

Fig. 5.1. If the breasts are very large and the glandular tissue is hard, it is best to transpose the nipple on an inferiorly based pedicle, as described by Robbins (1977)

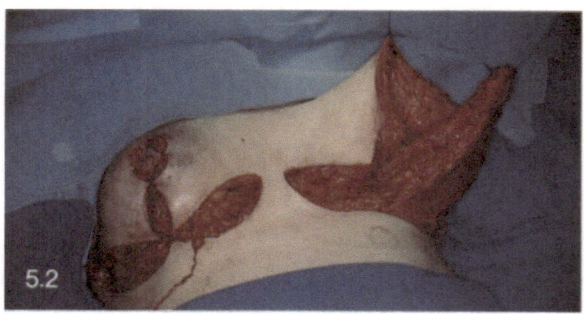

Fig. 5.2. Again, the inferior nipple pedicle should be patterned after the shape and size of the surgeon's hand

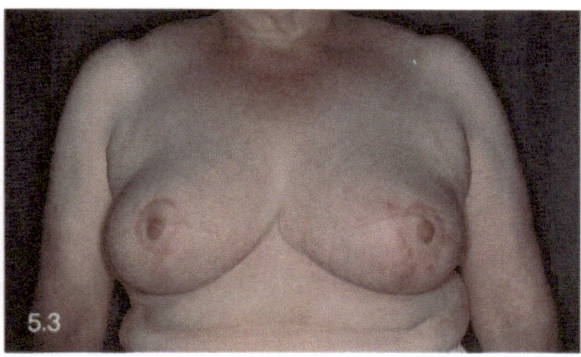

Fig. 5.3. Postoperative result

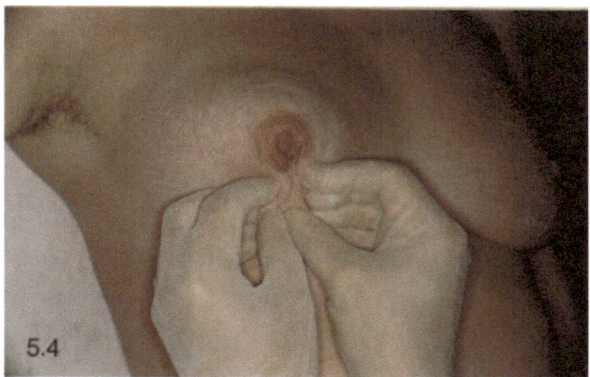

Fig. 5.4. If there is excessive fullness only in the lower brest quadrants, nipple elevation is not required

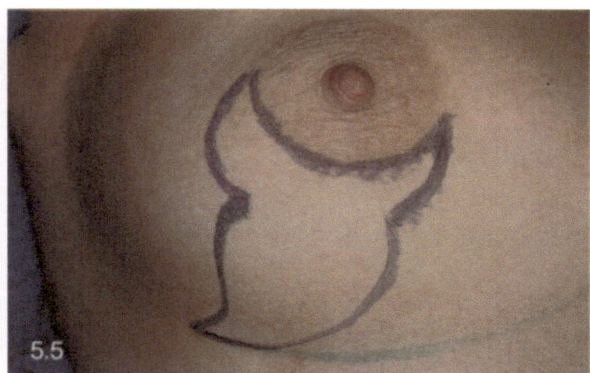

Fig. 5.5. A "devil's excision" is recommended for these cases

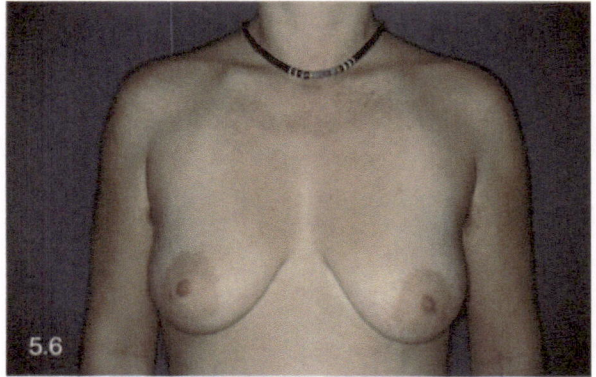

Fig. 5.6. Before mastopexy

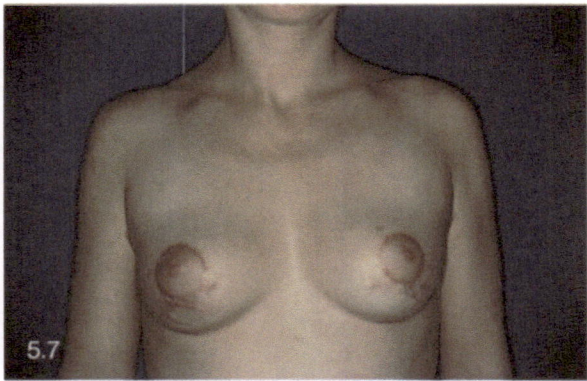

Fig. 5.7. Two weeks after mastopexy with an L-shaped incision and nipple transposition

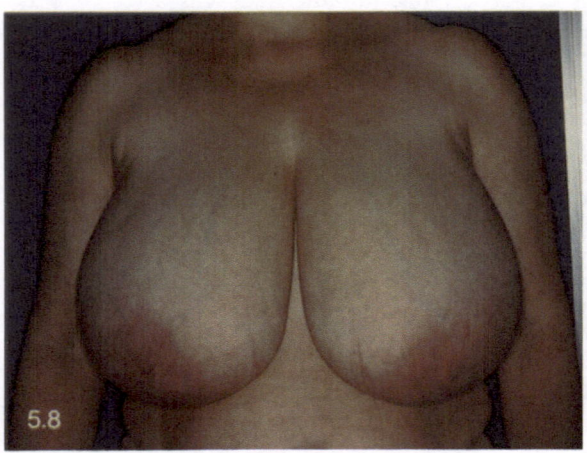

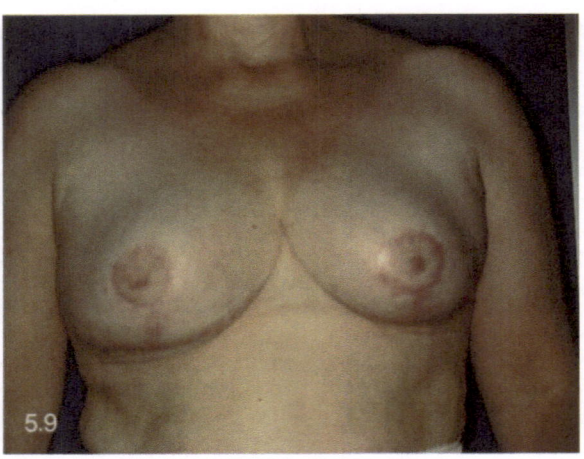

Fig. 5.8. Breasts this large can be reduced with nipple transposition by using the "open hand" pattern to fashion a long pedicle that will reach to the new site (see Fig. 4.17)

Fig. 5.9. Postoperative result

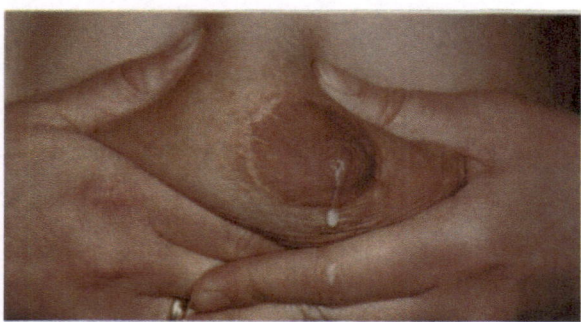

Fig. 5.10. Experience has shown that large breasts do not have good lactational function. Even so, the remaining superior third of the glandular tissue may be adequate for nursing

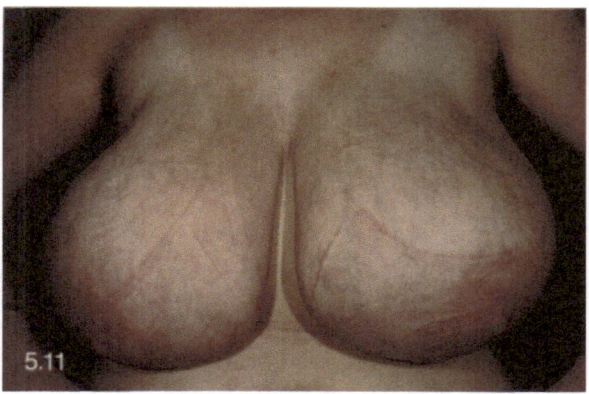

Fig. 5.11. In breasts that presumably will require the resection of more than 1000 g of glandular tissue, nipple reconstruction by free transplantation is advised

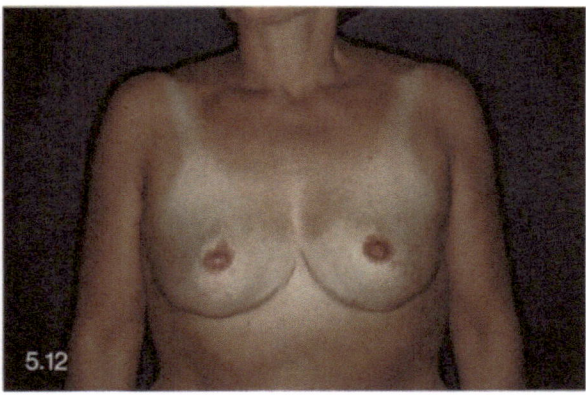

Fig. 5.12. Postoperative result one year later. The operation has transformed a matron (see Fig. 5.11) into an active, youthful-appearing woman

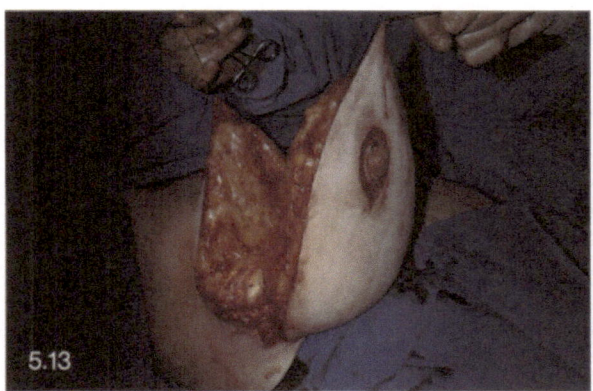

Fig. 5.13. The nipple-aerola complex is circumcised to the thickness of a full-thickness skin graft. This time the superior pattern marks are incised, and the resection proceeds horizontally

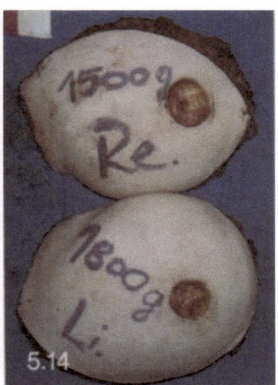

Fig. 5.14. The resected specimens

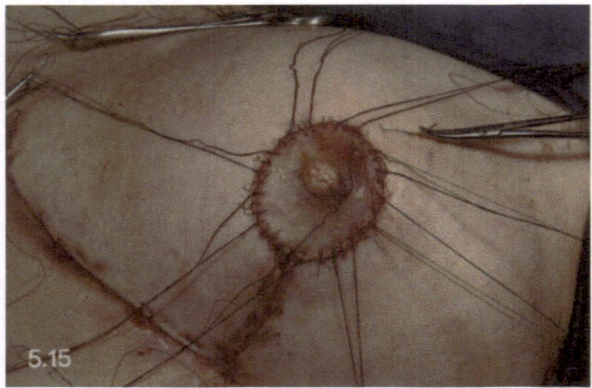

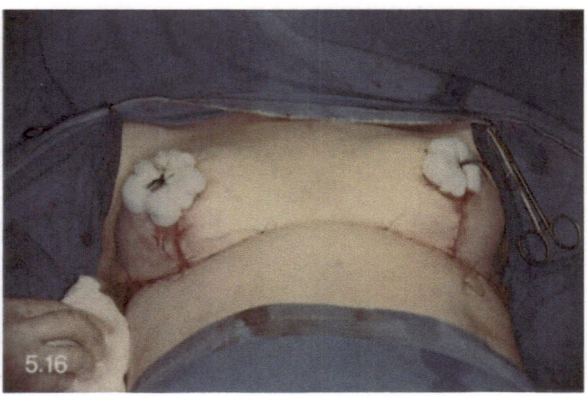

Fig. 5.15. The nipple-areola complex is sutured into its recipient bed. The complex can be transplanted as a full-thickness graft with little risk of superficial nipple slough

Fig. 5.16. Pressure is applied to the free grafts for 8 days with foam bolus dressings

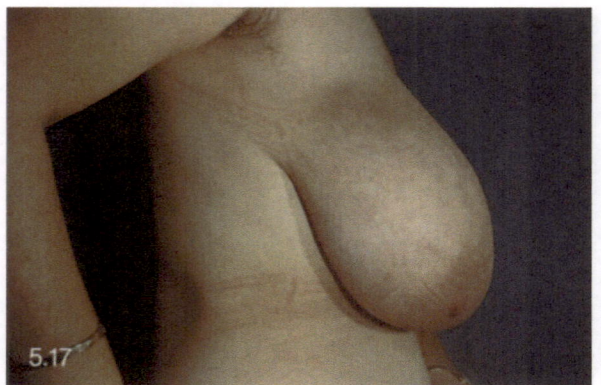

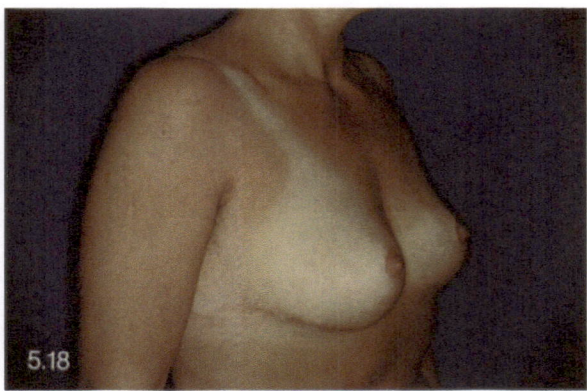

Fig. 5.17. Preoperative appearance of the patient in Fig. 5.11

Fig. 5.18. Postoperative appearance. Note the good projection of the nipples after free transplantation. Of course, lactation is sacrificed by this operation

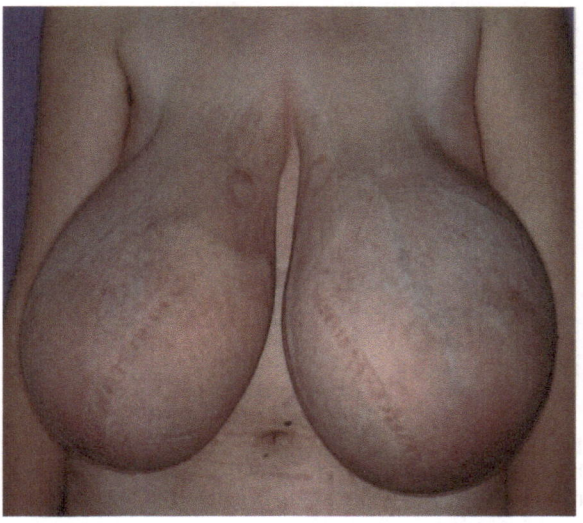

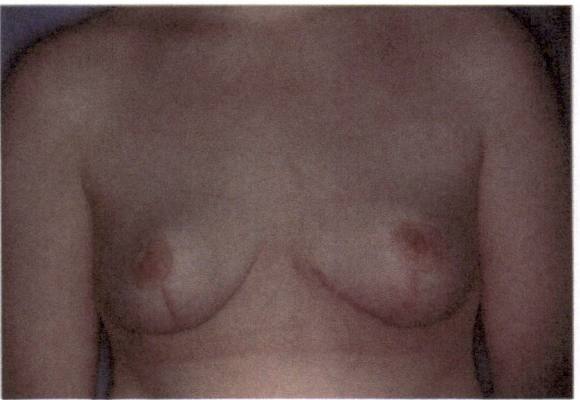

Fig. 5.20. Postoperative result after resection of 4270 g of the left breast and 3665 g of the right breast. The nipple-areola-complex had been transplanted as a free fullthickness graft

Fig. 5.19. Young woman 17 years of age showing juvenile gigantomasty

6 Corrective Operations

The most frequent complaints following reduction mammoplasty relate to hypertrophic scarring. Hypertrophic scars around the areola and on the inframammary crease can be quite conspicuous, especially in young women. The primary treatment of choice for a hypertrophic scar is compression, which is effectively administered by a tight-fitting brassiere whose transverse elastic exerts direct pressure on the inframammary scar. The bra should be worn day and night and generally can be discontinued after about three months. The residual scars, which may be up to 1 cm wide, can then be excised one year later as an ambulatory procedure. The best results are obtained by initially excising scar segments no more than 8 cm long, to avoid the restimulation of hypertrophic scarring. The remaining scars can then be excised six months later, again proceeding in small steps. The wounds are closed with two rows of intracutaneous sutures (Fig. 4.21) or with buried absorbable threads connected to an intracutaneous suture line.

Intralesional injections of triamcinolone (Volon-A) with a Dermojet device (Padgett) may lead to more rapid scar regression, but they leave wider residual scars that will still require excision at a later time.

Refinements in operating technique and the option of free nipple grafting, even in firm juvenile breasts, have largely eliminated the problem of nipple slough. If the nipple appears white or livid at the end of the operation, dextran 40 (Rheomacrodex) and pentoxifylline (Trental) may be given intravenously in an attempt to lower the blood viscosity (Fleige 1983). If nipple color has not improved within two hours, the areolar sutures and vertical suture line should be reopened to allow recovery of the bent nipple-areola complex. Five to eight days later the suture lines may be reclosed following a regimen of 250 ml dextran 40 and 150 mg pentoxifylline administered twice daily.

Fat necrosis, impaired wound healing, or hematoma formation are indications for early surgical intervention and secondary closure. We have had very good results with locally administered gentamycin for the prophylaxis of infection.

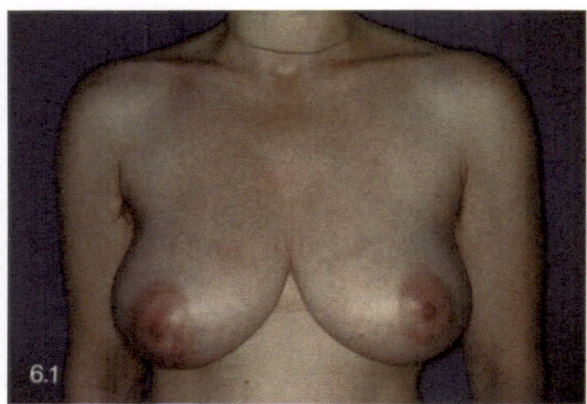 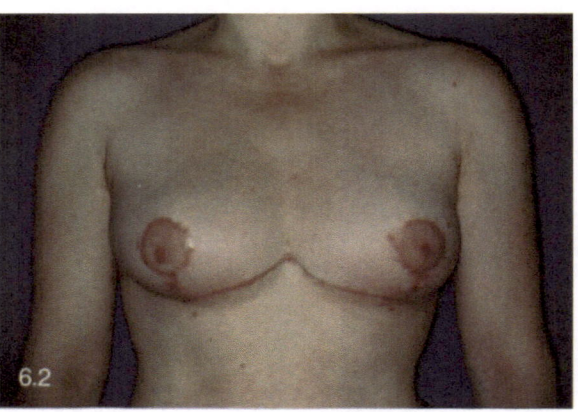

Fig. 6.1. Woman 28 years of age with moderate hypertrophy and ptosis

Fig. 6.2. Two months after reduction mammoplasty, scar hypertrophy is already apparent. In this case, unfortunately, the medial wounds of the two breasts were conjoined (see Fig. 4.10)

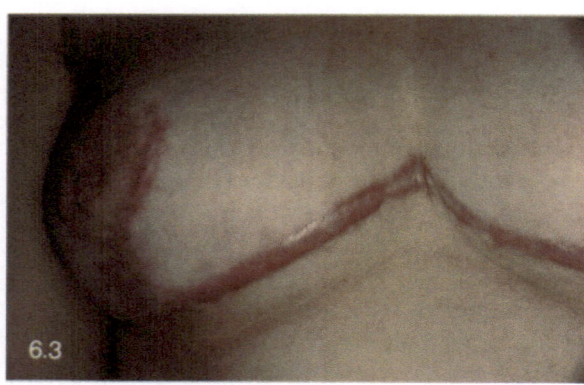

Fig. 6.3. One year later scarring is already regressive. However, this case illustrates the importance of keeping the inframammary scar as short as possible (see Fig. 4.9), even if there are "dog ears" requiring later removal by outpatient surgery. The pressure from a snug brassiere worn postoperatively prevents scar hypertrophy

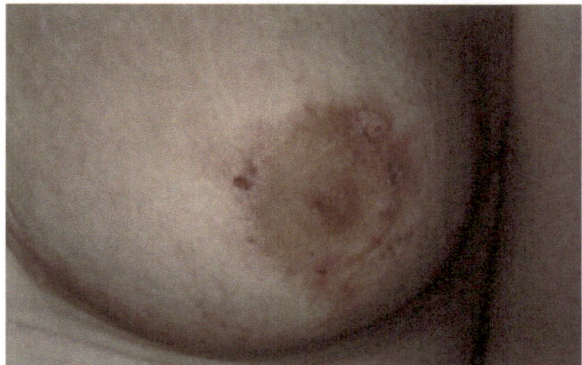

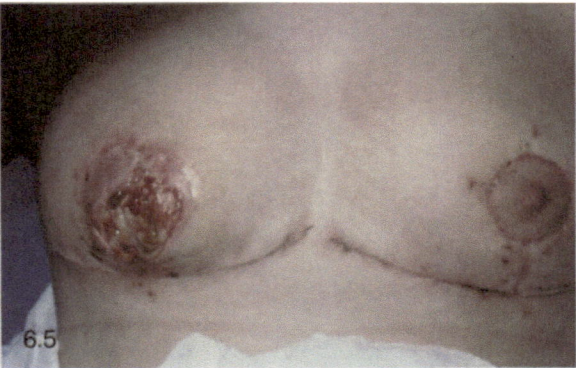

Fig. 6.4. Infected sebaceous cysts are relatively common and may completely encircle the areola by 6–12 months. Arising from Montgomery glands that were opened during deepithelization, they are adequately managed by early incision

Fig. 6.5. The most feared complication is nipple slough, which should not occur if correct plastic surgical principles are followed. Early debridement of necrotic areas and secondary sutures will greatly accelerate the healing process

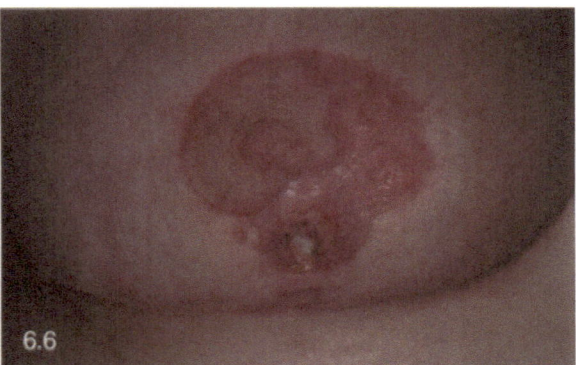

Fig. 6.6. At five weeks postoperatively, the defect left by the partial nipple loss is epithelized. The basic treatment after debridement would consist of an early secondary suture followed later by expansion of the areola

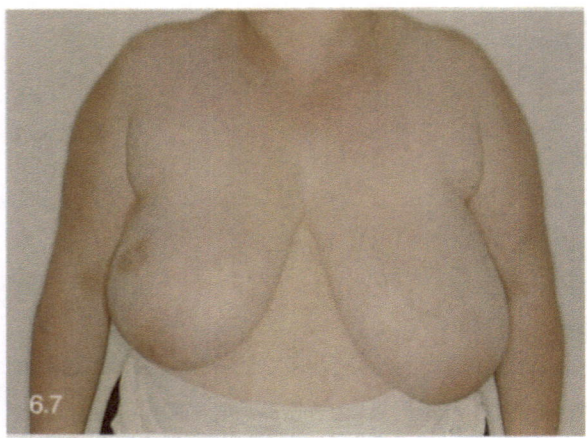

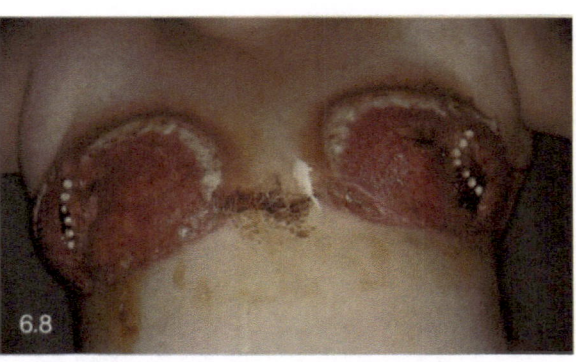

Fig. 6.7. Woman 23 years of age with juvenile mammary hyperplasia and obesity had a reduction mammoplasty elsewhere

Fig. 6.8. Postoperatively the patient developed a fulminant skin necrosis and superinfection *(Staphylococcus epidermidis!)* which showed all the features of pyoderma gangrenosum (=necrotizing vasculitis). The most likely cause was a vascular hyperergia to staphylococci toxins. The infection was managed by the implantation of PMMA beads. Though the patient was treated in our hospital with systemic cortisone, the necrotizing process continued to progress, necessitating a wide circumcision of the torpid borders

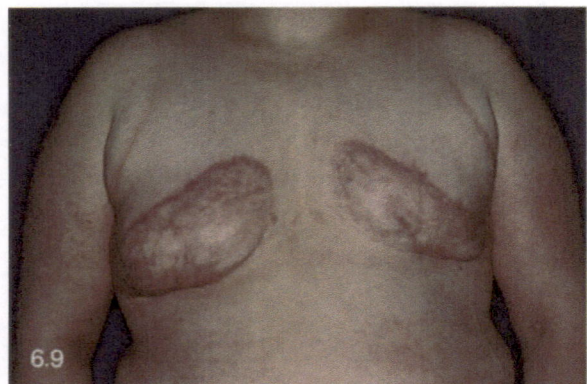

Fig. 6.9. Appearance two years after meshed skin grafting. For now, the patient has declined breast reconstruction by advancement of abdominal skin (Fig. 16.2) and nipple reconstruction

Lowering the nipples: The cosmetic result of a reduction mammoplasty stands or falls with the position of the nipples. The nipple sites should not be determined preoperatively by measuring from fixed landmarks (sternal notch, clavicle, upper arm) but should be based stricly ¡on the height of the inframammary crease (Fig. 4.4) (Lemperle and Höhler 1972). Through natural stretching of the skin, each mammary gland will sag back over the inframammary line, which encircles the chest like a high-waisted Empire gown (Fig. 4.3).

The only way to adjust nipples that are positioned too high is to cut around the nipples and lower them to a more prominent site on the new breast. The resulting defect can be closed obliquely (Fig. 6.11). Scar formation is generally satisfactory, as the candidates for this procedure tend to have weak connective tissues.

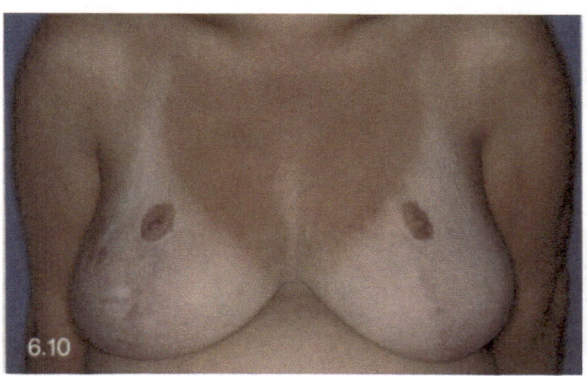

Fig. 6.10. In this case the markings for the new nipple sites were based not on the height of the inframammary crease (Fig. 4.3) but on fixed measurements (18 cm from the sternal notch). The breast mounds, placed too high at the time of operation, have sagged back to their natural position, leaving the nipples behind

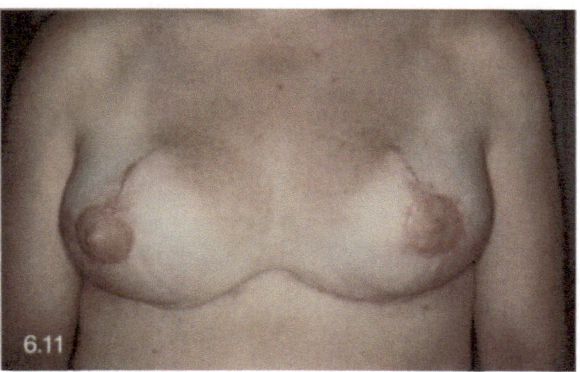

Fig. 6.11. The only solution is to circumcise the nipple-areola complexes and lower them 1.5 times the areolar diameter. The breasts (at 4 weeks postoperatively) will undergo some additional sagging

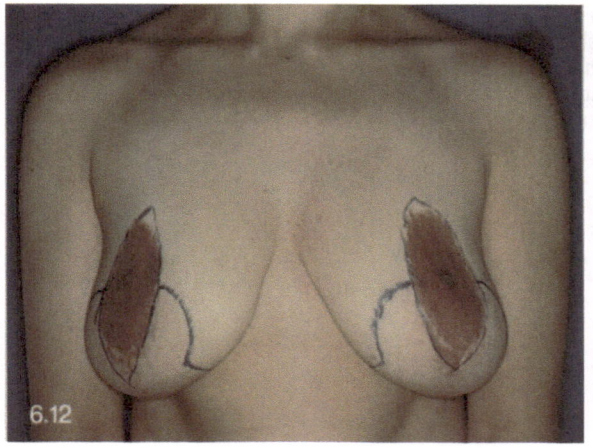

Fig. 6.12. Appearance after reduction mammoplasty: The nipple-areola complexes are positioned too high, and there is extreme areolar spreading

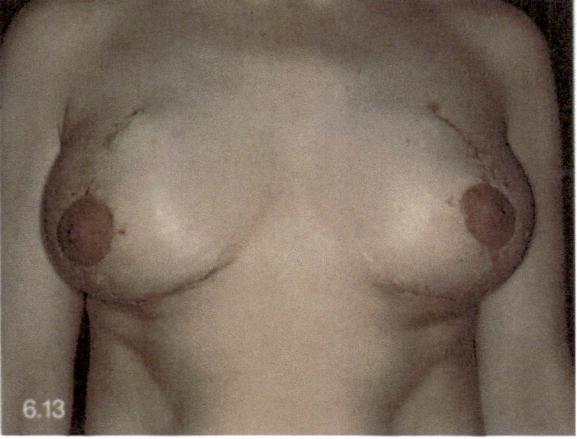

Fig. 6.13. The areolae have been circumcised, reduced, and transposed to a lower site. Further mastopexy in this case without repositioning the nipples would not have yielded a permanent result

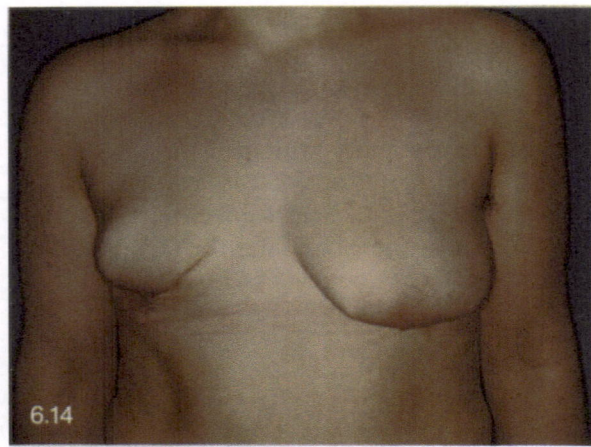

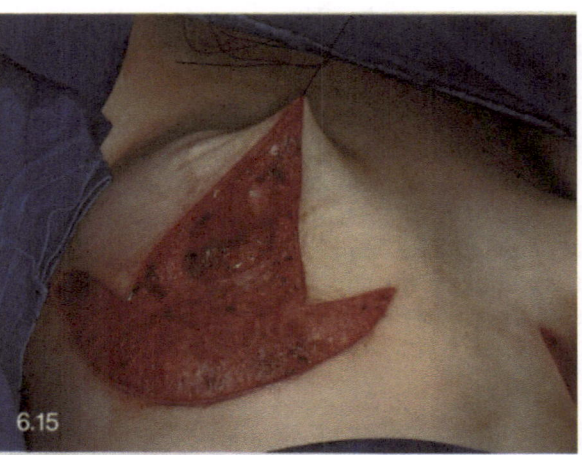

Fig. 6.14. Failed bilateral reduction mammoplasties in a 35-year-old woman

Fig. 6.15. The objective is to restore fullness to the right breast by using a deepithelialized thoracoepigastric flap

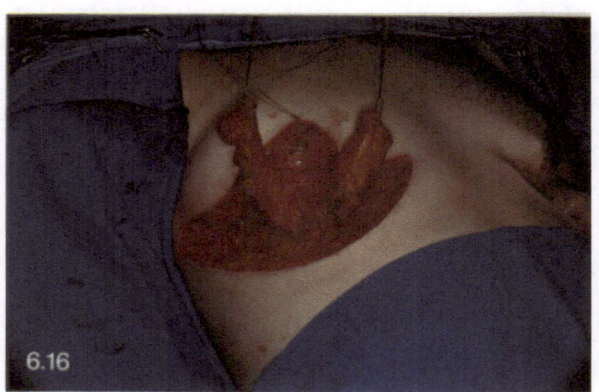

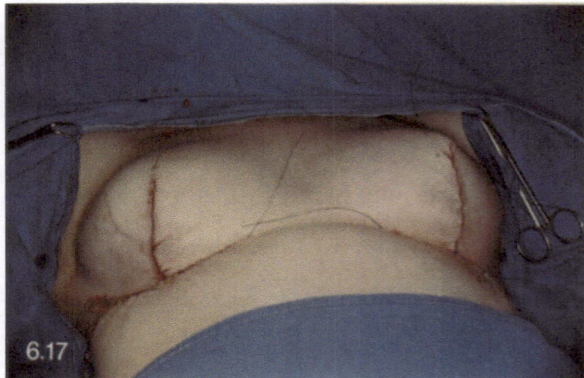

Fig. 6.16. Flaps supplied by the epigastric perforating vessels are developed on both sides

Fig. 6.17. A good breast mound is formed by closing the skin over the inset flap. The skin of the upper abdomen has been fixed to the intercostal muscles at the level of the inframammary crease with permanent simple interrupted sutures

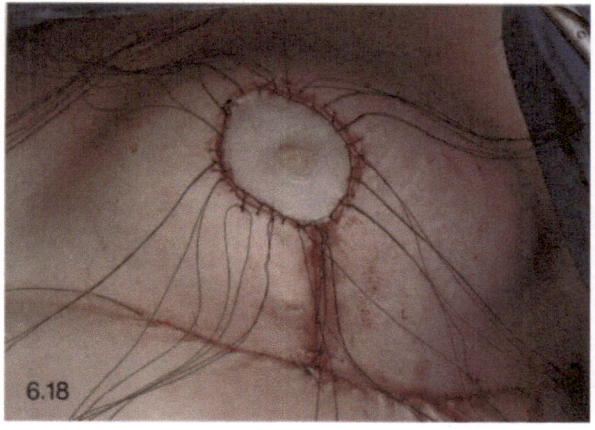

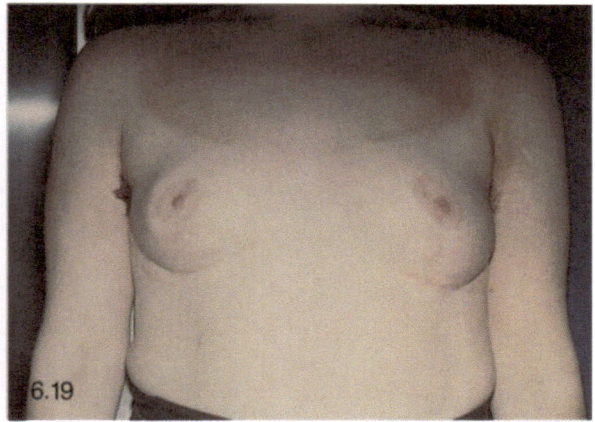

Fig. 6.18. The preserved left nipple was free-grafted to the breast. A right nipple was constructed from an excess peripheral areolar strip and a band of scar tissue

Fig. 6.19. Appearance five years later

References

Bolger WE, Seyfer AE, Jackson SM (1987) Reduction mammaplasty using the inferior glandula „pyramid" pedicle: experiences with 300 patients. Plast Reconstr Surg 80: 75–84

Fleige R (1983) Untersuchungen über die Wirkung von durchblutungsfördernden Pharmaka auf Hautlappenplastiken bei Ratten. Dissertation, Frankfurt

Höhler H (1978) Die Reduktionsmammaplastik der weiblichen Brust. Z Plast Chir 2: 68–91

Jaeger K, Schneider B (1982) Die Innervation und Durchblutung der Mamille im Hinblick auf die perimamilläre Inzision. Chirurg 53: 525–527

Lassus C (1987) Breast reduction: Evaluation of a technique - a single vertical scar. Aesthetic Plast Surg 11: 107–112

Lejour M, De May A, Duchateau J, Deraemaecker R (1987) Breast reductions with the SSS technique Transact. 9. Int. Congr. Plast. Surg, Delhi Tata. Mc Graw-Hill, New York, pp 368–370

Lemperle G, Höhler H (1972) Die Bedeutung der Inframammarlinie bei der Reduktions- und Augmentations-Mammaplastik. In: Schrudde J (Hrsg) Plastische Chirurgie. Pilgram, Köln, S 119–120

Maillard GF (1986) A Z-Mammaplasty with minimal scarring. Plast Reconstr Surg 77: 66–76

Marchac D, De Olarte G (1982) Reduction mammaplasty and correction of ptosis with a short inframammary scar. Plast Reconstr Surg 69: 45–55

McKissock PK (1972) Reduction mammaplasty with a vertical dermal flap. Plast Reconstr Surg 49: 245–252

Meyer R, Kesselring UK (1979) Various dermal flaps with L-shaped suture line in reduction mammaplasty. Aesthetic Plast Surg 3: 41–46

Pitanguy I (1967) Surgical treatment of breast hypertrophy. Br J Plast Surg 20: 78–85

Regnault P (1974) Reductionmammaplasty by the B technique. Plast Reconstr. Surg 53: 19–25

Robbins TH (1977) A reduction mammaplasty with areola-nipple based on an inferior dermal pedicle. Plast Reconstr Surg 59: 64–67

Strömbeck JO (1960) Mammaplasty: Report of a new technique based on the two-pedicle procedure. Br J Plast Surg 13: 79–90

Strömbeck JO (1964) Macromastia in women and its surgical treatment. Acta Chir Scand [Suppl] 341: 1–128

Wise RH (1956) A preliminary report on a method of planning the mammaplasty. Plast Reconstr Surg 17: 367–375

Part C

Developmental Anomalies

7 Amazon Syndrome, Poland's Syndrome

Indications

Developmental anomalies in the form of Amazon syndrome or Poland's syndrome should be corrected at the earliest possible age (between 10 and 15 years) to mitigate the effect of the deformity on the patient's self-image and her social and athletic development. Any subsequent corrections that may be needed, such as a change of implant or mastopexy, are an acceptable price to pay for an unencumbered puberty.

At the same time, one should always consider the tendency toward hypertrophic scarring in this young population. Procedures that require large incisions, such as the latissimus dorsi flap reconstruction, should be postponed until the end of the growth period (18 years).

The essential features (Fig. 7.4) of Poland's syndrome (Poland 1841) are:

1. aplasia of the pectoralis major muscle, and
2. hand deformities such as shortness of the fingers, syndactyly, and oligodactyly.

Additionally there may be:

1. unilateral mammary hypoplasia or aplasia in women, nipple dysplasia in men;
2. radiocubital synostosis; or
3. a transverse palmar crease.

Amazon syndrome (Mühlbauer and Wangerin 1977) refers strictly to hypoplasia or aplasia of one breast with no muscular defect (Fig. 7.1).

Technique

The simplest operation is always best. In simple Poland's syndrome, early augmentation of the hypoplastic breast will provide the necessary volume to fill a brassiere. Correction of the nipple position (Fig. 9.3) and mastopexy of the contralateral breast, if required, should be postponed until breast growth (puberty) is completed.

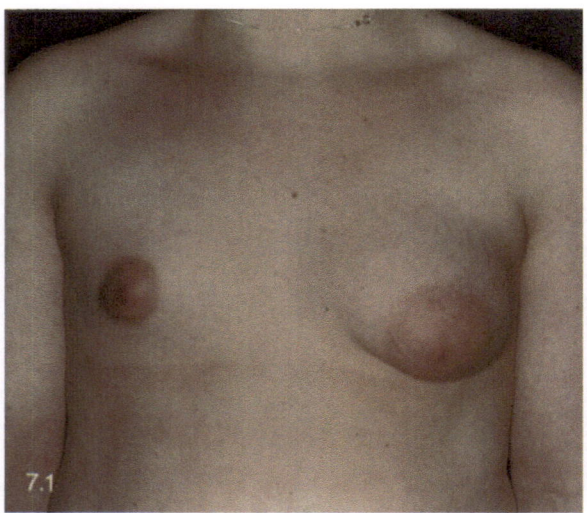

Fig. 7.1. Hypoplasia of the right breast (Amazon syndrome)

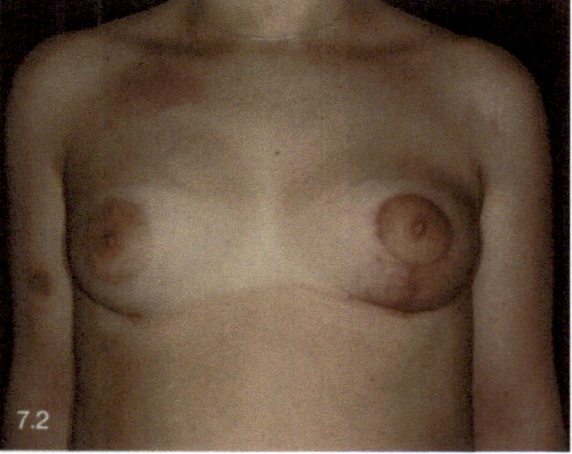

Fig. 7.2. Appearance after augmentation of the right breast with a 200-ml implant and a symmetrizing left mastopexy

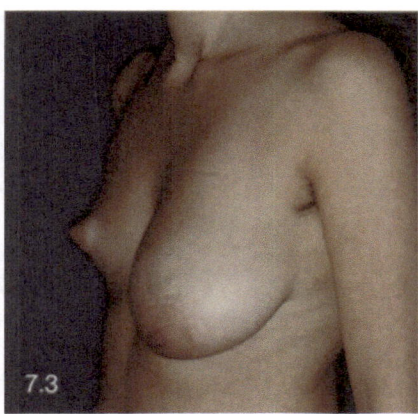

Fig. 7.3. Hyperplasia and ptosis of the left breast with a small right breast

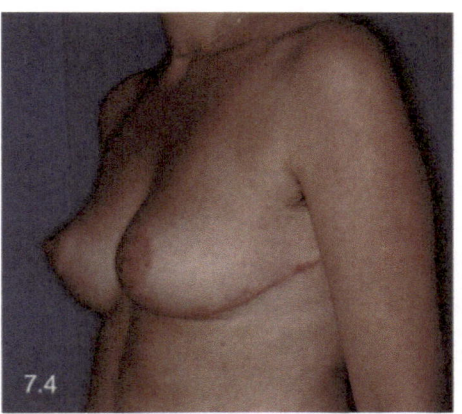

Fig. 7.4. Appearance after augmentation of the right breast with a 150-ml prosthesis and a left reduction mammoplasty

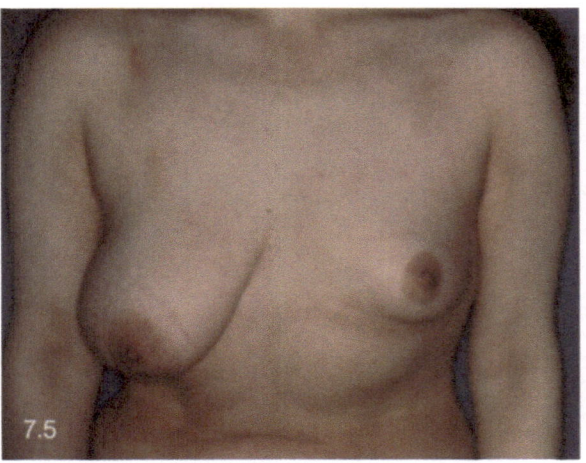

Fig. 7.5. Unilateral hyperplasia with a ptotic right breast

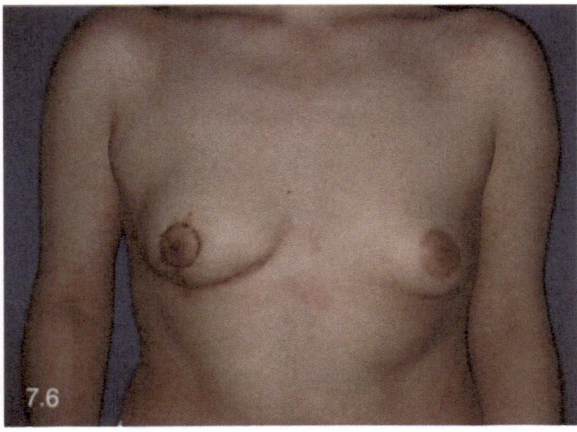

Fig. 7.6. Appearance after symmetrizing reduction of the right breast

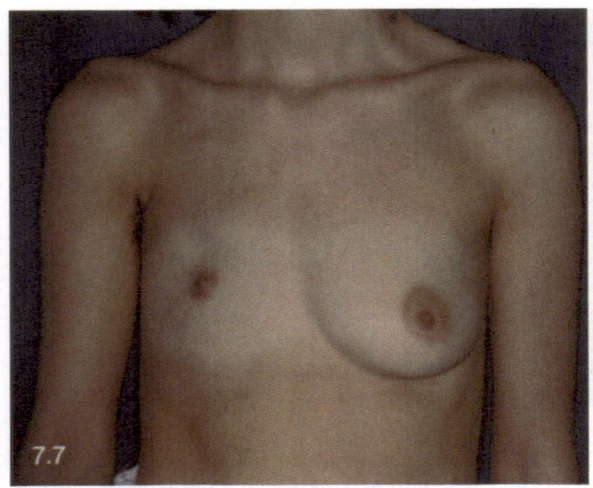

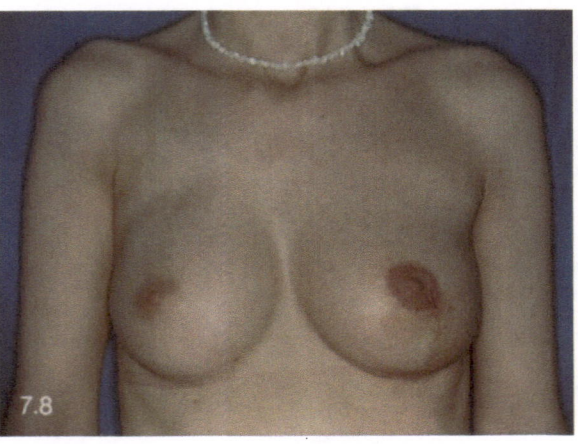

Fig. 7.8. Appearance after right breast augmentation with a 230-ml implant and a Maillard mastopexy of the left breast

Fig. 7.7. Poland's syndrome with a high right nipple, absence of the pectoralis major muscle, and syndactyly

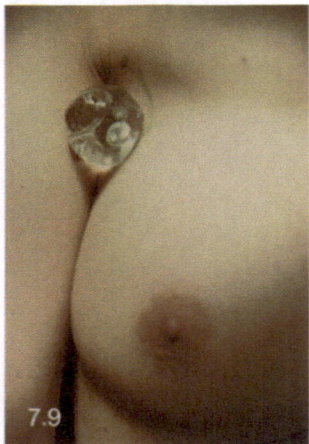

Fig. 7.9. The pectoralis defect on the anterior axillary line is aesthetically corrected with a 40-ml silicone implant

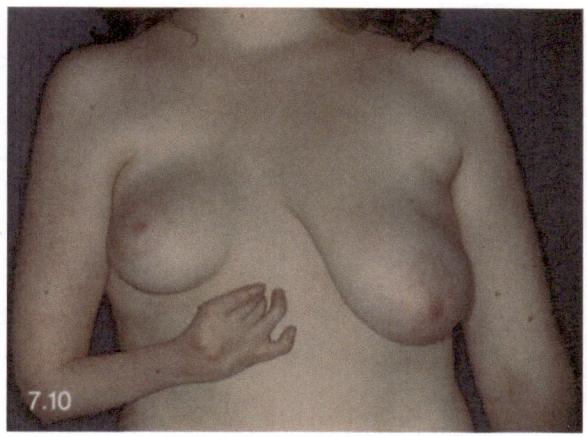

Fig. 7.10. Typical Poland's syndrome with absence of the pectoralis major muscle and hand deformity

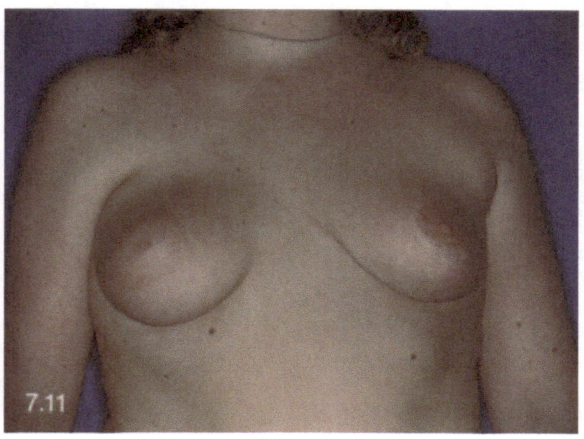

Fig. 7.11. Appearance after symmetrizing reduction of the left breast

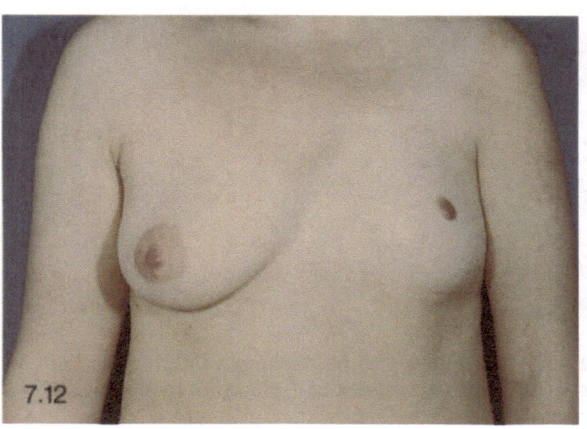

Fig. 7.12. Poland's syndrome with narrowness of the left shoulder

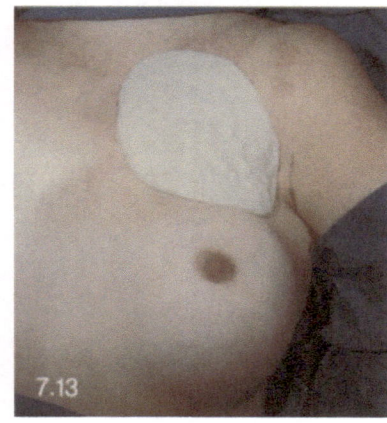

Fig. 7.13. RTV silicone elastomer (see Fig. 10.3) is molded externally to the pectoralis defect and implanted subcutaneously

Fig. 7.14. Appearance after simultaneous right mastopexy and left pectoralis reconstruction. The left nipple could be transposed medially and inferiorly (see Fig. 3.13)

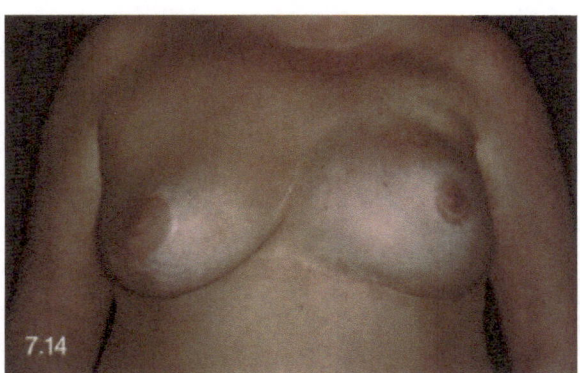

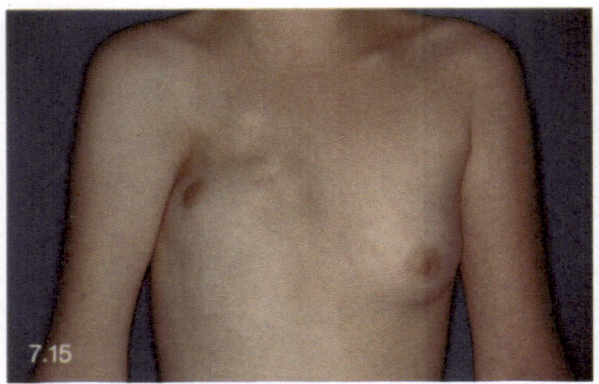

Fig. 7.15. Poland's syndrome with severe thoracic deformity

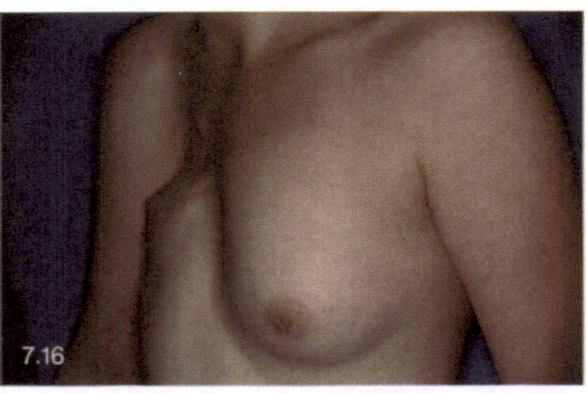

Fig. 7.16. The 2nd, 3rd, and 4th ribs are absent

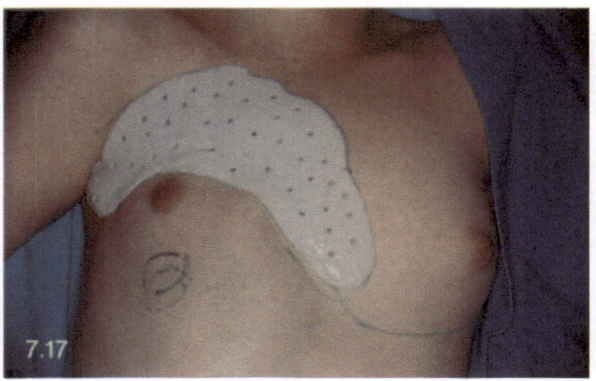

Fig. 7.17. The thoracic defect is reconstructed with an RTV silicone implant that was molded preoperatively (see Fig. 10.4)

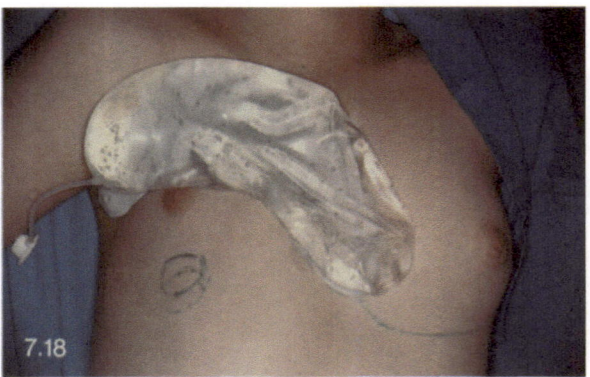

Fig. 7.18. To move the nipple-areola inferiorly, a kidney-shaped soft-tissue expander is placed over the silicone implant

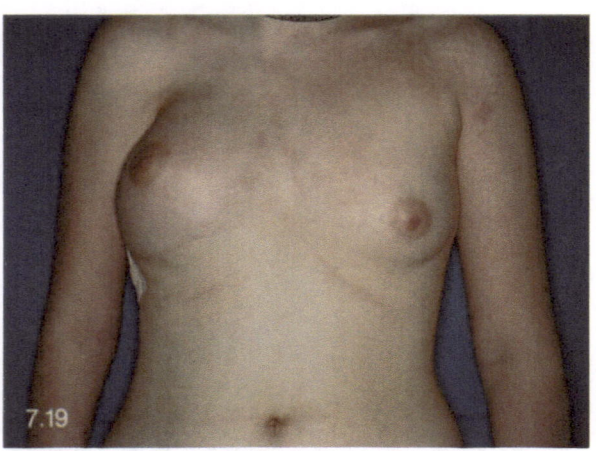

Fig. 7.19. The soft-tissue expander has been exchanged for a 150-ml implant. The stretched skin has shrunk again. Right nipple transposition can be performed at a later time (see Fig. 6.10)

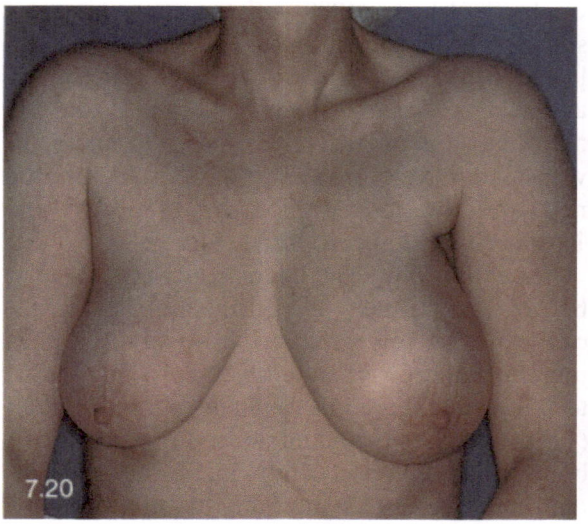

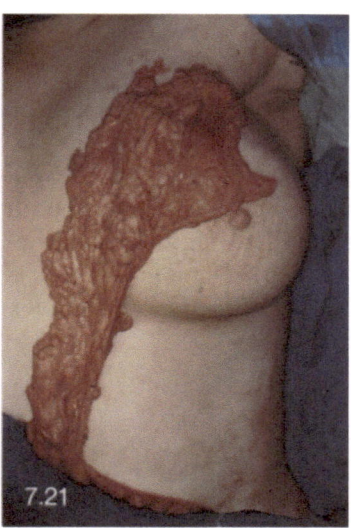

Fig. 7.20. Lymphedema of the left breast. This condition has progressed for five years as a result of Hodgkin's disease

Fig. 7.21. An omentoplasty is performed with the object of improving lymphatic drainage

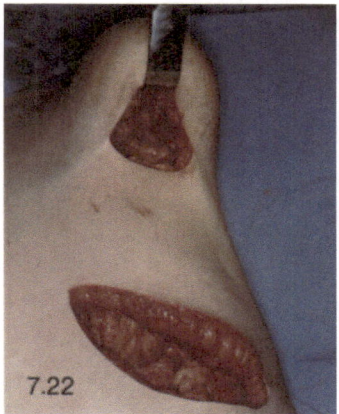

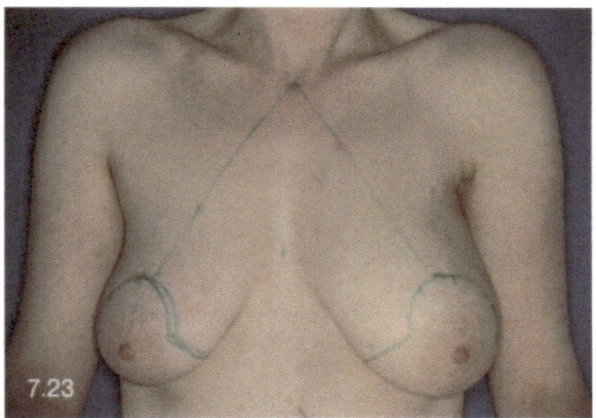

Fig. 7.22. Following division of the mammary gland into a superficial and deep layer, the omental flap is interposed

Fig. 7.23. Three months later the breast is markedly smaller, and the patient is ready for a reduction mammoplasty

8 Tubular Breast

A relatively rare congenital deformity, tubular breast has attracted the attention of plastic surgeons only in the last decade. It is caused by a hypoplasia of the lower quadrants of one or both breasts, with a correspondingly short distance between the nipple and inframammary crease (Fig. 8.10). Frequently the nipple-areola complex is protuberant (Fig. 8.1).

Technique

The surgical technique is adapted to the individual case. The periareolar "donut" mastopexy of Gruber and Jones (1980), using a pursestring closure of the wound margins, is certain to be followed by areolar spreading (Fig. 8.9), inasmuch as the nipple-areola complex became protuberant due to an underdeveloped corium unable to withstand tensile stresses. For this reason the new areolar circumference should not exceed 12 cm or that of the opposite side.

Generally, with a periareolar incision, the skin between the areola and inframammary crease can be sufficiently stretched at operation to permit the insertion of an implant. An alternative technique, described by Williams and Hoffmann (1981), is to free the glandular tissue in the upper breast quadrants posteriorly, incise the tissue radially, and advance it inferiorly to impart fullness to the lower quadrants (Fig. 8.11).

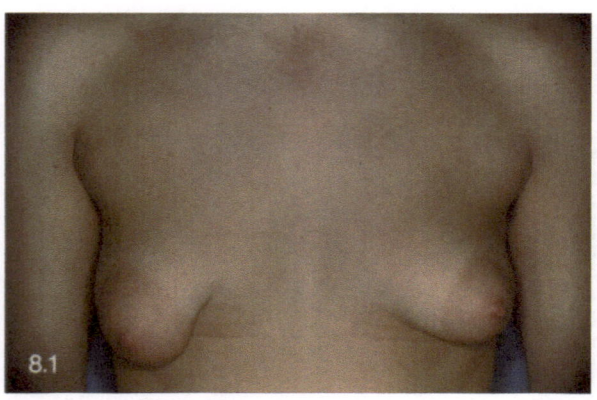

Fig. 8.1. Tubular breasts, more pronounced on the right side than on the left. The patient wanted symmetrical breasts but no augmentation

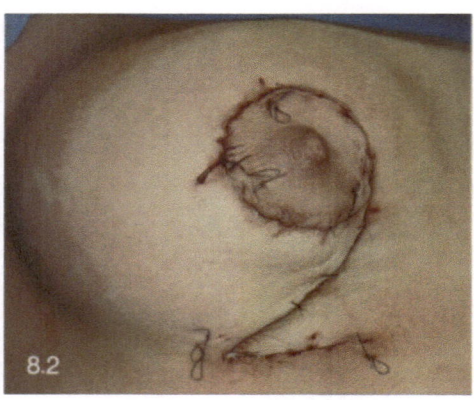

Fig. 8.2. Z-mastopexy of Maillard (see Figs. 15.8–15.14)

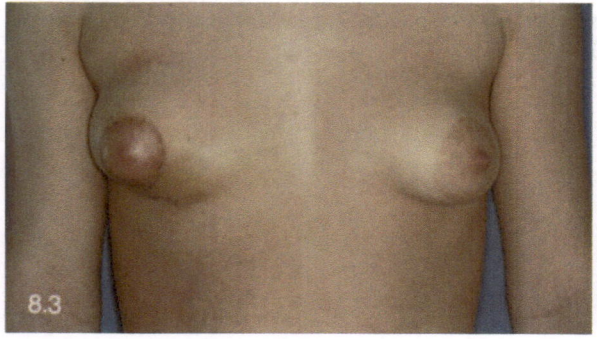

Fig. 8.3. Eight days postoperatively the breast still appears constricted by the Z-plasty

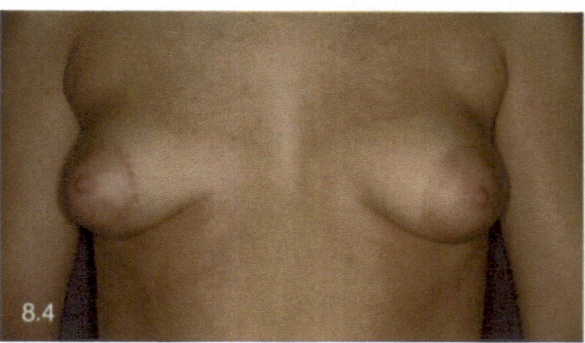

Fig. 8.4. Three months later, symmetry is achieved

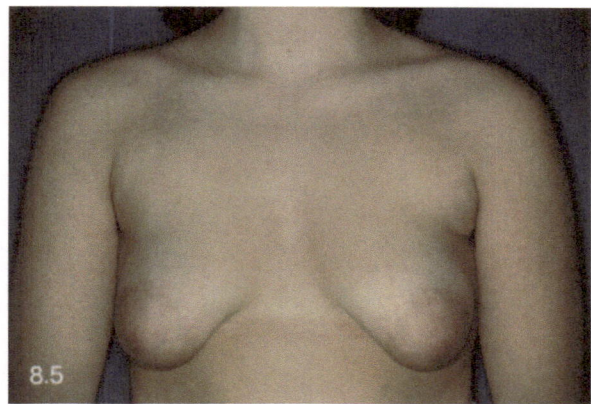

Fig. 8.5. Typical tubular deformity of both breasts

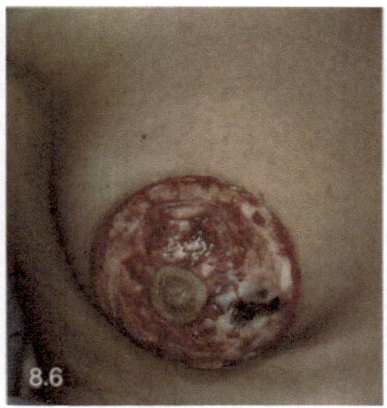

Fig. 8.6. Reduction and deepithelialization of the protuberant areola

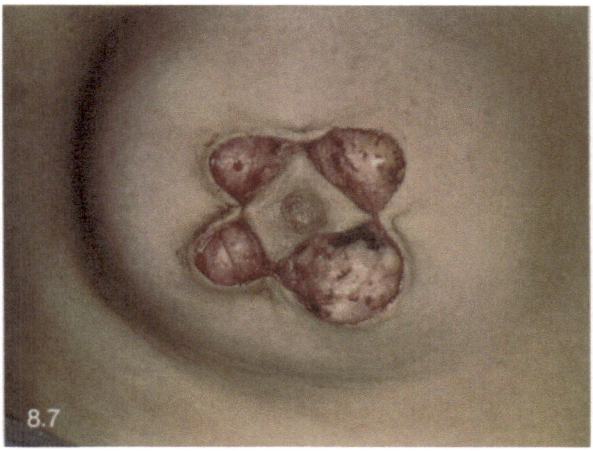

Fig. 8.7. Fixation of the wound edges with buried absorbable sutures

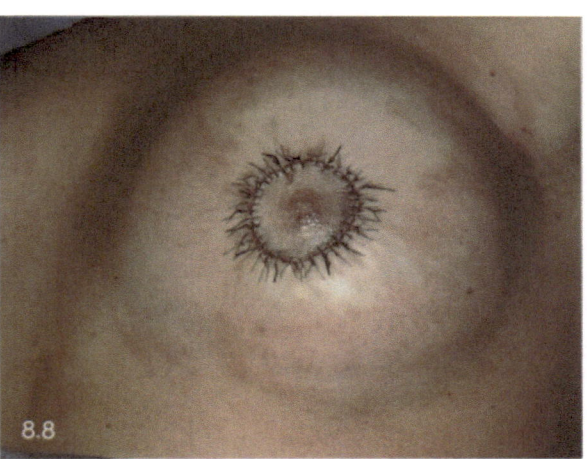

Fig. 8.8. The reduced areola is sutured to the wound
edges, which are pleated in pursestring fashion

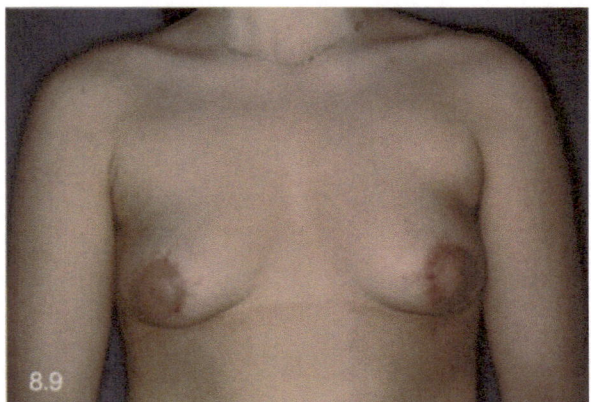

Fig. 8.9. One year later (see Fig. 8.5) there has been sepa-
ration of the wound edges with spreading of the areolae

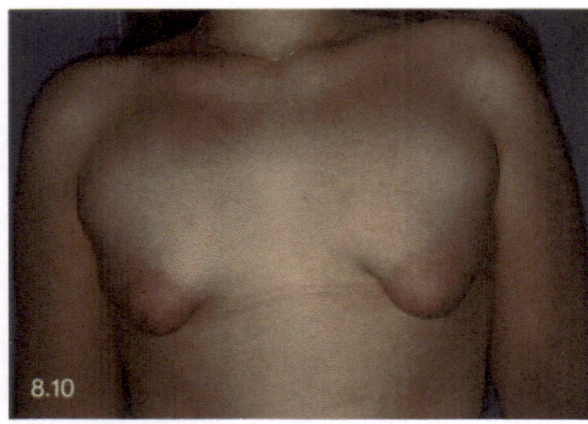

Fig. 8.10. Typical tubular breasts with absence of the lower quadrants

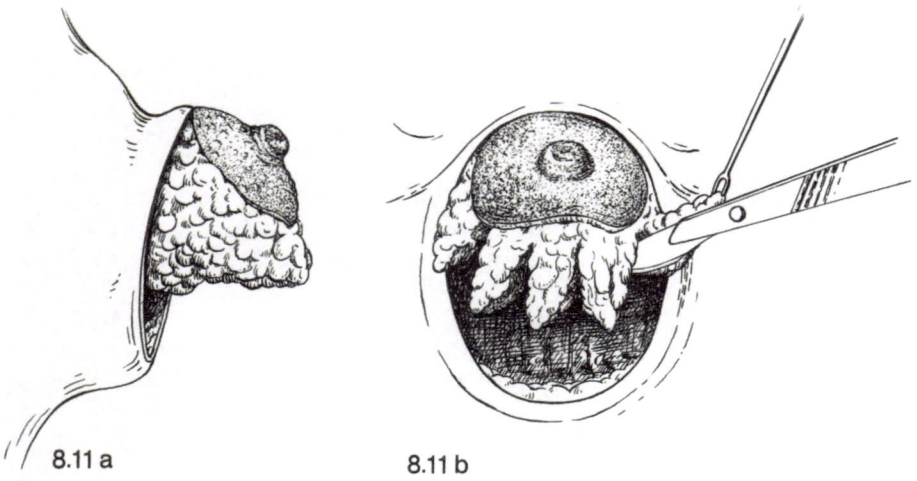

8.11 a   8.11 b

Fig. 8.11a, b. Following reduction of the areola, the glandular tissue is radially incised, swung into an inferior- ly dissected pocket, and fixed to the new inframammary crease (after Williams and Hoffmann 1981)

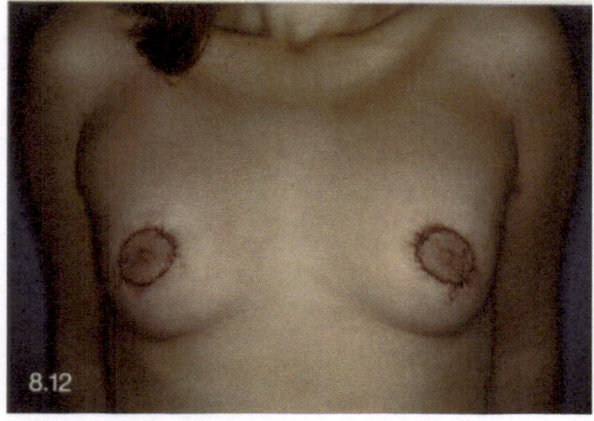

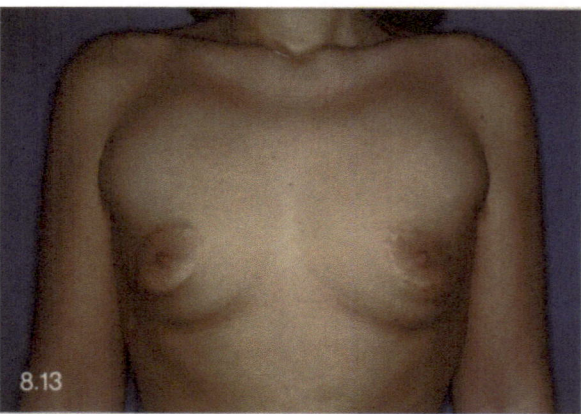

Fig. 8.12. Immediate postoperative result

Fig. 8.13. Appearance after three years

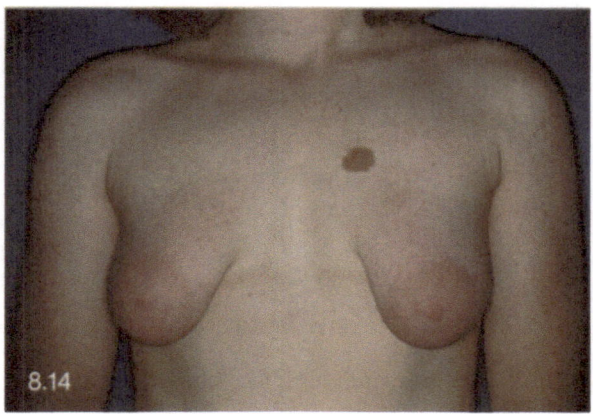

Fig. 8.14. Tubular breasts in an 18-year-old female

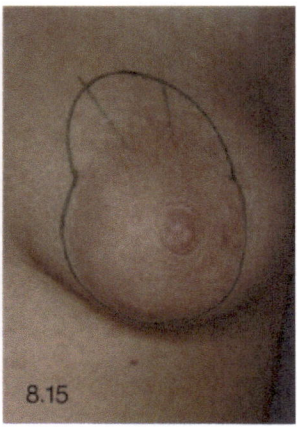

Fig. 8.15. Skin markings for the "B technique" of Regnault, which often encompasses only the areola

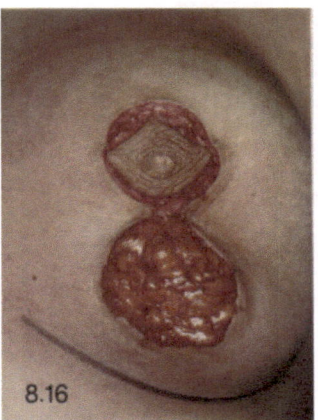

Fig. 8.16. The reduced areola is sutured into the superior half of the "B." The wound edges are apposed vertically or obliquely with resection of a small inferior "dog ear"

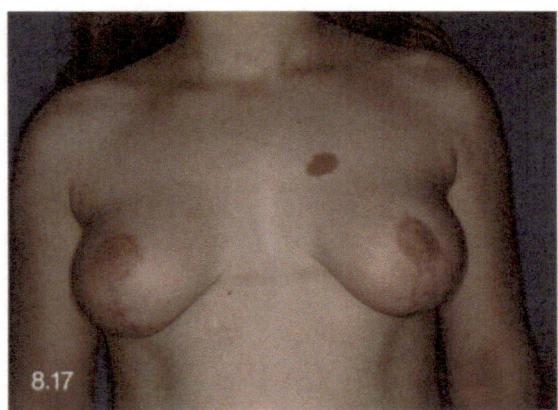

Fig. 8.17. Four months later

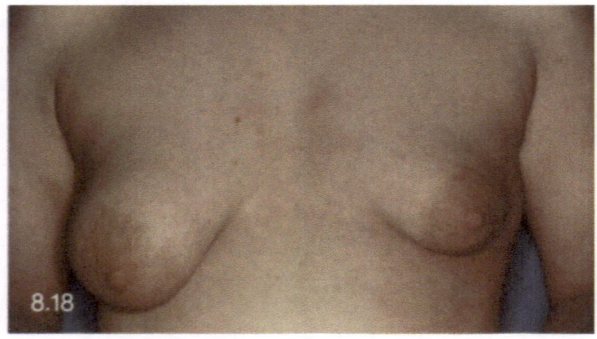

Fig. 8.18. Bilateral tubular breasts with left hypoplasia. The patient does not desire a silicone implant

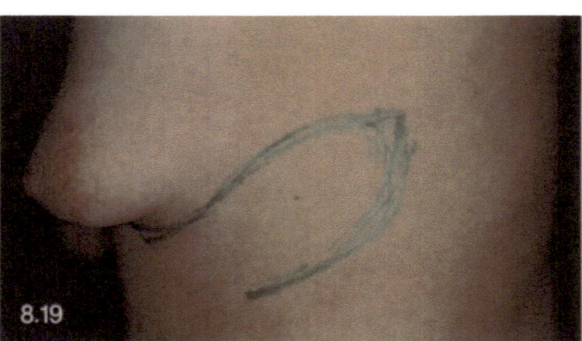

Fig. 8.19. Skin markings for a thoracoepigastric flap (see Fig. 17.2)

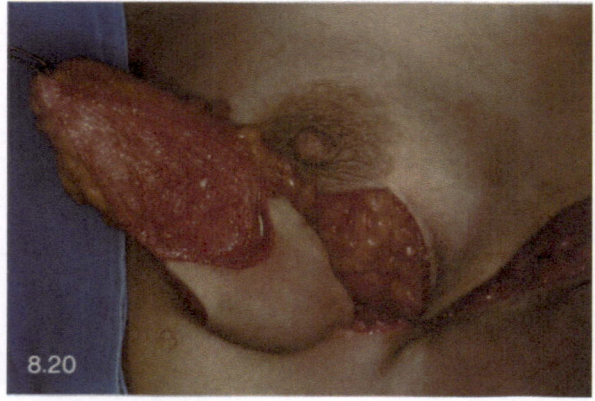

Fig. 8.20. Half of the flap is deepithelialized. The remaining half is used to increase the distance from the areola to the inframammary line (Exner)

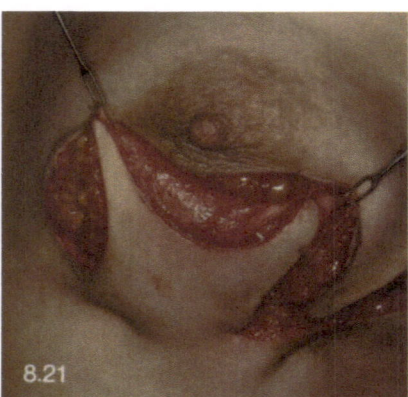

Fig. 8.21. Insertion of the deepithelialized portion of the flap

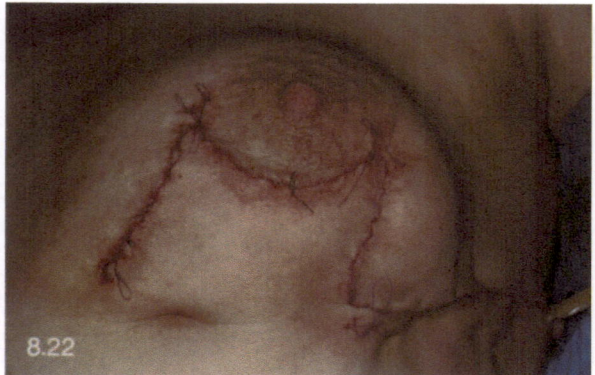

Fig. 8.22. Closure of the wound

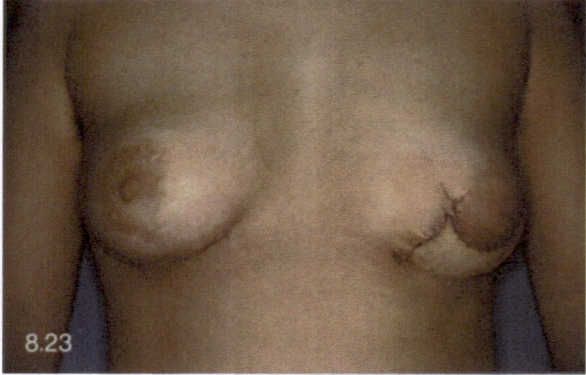

Fig. 8.23. Early postoperative result. A simultaneous right mastopexy was also performed

9 Nipple Anomalies

Indications

Unilateral or bilateral nipple retraction, either occurring in response to cold or touch or existing as a permanent condition, is relatively common and is rarely accompanied by eczema. The latter, of course, provides an absolute medical indication for surgery. Most patients, though, are young women who desire surgical correction for reasons of asymmetry or aesthetics.

The milk ducts in this deformity are surrounded by a heavy layer of connective tissue which causes a relative shortening of the ducts during breast growth. Since skeletalization of the individual milk ducts would be dangerous as well as tedious, complete division of all the ducts is the only recourse (Fig. 9.14), although naturally this destroys the possibility of subsequent lactation.

Technique

Various complex techniques have been described, but none claiming to preserve lactation are successful. The nipple consists of 12–20 lactiferous ducts surrounded by radial and concentric bundles of smooth muscle fibers – the areolomamillary muscles. A superficial and deep plexus of nerves and arterial vessels supply the nipple.

As in all plastic surgery, the simplest method is often the best: The nipple is pulled forward with a sharp hook and slit into halves to gain deep access for transecting the milk ducts as far as the areolar skin (Fig. 9.14).

If the patient is also considering augmentation mammoplasty, the latter should be done first since the pressure of the implant may be sufficient to effect and maintain eversion of the nipple.

Complications

Eccentric indrawing of the operated nipple is possible only if one of the shortened milk ducts has not been divided. Both nipple halves must remain standing after division of the ducts.

We have not encountered any blood-flow problems sufficient to cause superficial necrosis, nor have any of our patients experienced a loss of deep sensation.

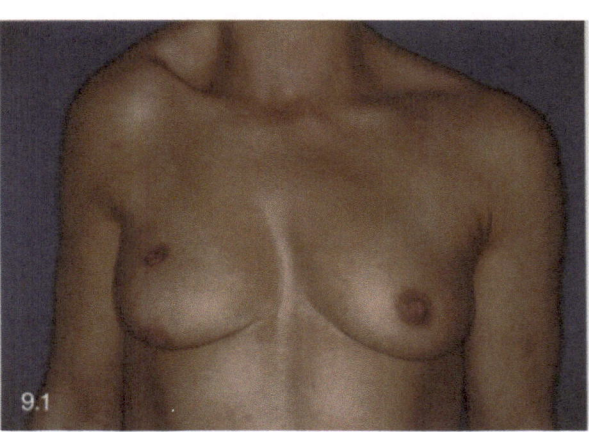

Fig. 9.1. Accessory right nipple with congenital elevation of the shoulder

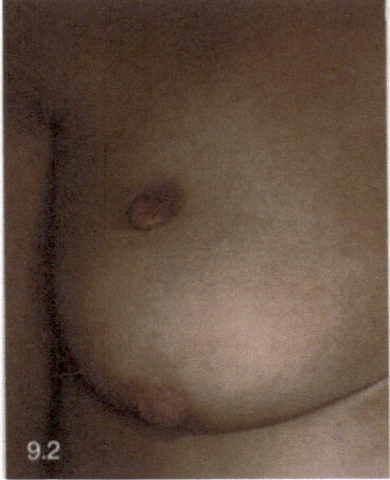

Fig. 9.2. Most of the glandular tissue appears to emerge at the lower nipple

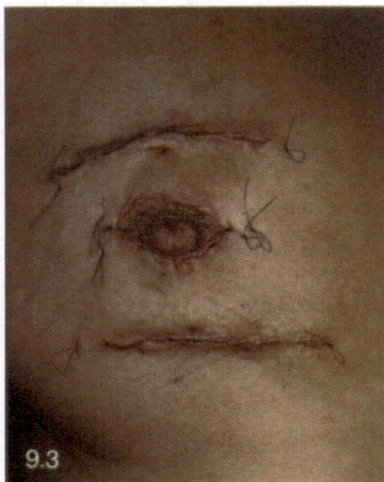

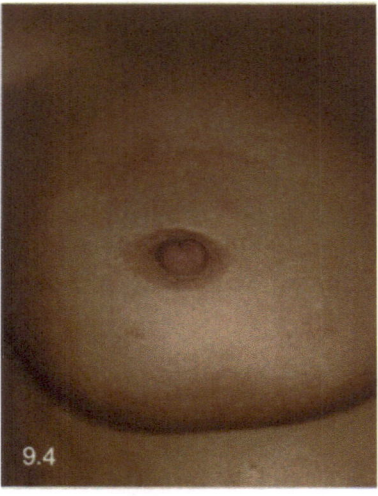

Fig. 9.3. The upper nipple is excised and discarded, and the lower nipple is transposed into an opening between the two nipples. This required mobilizing the inferior half of the mammary tissue. The old nipple sites are closed with intracutaneous sutures

Fig. 9.4. Appearance four years later

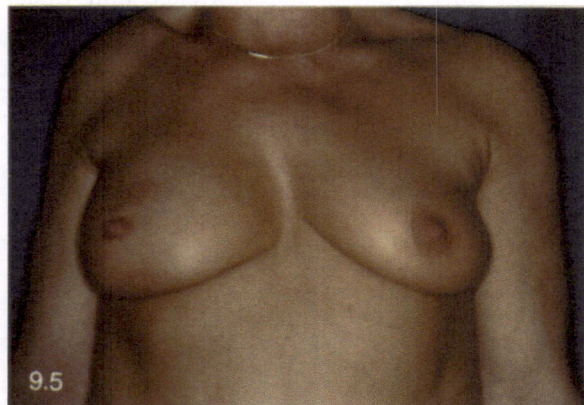

Fig. 9.5. The right areola could be expanded eccentrically to match the healthy side

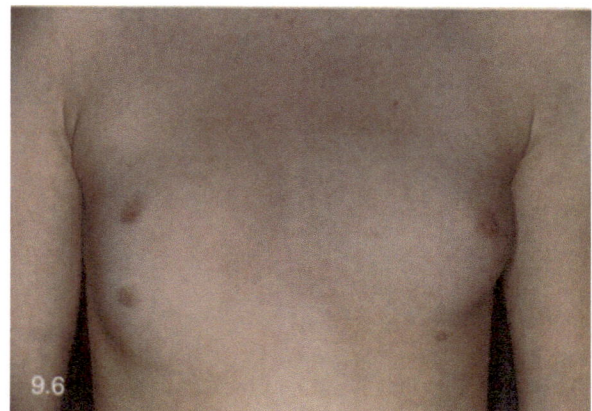

Fig. 9.6. Duplication of the right nipples. Each areola is approximately half as large as on the left side

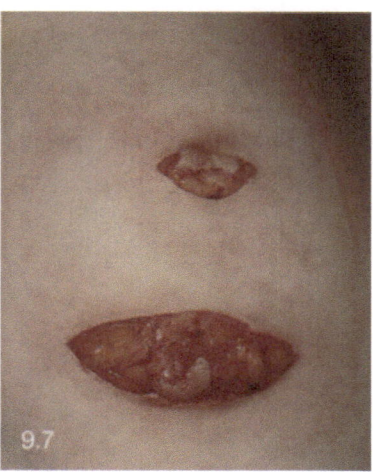

Fig. 9.7. The upper areola is opened by a downward radial incision, the lower areola by an upward incision. The inferior mammary tissue is mobilized posteriorly and anteriorly

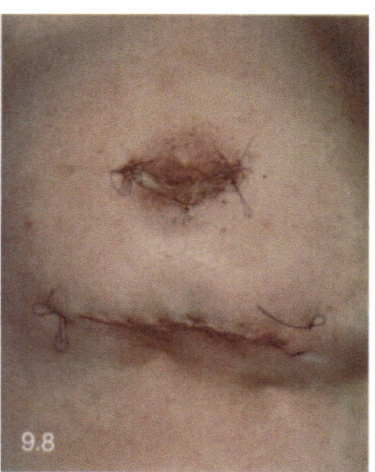

Fig. 9.8. The lower areola is spread out, transposed superiorly, and sutured to the upper areola to form a single complex

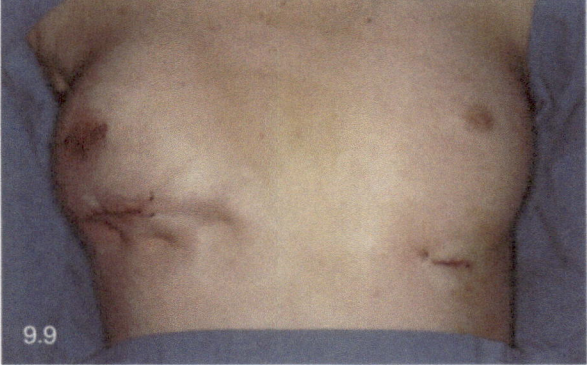

Fig. 9.9. Immediate postoperative view. A small accessory nipple on the left side was also removed

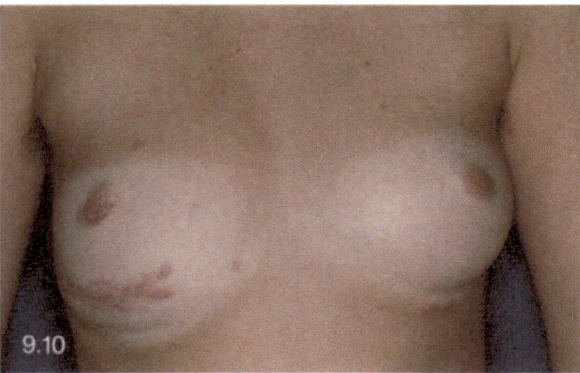

Fig. 9.10. Two years after operation. The right inframammary crease requires refixation

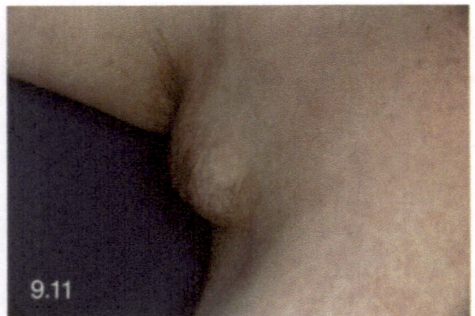

Fig. 9.11. Accessory preaxillary breast tissue in a 38-year-old woman who underwent massive weight reduction

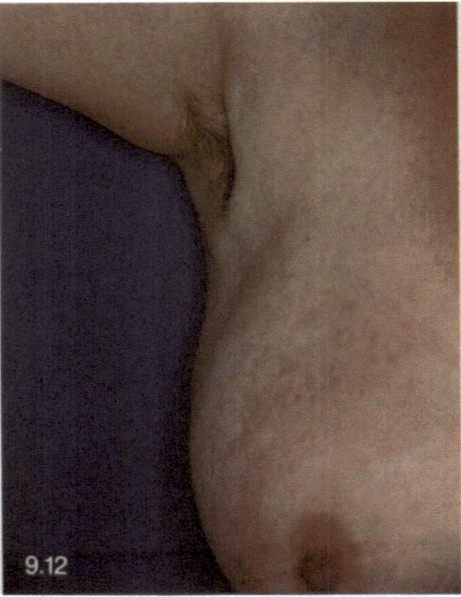

Fig. 9.12. The accessory tissue was removed along with a spindle-shaped piece of skin

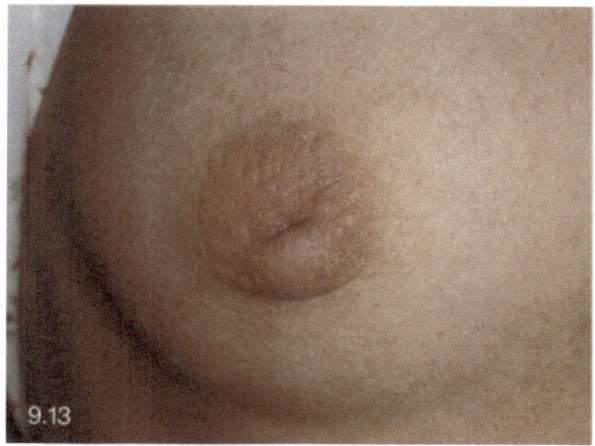

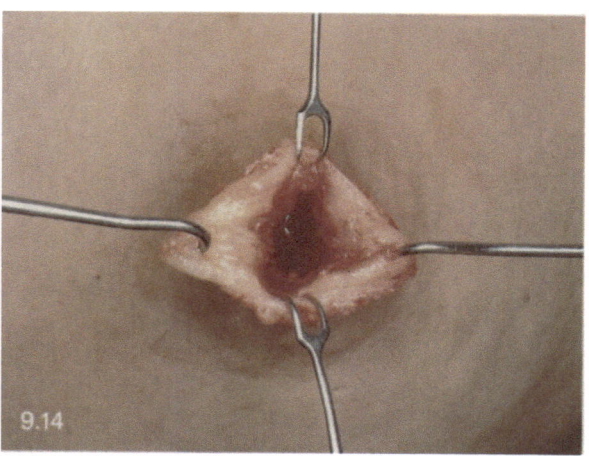

Fig. 9.13. Retracted nipple that is unresponsive to stimuli and therefore prone to eczema

Fig. 9.14. Through a 1-cm-long incision in the retracted nipple, the 8–12 shortened milk ducts are transected at a depth of about 1 cm, allowing the nipple to be everted. The eversion can be reinforced with a deeply placed purse-string suture of absorbable material (hemostasis is unnecessary). The skin is closed with several sutures, and a foam ring is placed around the erect nipple for several days to bolster the repair

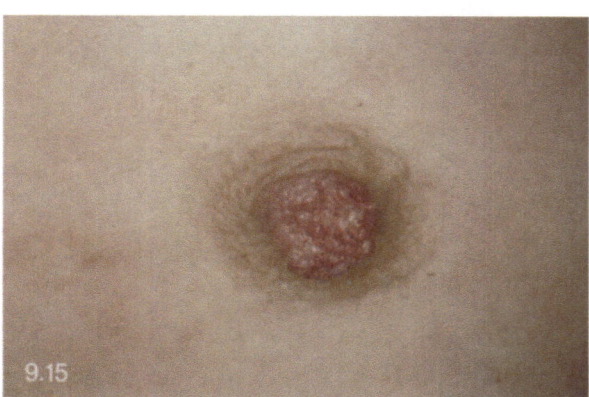

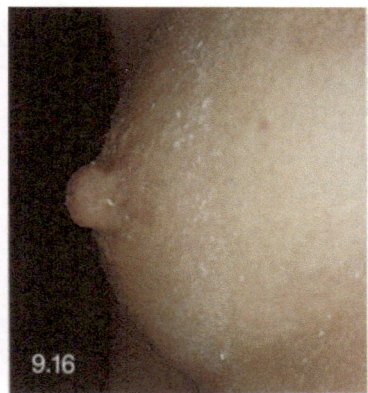

Fig. 9.15. Immediate postoperative result

Fig. 9.16. Result at eight days

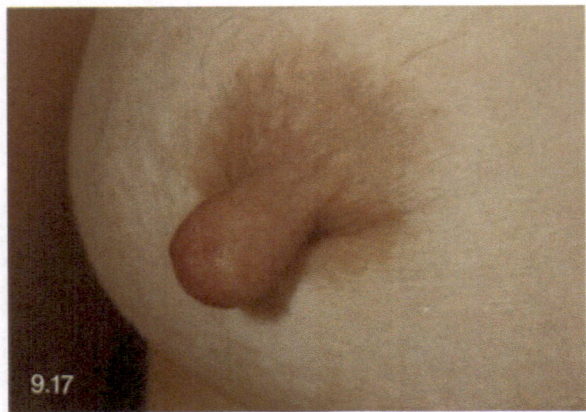

Fig. 9.17. Nipple hyperplasia. The nipple can simply be amputated at the desired level while in the extended condition. The wound may be closed concentrically with simple interrupted sutures or it may be left open, since deepithelialization [sic] proceeds from the lactiferous ducts

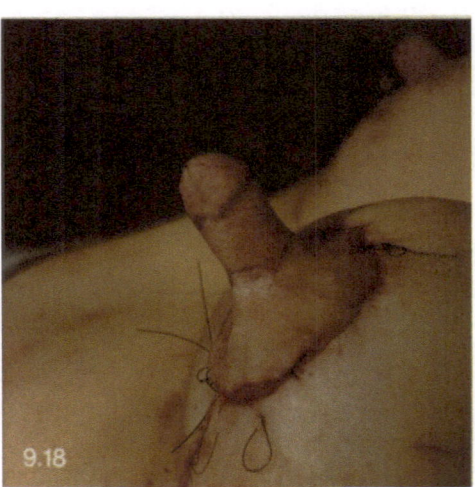

Fig. 9.18. Another technique is to telescope the long nipple upon itself after deepithelializing a ring-shaped area 1 cm wide

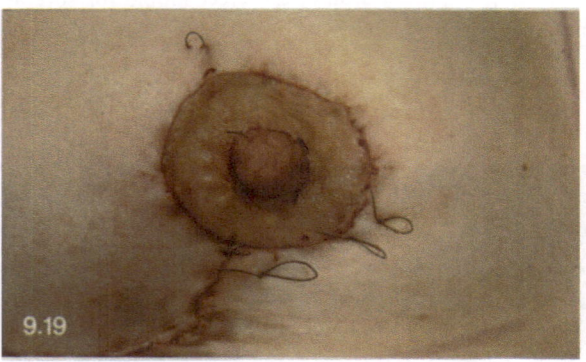

Fig. 9.19. The shortened nipple is fixed to the areola with simple interrupted sutures

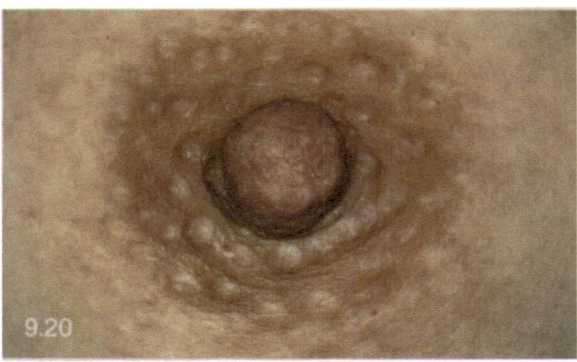

Fig. 9.20. Hyperplasia of Montgomery's glands, which the patient finds objectionable

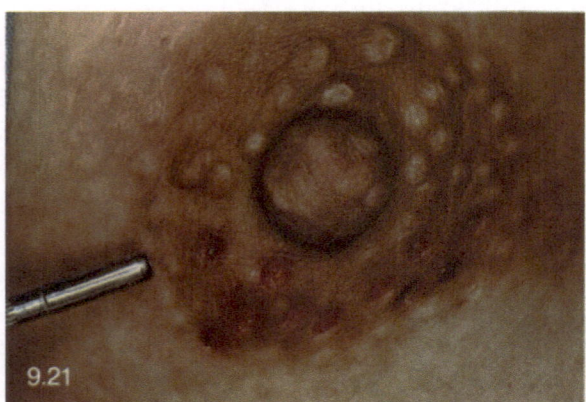

Fig. 9.21. The most conspicuous of the glands can be directly excised with a trephine

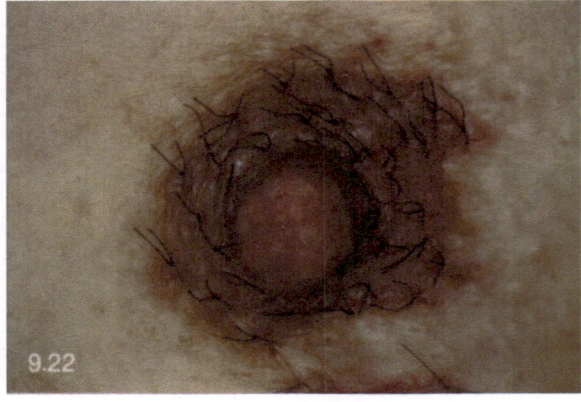

Fig. 9.22. Closure of the wound edges in concentric lines with simple interrupted sutures

10 Funnel Chest

Indications

Funnel chest tends to affect women less frequently than men. Only 5% of patients with the deformity require operative repair for physiological reasons. All others are operated for psychological need, in which case a silicone implant is placed subcutaneously to restore the chest-wall contour.

With a prevalence of 1:2000, funnel chest is not a rare deformity, though its physiological effects tend to be greatly overstated. A reduced vital capacity cannot be improved by elevating the depressed area, and the familiar ECG changes (p-dextrocardiale) are usually based on a torsion of the cardiac axis rather than a compromised ejection volume. Spinal problems are unlikely to develop unless the deformity is extreme.

Because most patients with funnel chest show no pathological symptoms, the simplest type of aesthetic procedure should be selected.

The best time for operation is at 5-6 years of age, before the child enters school. Often, however, the deformity is not noticed until it becomes obvious during puberty as a result of breast growth, so operative treatment will not be necessary until that time.

Technique

In 1972, Dow Corning Corporation introduced a new product called RTV Silastic 382 Medical Grade Elastomer (Fig. 10.2). This self-curing ("Room Temperature Vulcanizing") silicone rubber is formed by mixing the light-gray, syrupy, basic polymer of dimethylpolysiloxane with the clear catalyst, stannous octoate. The time needed for complete cross-linking depends on the amount of catalyst added. Thus, when 5 drops of catalyst are added to 20g of basic polymer at room temperature, the elastomer will cure completely within 5 minutes. In contrast to other polymers such as acrylate adhesives or Palacos, the curing process does not generate heat.

Once vulcanization is complete, the elastomer is as chemically inert as any other medical silicone product. It is nontoxic, nonallergenic, and causes no foreign-body reaction. As in augmentation mammoplasty, a fibrous capsule forms around the implant. Nevertheless, marketing of the elastomer in the U.S. was suspended in 1987 because of FDA objections to the tin content of the product.

Shortly before operation the patient is placed in the supine position, and the chest-wall depression is filled with water. The water is then weighed to determine the correct amount of RTV silicone to be mixed with the catalyst. The syrupy mixture is then spread into the depression, which is thinly smeared with petroleum jelly, and allowed to cure for 2-5 min. The hardened implant is then removed and sterilized in an autoclave. To optimize the chest contour, the front surface of the implant can first be lightly carved out with a scalpel to reproduce the slight concavity of the natural sternum with respect to the ribs. A leather hole punch is then used to make 20-40 perforations in the implant, both to reduce the weight of the implant and to encourage its fixation by fibrous tissue ingrowth (Fig. 10.4).

In children and men, the implant may be inserted through an approximately 6-cm-long incision below the xiphoid that follows the major abdominal skin lines. In women, an inframammary incision can be used. From there the skin overlying the sternum is bluntly undermined by scissor and then finger dissection, and thorough hemostasis is achieved with the aid of a cold-light retractor. A suction drain is placed behind the implant and left for 6-10 days, since wound secretions are apt to be heavy. Antibiotics may be instilled for several hours if there is reason to suspect *Staphylococcus epidermidis* infection.

Complications

Serum may still collect after removal of the suction drain, and approximately one-third of patients must return to have the fluid aspirated. The prolonged exudation is probably caused by friction between the implant and sternum at the start of each respiratory excursion. The persistence of secretions for more than two weeks should raise suspicion of *Staphylococcus epidermidis* infection, and gentamycin or another suitable antibiotic should be instilled.

Funnel chest in women may be associated with mammary hypoplasia, in which case the simultaneous implantation of a silicone gel prosthesis (preferably through a separate axillary in-cision) will provide further aesthetic enhancement (Figs. 10.8–10.10).

If the implant is found to be too large or too small, this can be corrected fairly easily by inserting another implant below the first or by cutting off projecting edges. Ease of adjustment is a major advantage of the self-curing silicone rubber prosthesis. This advantage is lacking in silicone-gel-filled prostheses fabricated by the manufacturer from plaster casts, though at present this is the only approved method that is available.

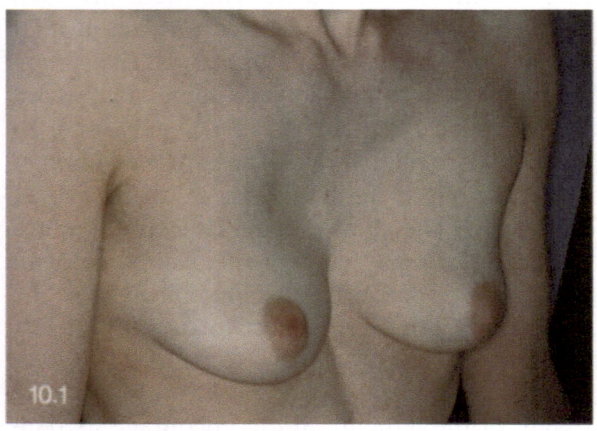

Fig. 10.1. Extreme funnel chest with no associated pathology

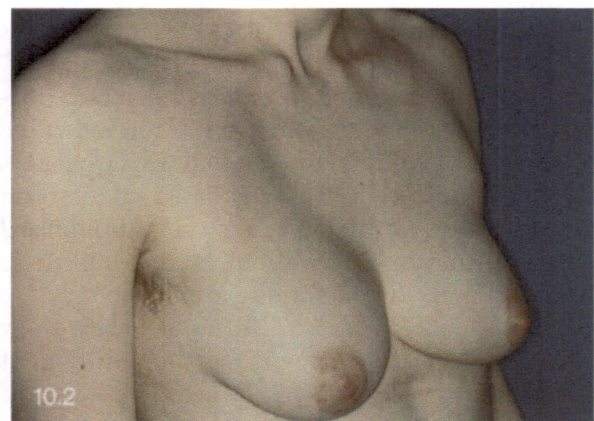

Fig. 10.2. Postoperative result

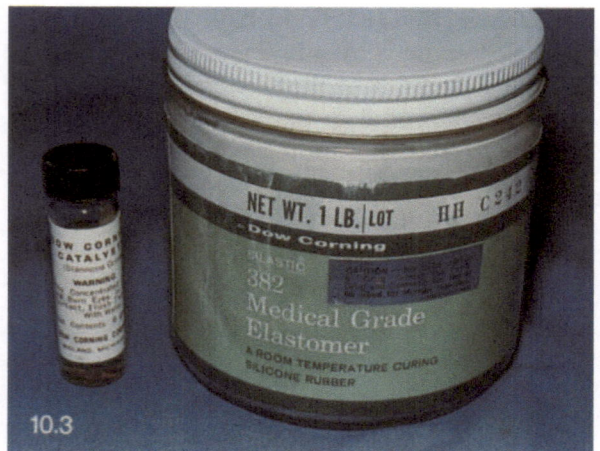

Fig. 10.3. RTV ("Room Temperature Vulcanizing") silicone elastomer from Dow Corning, shown with its stannous octate catalyst. (This product is no longer marketed in the U.S.)

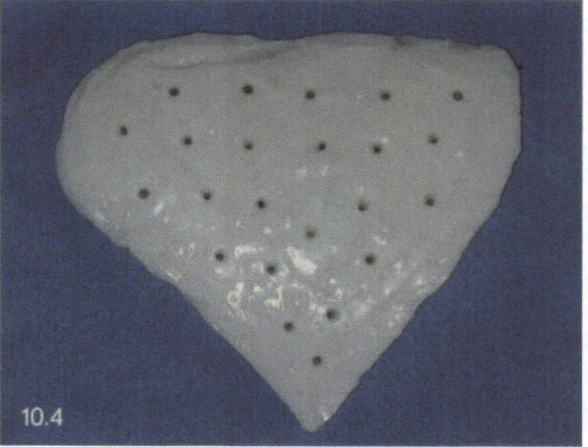

Fig. 10.4. The preoperatively molded implant is sterilized and inserted through an incision on an inframammary crease

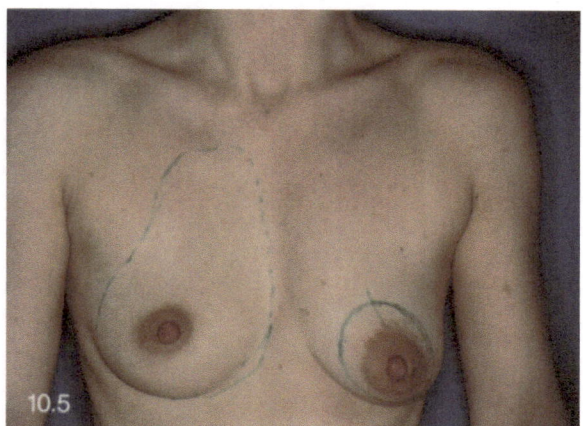

Fig. 10.5. Lateral funnel deformity encompassing the second through sixth ribs on the right side

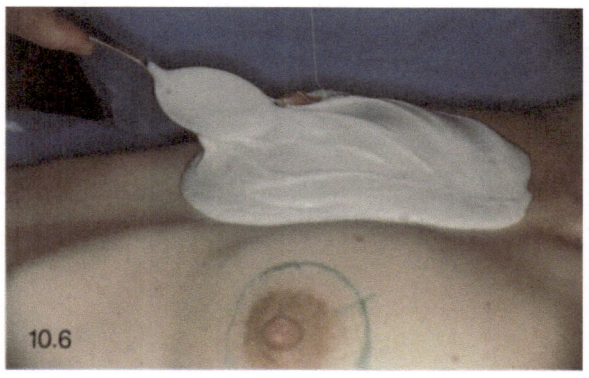

Fig. 10.6. The syrupy silicone-catalyst mixture is spread into the depressed area. Curing takes about 2-10 min

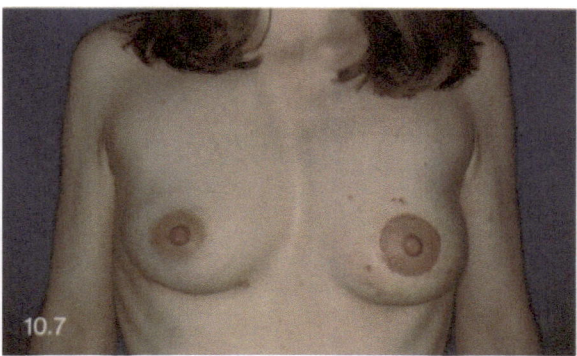

Fig. 10.7. The molded implant was inserted through the right inframammary crease. The left nipple-areola complex was simultaneously raised

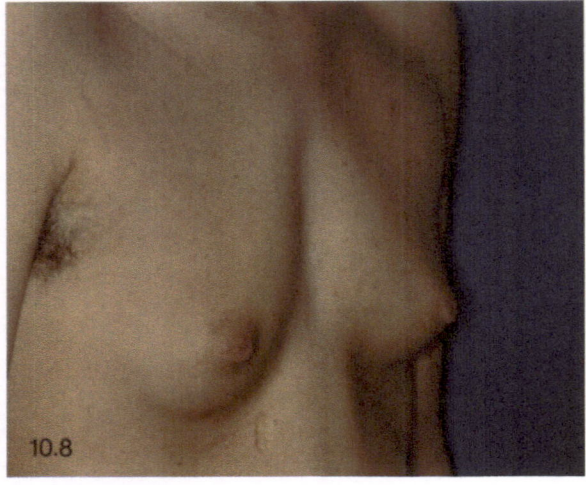

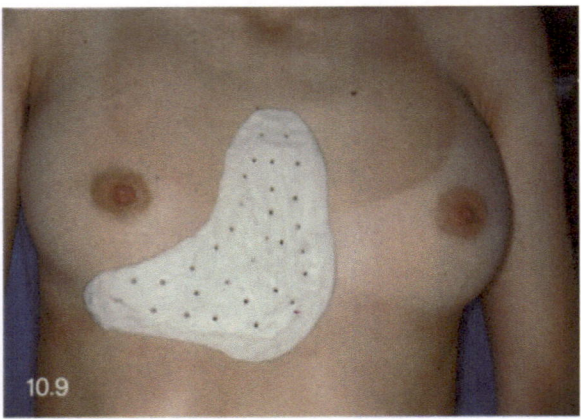

Fig. 10.9. An implant similar to this one was molded to the deformity and inserted through the right inframammary crease

Fig. 10.8. Unilateral depression involving the seventh through tenth ribs on the right side

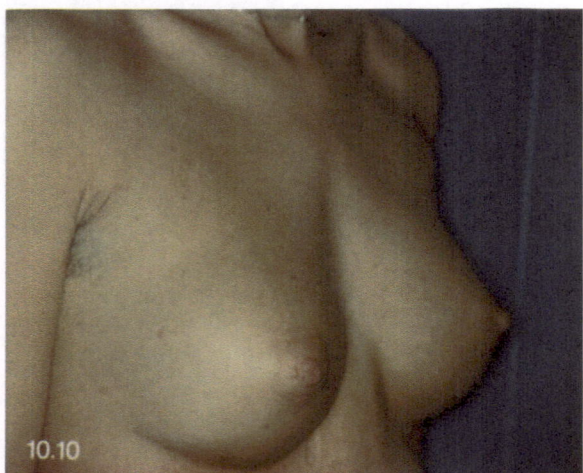

Fig. 10.10. Concurrent augmentation of both breasts with 150-ml implants

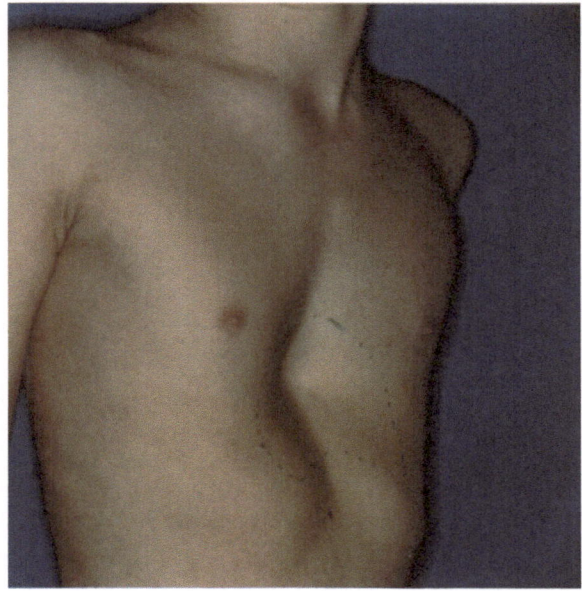

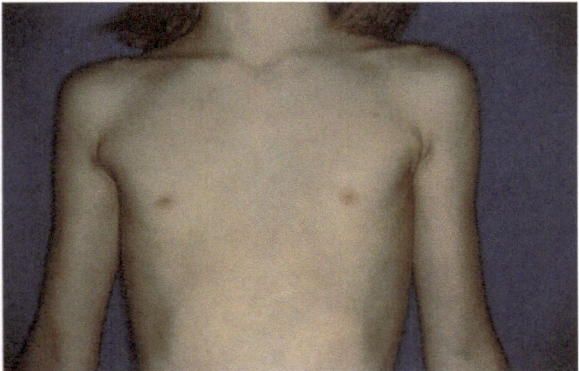

Fig. 10.12. Eight-year-old girl following implantation of an RTV silicone prosthesis

Fig. 10.11. A good time to correct the deformity is before the child enters school, as this will avoid body-image problems that may arise in swimming and other sports

11 Gynecomastia and Transsexuality

Gynecomastia

Hypertrophy of the male breast through enlargement of the mammary gland requires distinction from false gynecomastia caused by fat accumulation in the obese male. True gynecomastia is based on a predominance of estrogen relative to testosterone or an overresponsiveness of estrogen receptors in the male breast bud to female sex hormones. Any depression of testosterone synthesis leads to a relative predominance of estrogen and thus to enlargement of the breast. This condition is encountered in Klinefelter's Syndrome, in primary hypogonadism, following orchitides, and during chronic hemodialysis. Overproduction of estrogen can result from feminizing tumors of the testes, hepatic cirrhosis, and estrogen therapy for prostatic carcinoma. Thyrostatic drugs also can cause gynecomastia in some patients. A substantial percentage of adolescent males between the ages of 10 and 17 develop slight unilateral or bilateral hypertrophy of the mammary gland that is considered a normal phenomenon of puberty; involution generally occurs within a few months. If the hypertrophy persists for more than 6-12 months and hormonal dysfunction is excluded, surgical reduction is advised.

Technique

With fatty breast enlargement, liposuction through short, relatively small-gauge cannulas may be sufficient therapy (Fig. 11.8) (Courtiss 1987). The cannula should be inserted at the posterior axillary line or through a small transverse incision on the upper abdomen.

If aspiration is not sufficient, the remaining glandular tissue and connective-tissue septa must be resected, following liposuction, through an intra- or periareolar incision (Fig. 11.6).

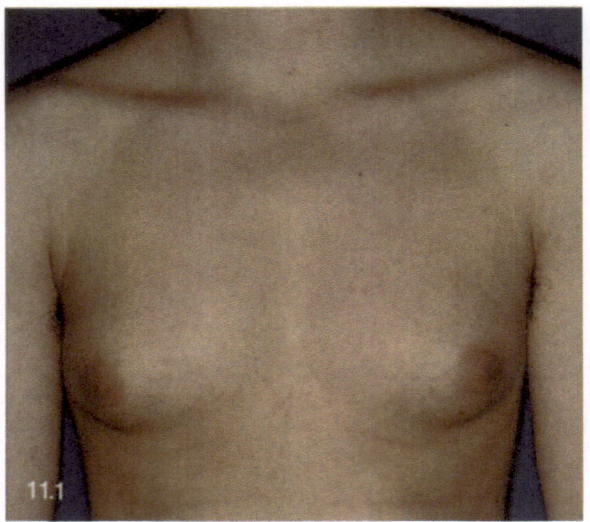

Fig. 11.1. Gynecomastia in a male with a normal hormonal status

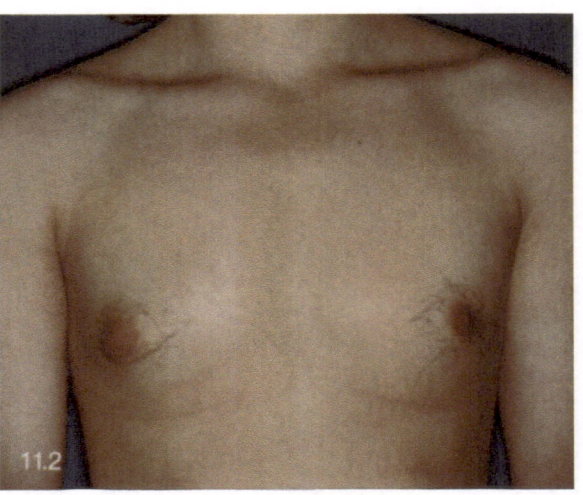

Fig. 11.2. Appearance after subcutaneous mastectomy

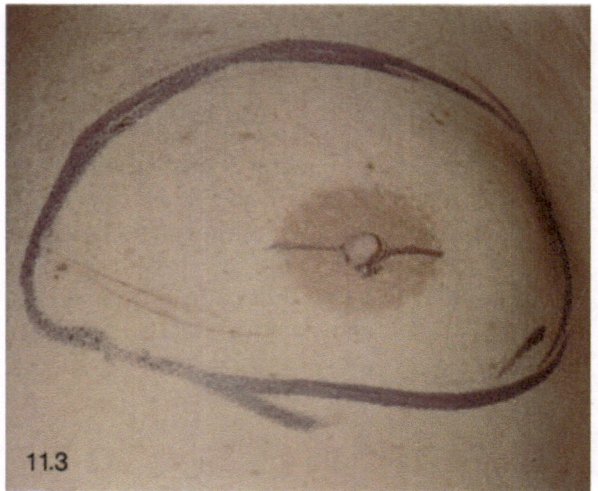

Fig. 11.3. With the patient seated, the extent of the mammary tissue resection is outlined on the skin. The incision should always be trans- or periareolar; it should never be placed outside the areola

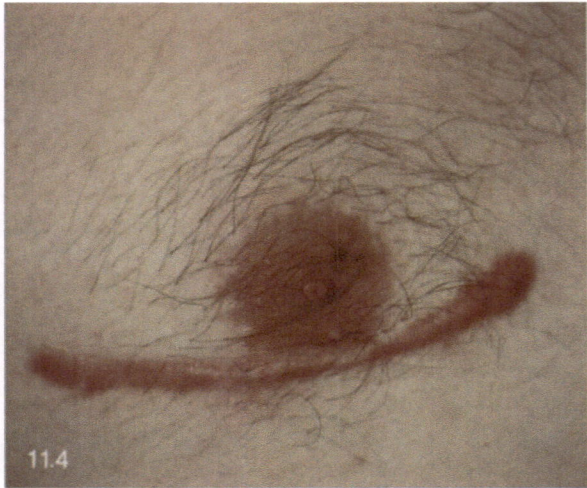

Fig. 11.4. Scar hypertrophy does not occur within the areola owing to the extreme thinness of the cutis, as in the .eyelids. This scar could have been avoided

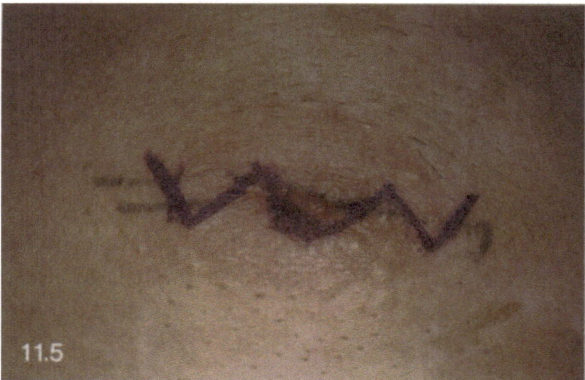

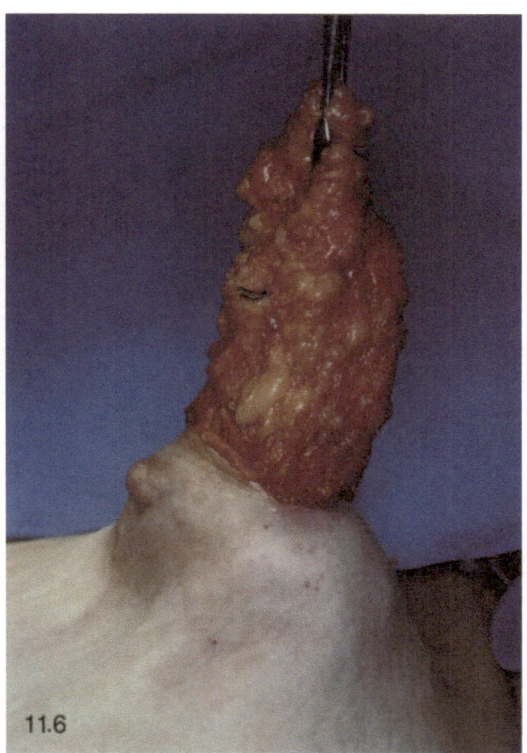

Fig. 11.5. The interruption of a scar by incisions leads to lengthening of the scar. This zig-zag incision can be lengthened laterally as required by adding another "V," and a relatively large mammary gland can be delivered through it

→

Fig. 11.6. During dissection of the mammary gland, care is taken to leave sufficient tissue beneath the areola so that that area will not become indrawn. The gland body is freed from the skin by sharp, eccentric dissection with a strong scissors, the fat-pad thickness of the surrounding skin serving as a guide to the depth of the dissection. When the gland body has been mobilized as far as the pectoral muscle, it can usually be bluntly stripped from the pectoralis fascia by upward traction

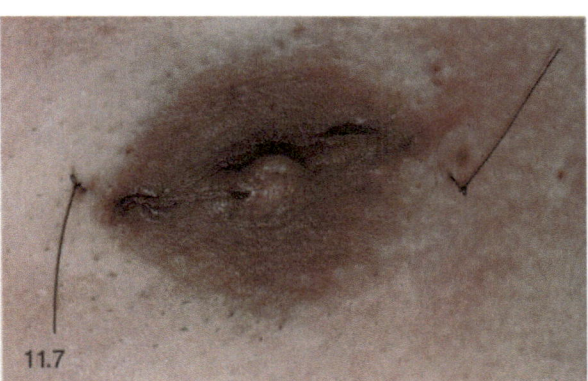

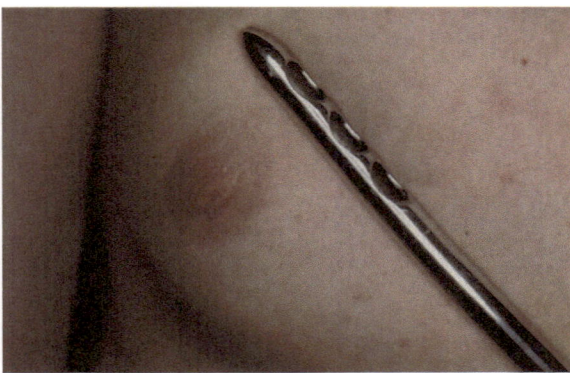

Fig. 11.7. After placement of a suction drain for 6–8 days (!), the incision is closed with a deep row of simple interrupted sutures and intracutaneous sutures. It is better for the threads to emerge at sites *inside* the areola

Fig. 11.8. In adipose gynecomastia (e. g., following estrogen therapy for prostatic carcinoma), the excess tissue can be aspirated with a cannula

Transsexuality

The transsexual individual, while unequivocally male or female in terms of chromosome makeup, hormonal status, genitalia, physique and pilosity, has the conviction that he or she is, in every significant respect, a member of the opposite sex. There are some 5000 transsexuals in Germany, approximately two-thirds of whom are anatomically male.

Feminizing hormonal therapy can produce moderate results in transsexual males who seek to bring their anatomy into conformity with their self-image. Estrogen therapy can elicit varying degrees of breast development and can even round out the angular male body contours, although it cannot eliminate beard growth or the Adam's apple, and it does not alter the skeletal build.

The effects of high testosterone doses in females are rather dramatic: The facial and body hair often become heavier than in the average male, the voice deeper, and the limbs more pronounced, while the muscular and subcutaneous

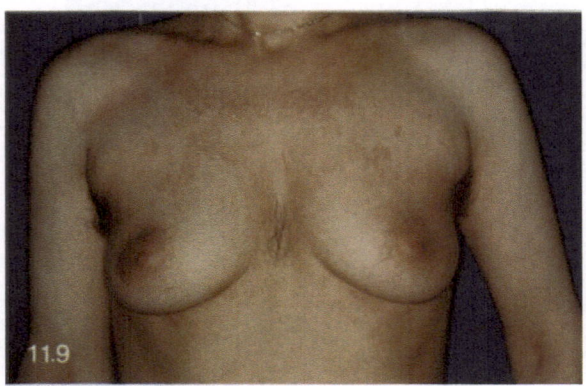

Fig. 11.9. Female transsexual

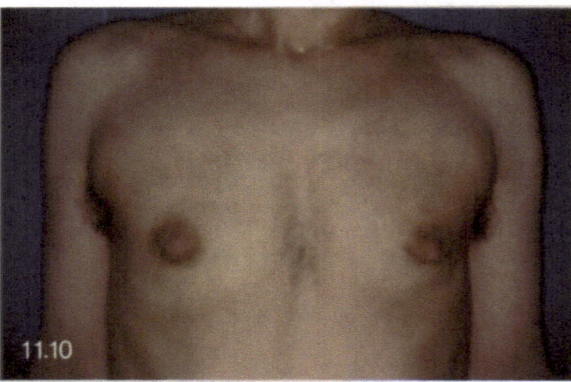

Fig. 11.10. Subcutaneous mastectomy without reduction of the skin envelope

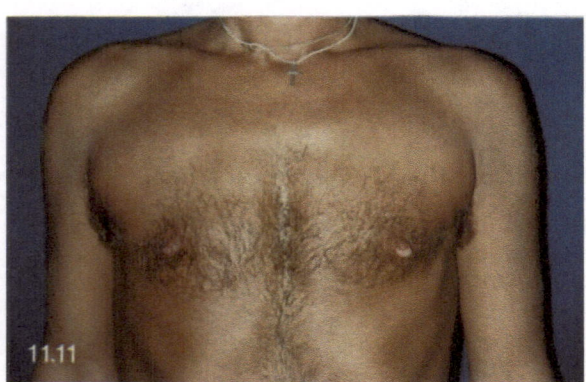

Fig. 11.11. One year after virilizing hormonal therapy. The effects on hair growth, skeletal growth, and muscular development are striking

tissues become virilized and the clitoris hypertrophies, often to the size of the small finger. However, hormonal therapy does not produce an involution of mammary tissue already present, so most female transsexuals will request a subcutaneous mastectomy in addition to sex-transforming genital surgery.

While augmentation by the transaxillary approach is generally very effective in women owing to the natural laxness of the skin and subcutaneous tissues under the influence of female hormones, subcutaneous mastectomy in the female transsexual can pose difficulties depending on the breast size. Skin reduction should never be done at initial surgery because the breast skin in young women, being remarkably elastic, is extremely prone to contracture (Fig. 11.10). We found that only 4 in 18 female transsexuals required a circumferential skin reduction from 6 to 12 months after their primary operation.

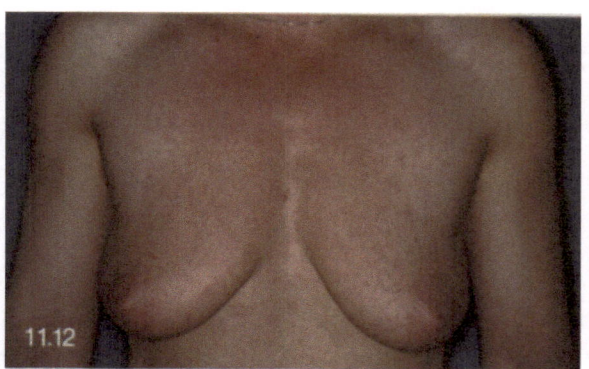

Fig. 11.12. Female transsexual

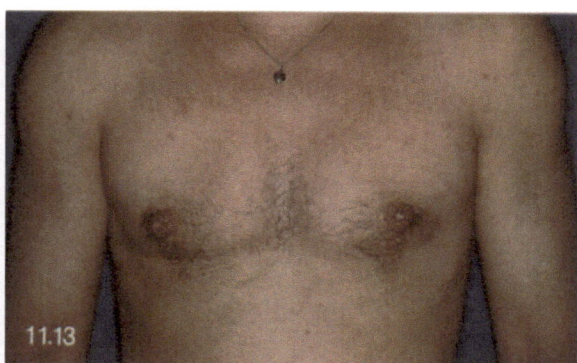

Fig. 11.13. Two years after subcutaneous mastectomy (without skin reduction) and treatment with male hormones

12 Burn Contractures

Third-degree burns of the anterior chest wall are relatively common in small children who burn themselves by dragging a container of scalding hot liquid off the table or stove. If the nipple is still intact and the breast bud is not removed when necrotic areas are debrided, the breast will develop during puberty only to the limit allowed by the cicatricial and grafted tissues.

If there are no contractures that restrict the range of shoulder motion, operative treatment should be delayed until the onset of breast development. At that time the most effective techniques rely on the use of rotating flaps, full-thickness skin grafts from the groin (where up to palm-size grafts can be harvested), and split-thickness skin grafts for larger defects. We are constantly impressed by the size of the defect that forms when the burned chest area is incised, and we are equally amazed by the development of a complete breast within a few weeks after release of the scarred skin and coverage of the resultant defects with split-thickness skin, full-thickness skin, or rotating flaps.

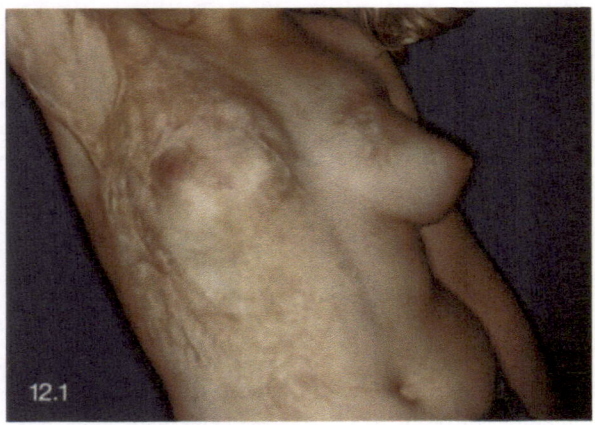

Fig. 12.1. Inhibition of breast growth on the right side due to a third-degree burn in early childhood

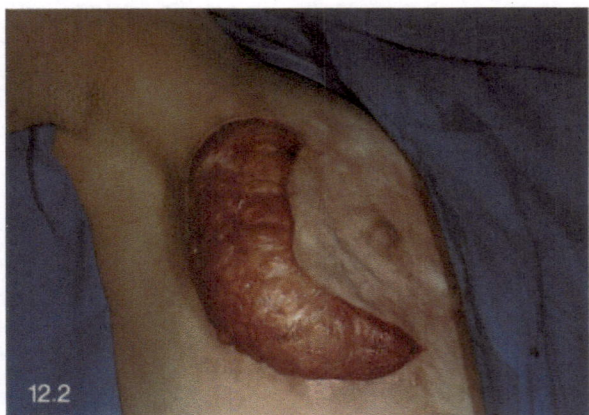

Fig. 12.2. There is a rapid herniation of mammary tissue when the burn contracture is incised

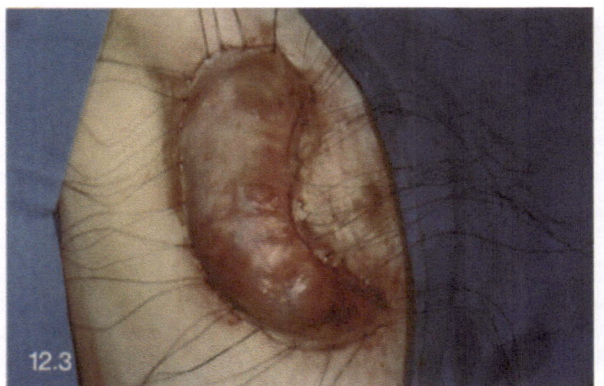

Fig. 12.3. The resultant defect is covered with a split-thickness skin graft (a better aesthetic result can be achieved with sull-thickness skin from the groin). The graft is attached with simple interrupted sutures

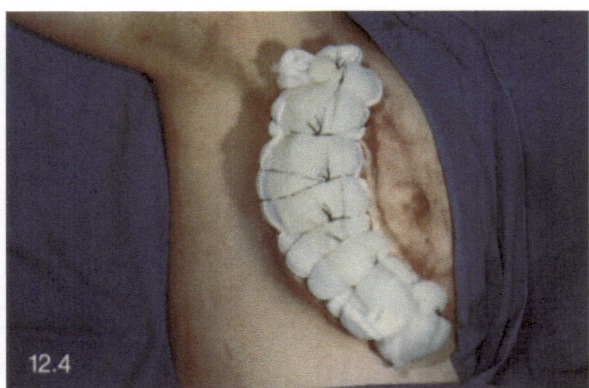

Fig. 12.4. A foam bolus pressure dressing is worn for the next eight days

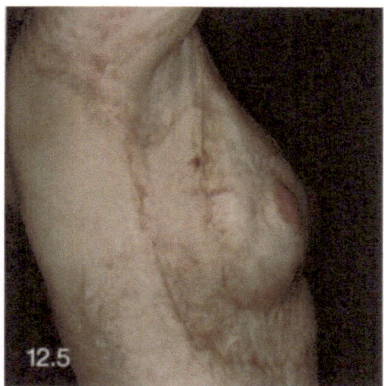

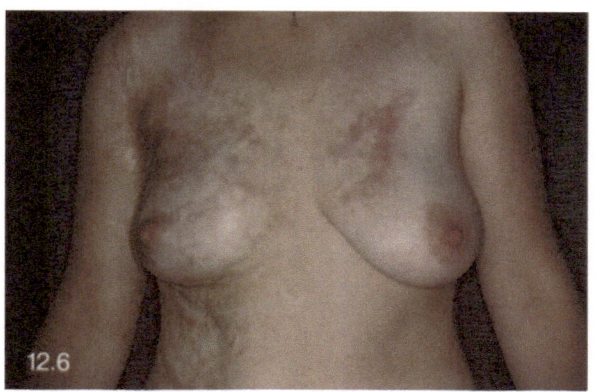

Fig. 12.5. Result at two months: The nipple is correctly positioned, and the mammary tissue is free to expand

Fig. 12.6. Satisfactory appearance 12 years later

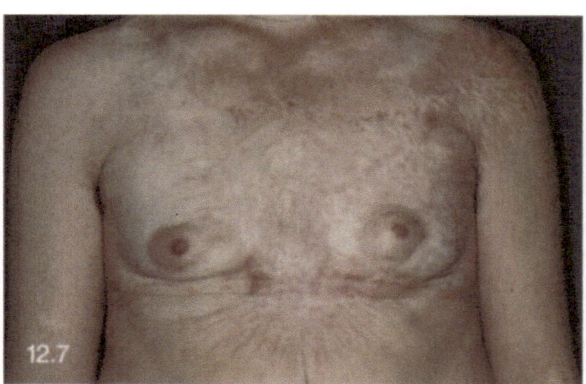

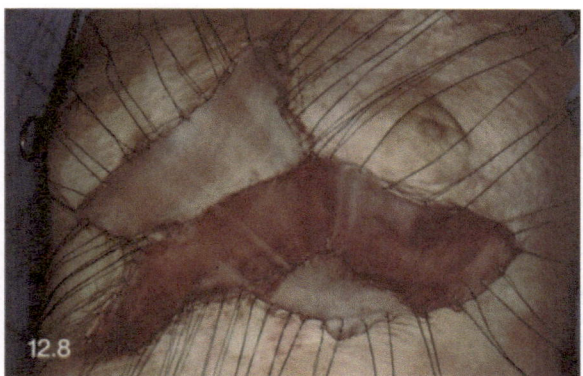

Fig. 12.7. Both breasts are medially displaced as a result of burn contractures

Fig. 12.8. A simple H-shaped incision produces a defect measuring 30x20 cm, which is grafted with split-thickness skin from the buttock

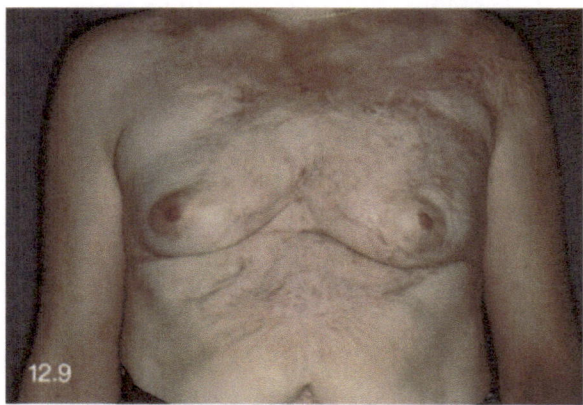

Fig. 12.9. Result one year later

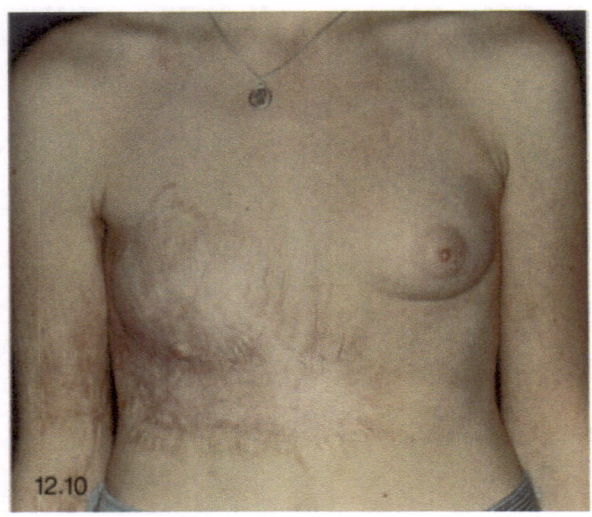

Fig. 12.10. The right breast has been drawn inferiorly by a sheet of scar tissue

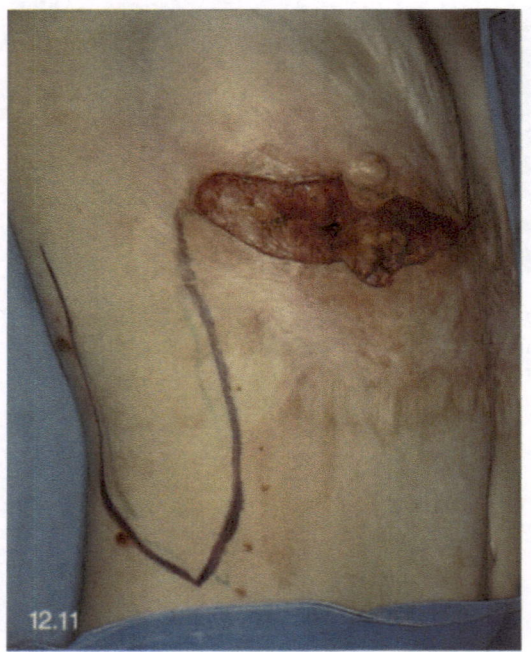

Fig. 12.11. The breast and nipple have retracted upward following a horizontal, infraareolar incision. The resulting defect is covered with a lateral vertical chest flap. A flap procedure should be done whenever possible, since a pedicled flap will expand with breast growth

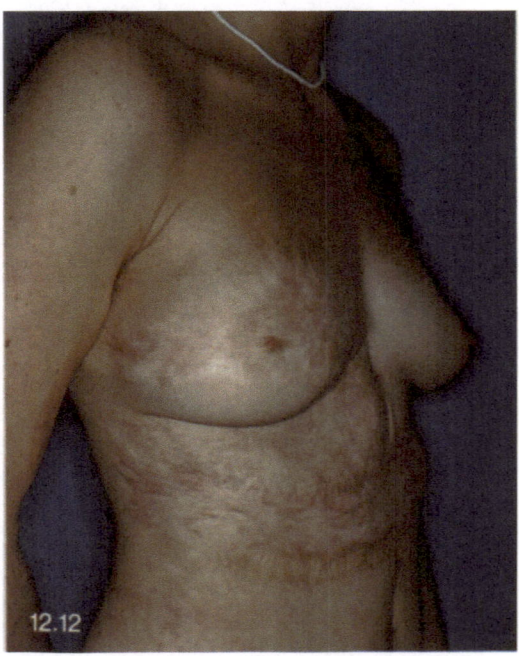

Fig. 12.12. Optimum aesthetic result

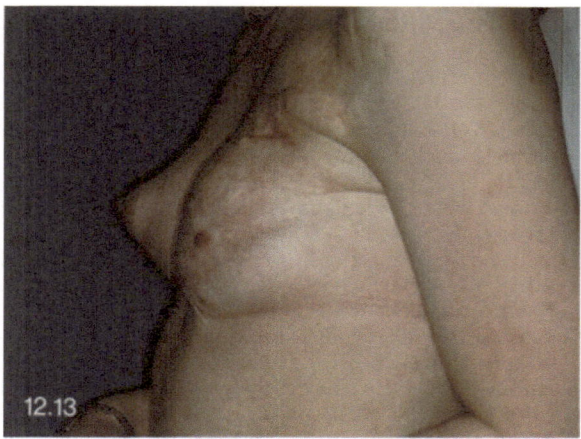

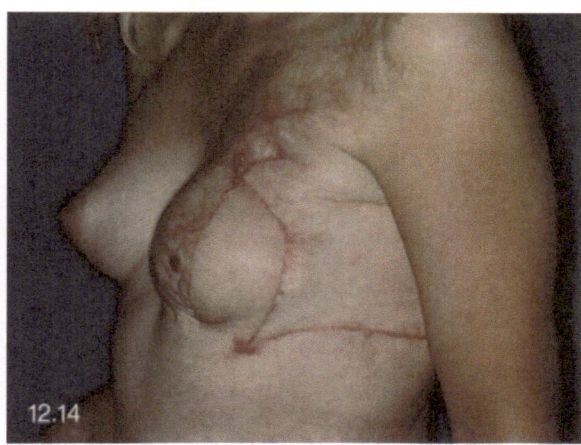

Fig. 12.13. This flat breast is kept from expanding by the overlying scar tissue from an old burn

Fig. 12.14. A horizontal flap is transferred from the lateral chest wall to cover both lateral quadrants of the left breast. A simultaneous Z-plasty is done to interrupt a band extending from the breast to the shoulder

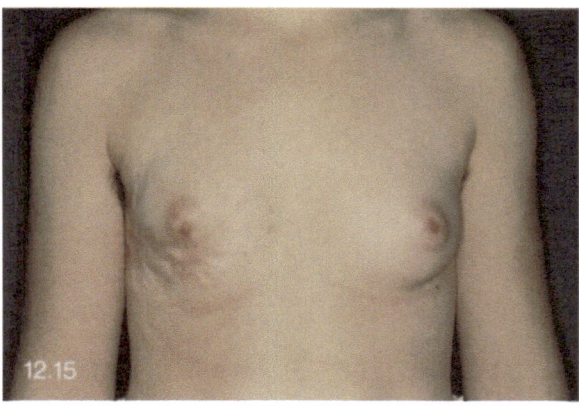

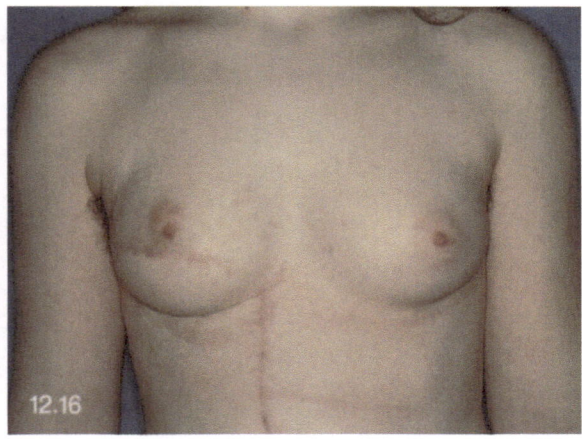

Fig. 12.15. Growth of the right breast has been inhibited by scar traction

Fig. 12.16. A vertical epigastric flap (see Fig. 18.2) has been swung horizontally into the skin defect created by incision of the scar, with a perfect result

References

Bass CB (1978) Herniated areola complex. Ann Plast Surg 1: 402

Broadbent TR, Woolf RM (1976) Benign inverted nipple. Transnipple areolar correction. Plast Reconstr Surg 58: 673–677

Courtiss EH (1987) Gynecomastia: Analysis of 159 patients and current recommendations for treatment. Plast Reconstr Surg 79: 740–759

Davidson BA (1979) Convention circle operation for massive gynecomastia to excise the redundant skin. Plast Reconstr Surg 63: 350

Gasperoni C, Salgarello M, Gargani G (1987) Tubular breast deformity: a new surgical approach. Eur J Plast Surg 9: 141–145

Gruber RP, Jones HW (1980) The „donut" mastopexy: indications and complications. Plast Reconstr Surg 65: 34–38

Hoffmann S (1982) Two stage correction of the tuberous breast. Plast Reconstr Surg 69: 169

Kraybill WG, Kaufmann R, Kinne D (1981) Treatment of advanced male breast cancer. Cancer 47: 2185–2189

Lemperle G, Exner K (1983) Die Behandlung der Trichterbrust mit RTV-Silikon-Implantaten. Handchirurgie 15: 154–157

Mühlbauer W, Wangerin K (1977) Zur Embryologie und Äthiologie des Poland- und Amazonen-Syndroms. Handchirurgie 9: 147–151

Oelsnitz G von (1983) Die Trichter- und Kielbrust. Bibliothek für Kinderchirurgie. Hippokrates, Stuttgart

Poland A (1841) Deficiency of the pectoral muscles. Guys Hosp Rep 6: 191

Vandenbusche F (1984) Asymmetries of the breast. A classification System. Aesthetic Plast Surg 8: 27

Williams G, Hoffmann S (1981) Mammaplasty for tuberous breasts. Aesthetic Plast Surg 5: 51–56

Part D

Breast Carcinoma

Each year, approximately 25,000 women in Germany develop carcinoma of the breast. This means that 1 woman in 15 must face ablative breast surgery in her lifetime. Although the number of tumors detected at an early stage has increased in recent years, half of all patients still die from distant metastases. In theory, the remaining half would be candidates for breast reconstruction.

Unfortunately, the therapeutic and adjuvant chemotherapy of breast carcinoma has not been as successful as was expected a decade ago. Metastases that were seeded at the time of operation are not destroyed by chemotherapy, only inhibited in their growth. Once the therapy is discontinued, the foci may grow very aggressively in the ensuing 6–12 months and lead to death within a short time.

Radiotherapy, which 10 years ago was largely abandoned as an adjuvant therapy for the prevention of local recurrence, kills no more than half of locally implanted cancer cells. Assuming a maximum local recurrence rate of 16%, the rate after postoperative local radiotherapy is still 8%!

Counseling

We do not approve of "radical" counseling, for it offers the patient nothing but anxiety, uncertainty, and hopelessness. Which of us could live with the truth? Therefore we tell the patient only what she needs to know ("It was breast cancer, but...") and will benefit from hearing. We became doctors to improve the quality of life, i. e., to project optimism and foster hope. Only those who have hope in the future truly live; those without hope merely exist.

What can a patient with knowledge of her lung metastases do about it? Though it has been said that the human will can move mountains, several psychological studies in recent years have shown that this is not true when it comes to influencing cancer growth.

Most women with breast cancer are already suffering enough from the burden of having the disease. Once systemic spread has commenced, the medical arts should be applied in a way that will help the patient live a psychologically unencumbered life for as long as possible.

The attending oncologist is responsible for maintaining a close, continuous follow-up so that any recurrence or metastasis can be promptly referred for surgery, chemotherapy, hormonal therapy or irradiation.

"Breast-Conserving" Therapy

The breast-conserving treatment of breast cancer, consisting of tumor excision with a margin of putatively healthy tissue combined with radiotherapy to the whole breast and a booster dose to the tumor bed, has been practiced with increasing frequency during the last decade (Veronesi 1986; Harder et al. 1988; Kubli 1988). It remains to be seen, however, whether this approach is the way of the future. Because the rate of local recurrence is already high with breast-conserving surgery and is expected to rise even further [Fisher (1986) reports 6% with and 24% without radiotherapy], we intentionally disregard breast conservation in this book. The 20%–30% incidence of multicentricity of breast cancer makes us extremely reluctant to leave behind mammary tissue that could just as well be replaced with a silicone implant. We should also recall that the value of prophylactic irradiation was widely questioned by the mid-1970s and came to be rejected by most therapists. Why should it suddenly be more effective today? Our first priority in the treatment of breast cancer must be the safety of the patient; the beauty of the retained or reconstructed breast is a secondary concern.

A retrospective study in 101 patients with early breast carcinoma (Fallowfield et al. 1986) showed that women treated by local excision and radiation experienced greater postoperative anxiety and depression than women who underwent simple mastectomy. The patients' main concern was whether they had received the "right" operation and whether all the cancer had been removed. By no means all women who receive a breast-conserving operation desire that type of surgery, and local excision does not protect patients from psychiatric morbidity.

13 Excisional Biopsy and Simple Mastectomy

Our standard operation for stage I or II breast carcinoma is a transverse mastectomy with exenteration of the axilla as described by Patey (Patey and Dyson 1948). Only when breast cancer is advanced do we perform an oblique "radical mastectomy" with removal of the pectoralis major muscle as advocated by Halsted in 1894 and Rotter in 1896.

A major advance in the operative treatment of breast cancer during the last 10 years is the practice, at many centers, of tailoring the procedure to the *stage* of the tumor and its location. This results in a more aesthetically pleasing ablative result and facilitates breast reconstruction.

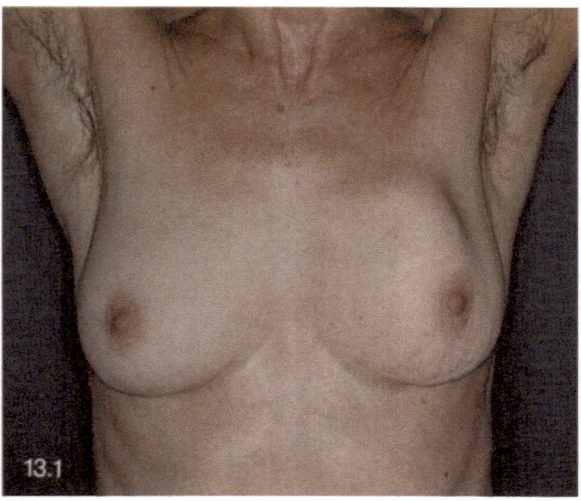

Fig. 13.1. Visible mass in the left breast. In cases where the patient has become aware of a nodule, it can be determined with approximately 90% accuracy whether the tumor is benign or malignant on the basis of palpable findings, mammography, and the patient's age and history. The patient should be counseled accordingly and apprised of the various needs and options that exist. If there is the least suspicion of malignancy, general anesthesia is indicated

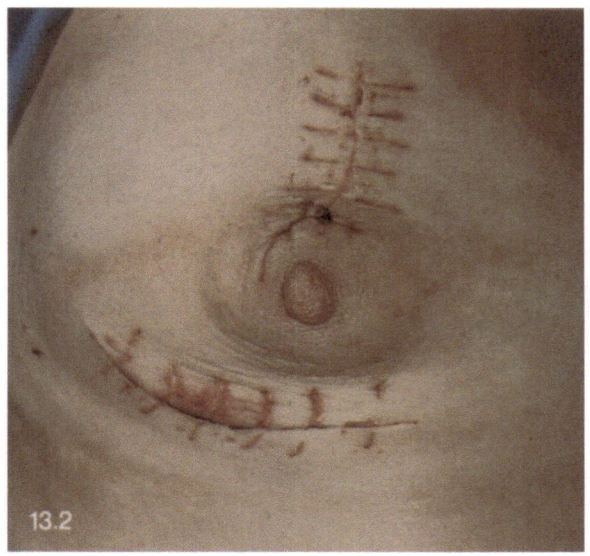

Fig. 13.2. Multiple suspicious nodules are uncommon. Generally they can be removed through a periareolar or inframammary incision. Radial breast incisions, prone to hypertrophic scarring, should be avoided. In young women intradermal sutures should be used on the breast to eliminate the "chicken ladder" that will perpetually remind her of the surgeon's handiwork

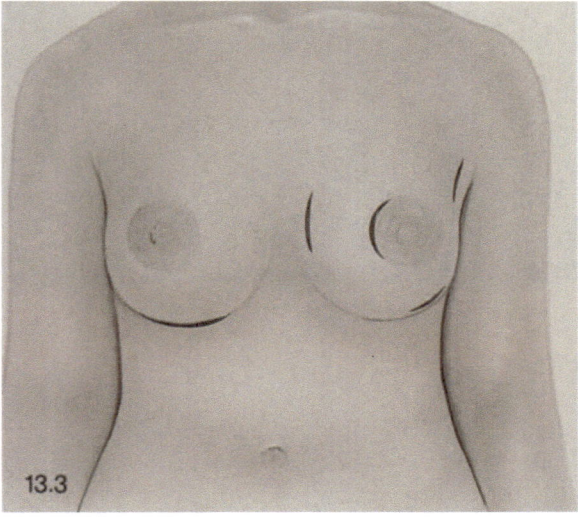

Fig. 13.3. The periareolar and inframammary incisions give access to any site in the normal-sized female breast. If the tumor is most likely benign, it can be reached through a long subcutaneous tunnel. However, a lesion that may be malignant should be approached as directly as possible

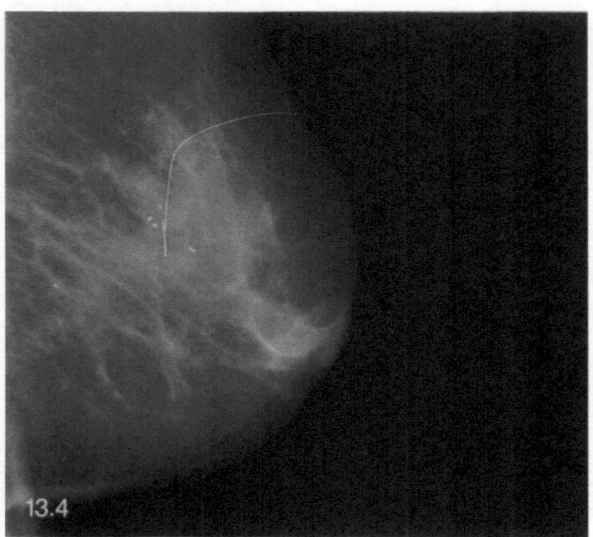

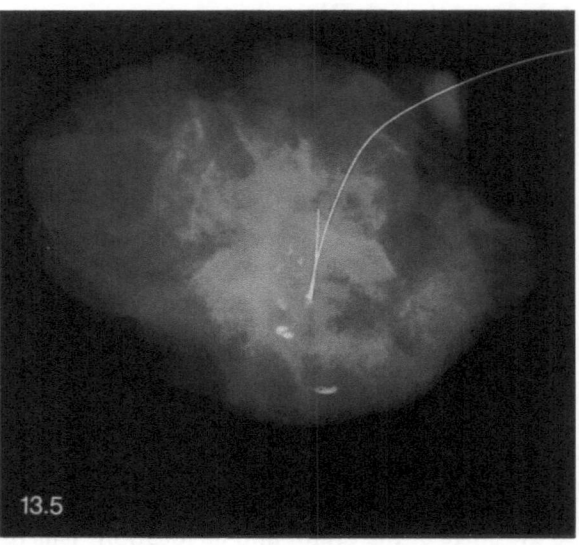

Fig. 13.4. If mammography reveals microcalcifications that are not palpable, preoperative needle localization can be performed to guide the excision

Fig. 13.5. Microcalcifications that are nonpalpable and distant from the nipple should be marked preoperatively by the radiologist. Otherwise, at operation, the surgeon can compress the breast vertically and horizontally as in the mammographic compression device and locate the suspicious area using a centimeter rule. Intraoperative specimen radiography is routinely performed

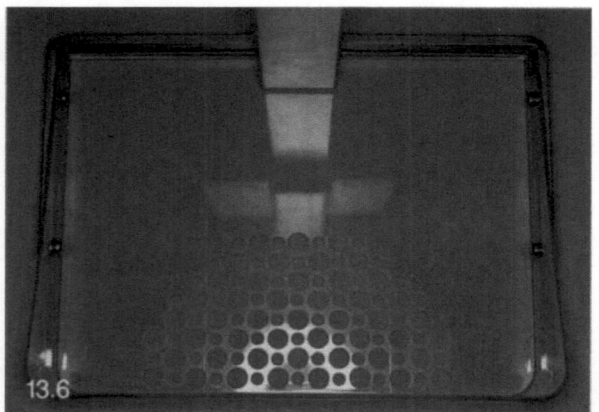

Fig. 13.6. Siemens has developed a special mammographic cone with grid-like perforations through which the tumor can be localized and the needle, armed with a harpoon wire, can be inserted

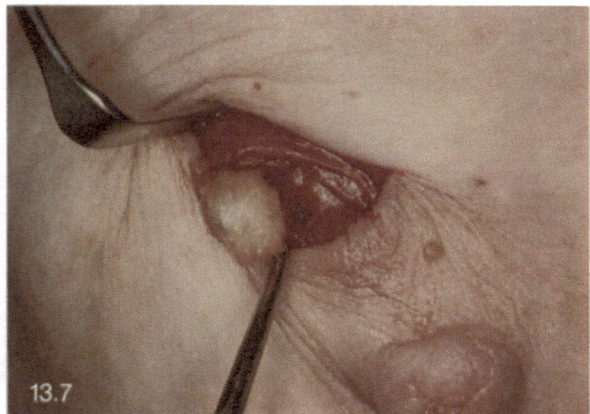

Fig. 13.7. Small fibroadenoma delivered through a peri-areolar incision from a distance of 4 cm. A tumor should never be grasped with a forceps, but if possible should be engaged at its edge with a sharp hook. Potentially malignant tumors should not be grasped with any kind of instrument, as this might seed cancer cells into the lymph

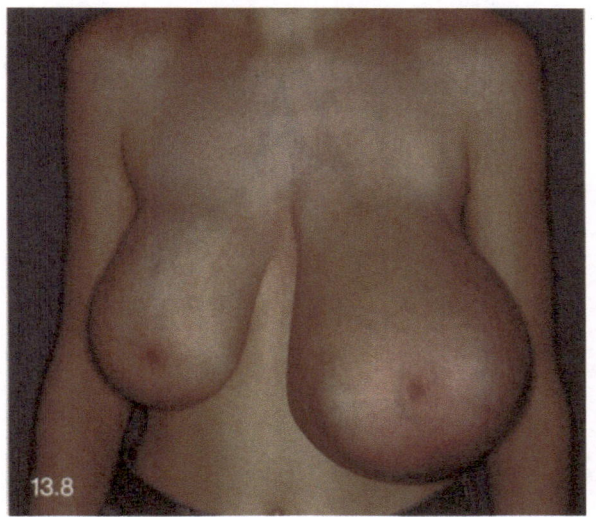

Fig. 13.8. Juvenile fibroadenoma in a 16-year-old girl

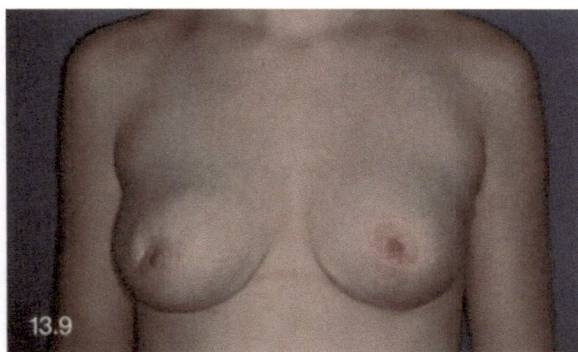

Fig. 13.9. One year after tumor removal and bilateral reduction mammoplasty

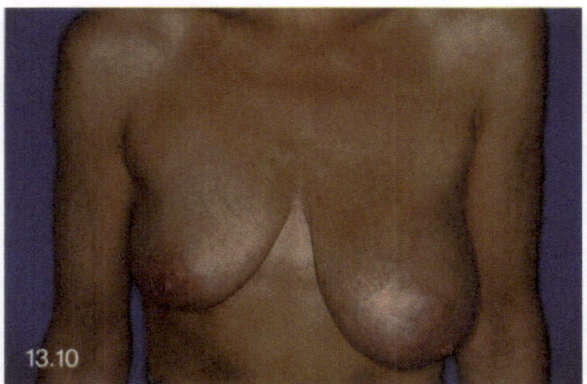

Fig. 13.10. Benign cystosarcoma phyllodes, which had been developing for 15 months

⟶

Fig. 13.11. A cystosarcoma phyllodes need only be extirpated at initial surgery, at which time the tumor bed is resected to a depth of 1 cm. If the tumor recurs, subcutaneous mastectomy is indicated along with very close follow-up, since these tumors can undergo malignant transformation within a period of months

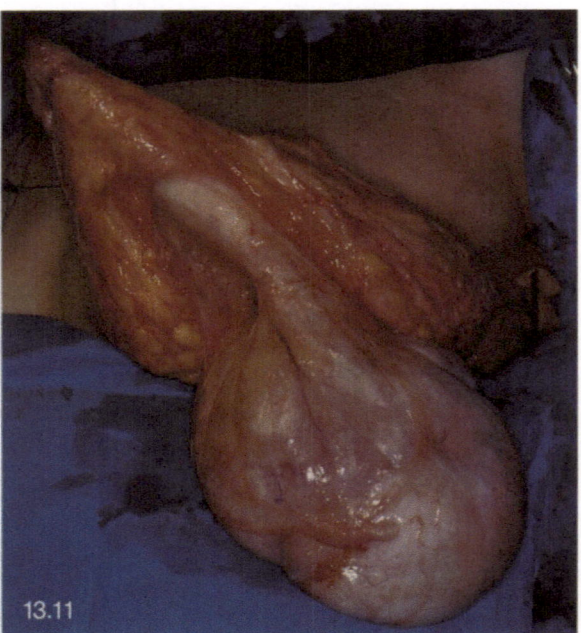

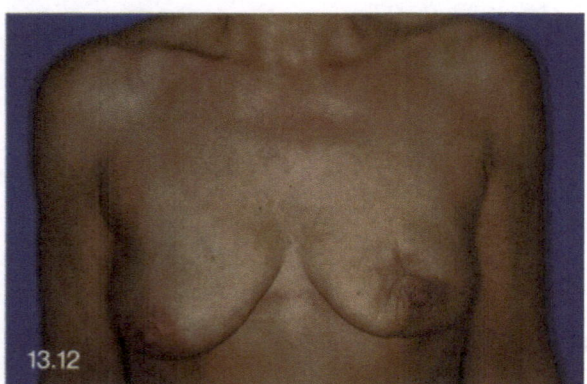

Fig. 13.12. After 2 months the skin has contracted to its former size (see Chap. 19, Tissue Expanders)

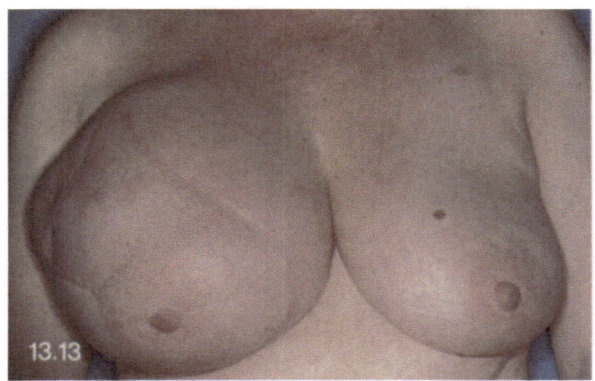

Fig. 13.13. Fourth recurrence of cystosarcoma phyllodes

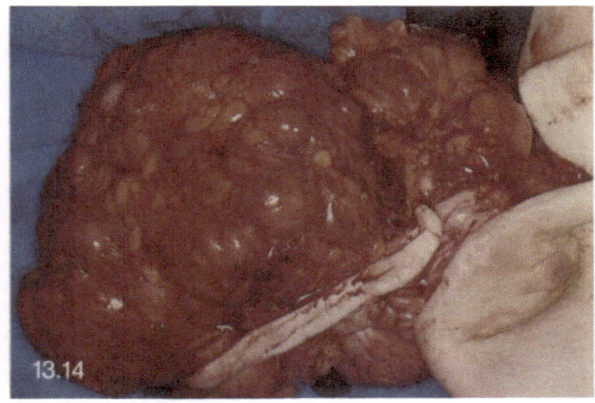

Fig. 13.14. The tumor is excised with a margin of healthy tissue, preserving the nipple-areola complex

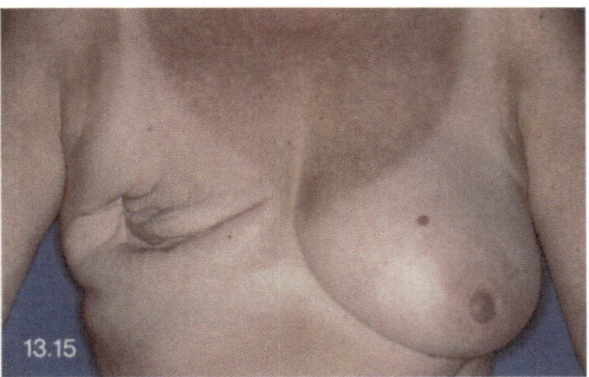

Fig. 13.15. At two years the patient shows no evidence of disease (cf. Fig. 20.14)

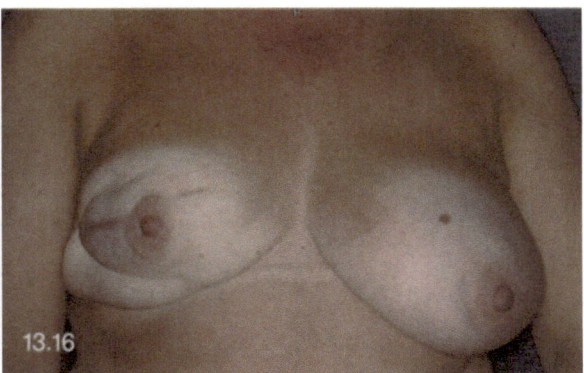

Fig. 13.16. The breast has been reconstructed with a bilumen silicone implant. The insertion of a larger prosthesis and a symmetrizing left breast reduction are proposed

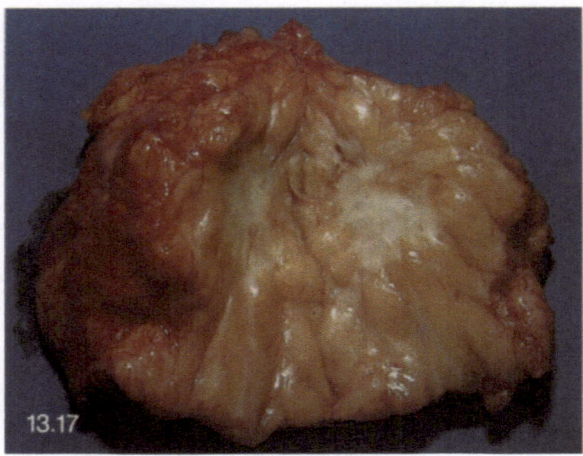

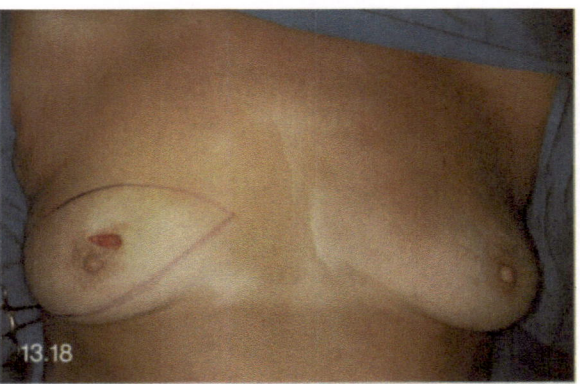

Fig. 13.17. Widely excised scirrhous carcinoma. No residual tumor cells should be found in the cavity left by the excision

Fig. 13.18. Simple mastectomy for a centrally located tumor necessitating removal of the nipple-areola. The axillary dissection can also be performed through this approach

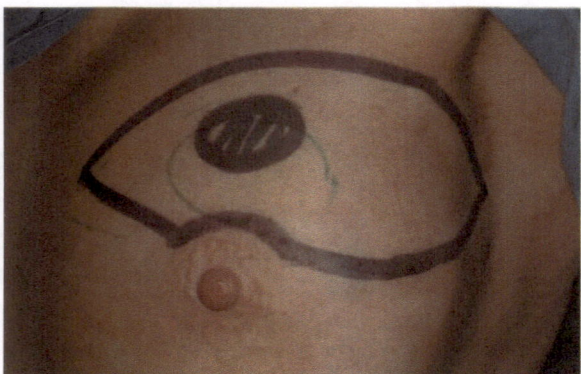

Fig. 13.19. If the tumor is above the areola in a ptotic breast, the resection can include a supraareolar ellipse of skin, permitting elevation of the nipple-areola to a more prominent site. Complete removal of the mammary gland is always indicated for cancerous and precancerous disease

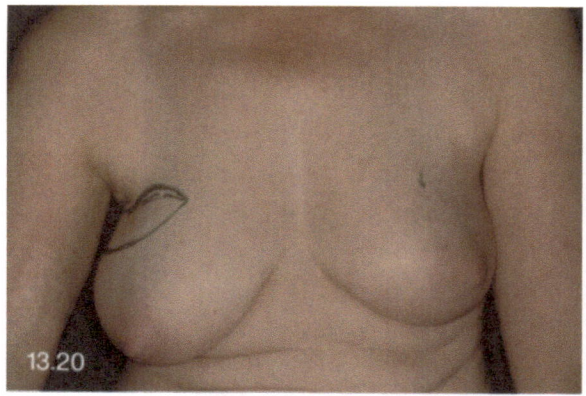

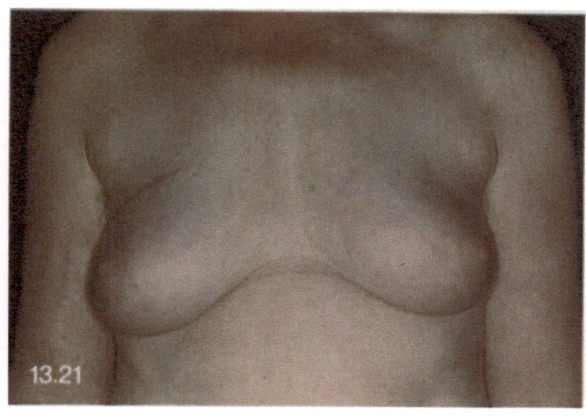

Fig. 13.20. A small carcinoma in the upper outer quadrant of the left breast was removed by quadrantectomy with an elliptical skin excision. As this improved the breast shape, a similar excision was performed on the right side. Of course, this can succeed only if scar formation is good

Fig. 13.21. The aesthetic result is satisfactory, but the patient is still considered high-risk because of the large amount of breast tissue that remains. Although tumorectomy with postoperative irradiation is commonly practiced, we do not advocate it because fibrosis of the irradiated mammary tissue is frequent and can make follow-up extremely difficult

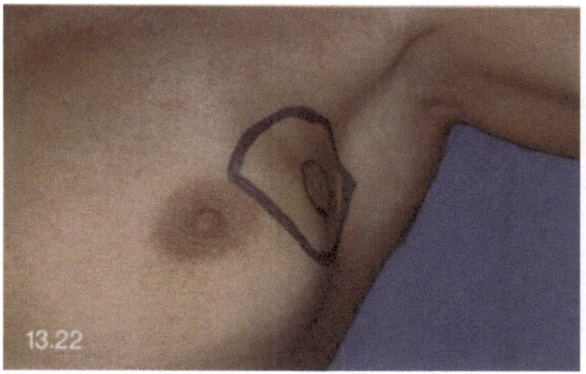

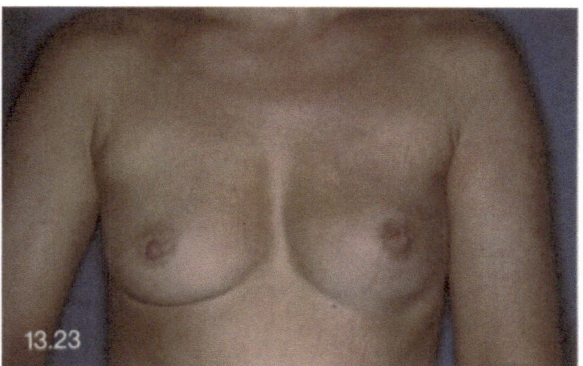

Fig. 13.22. Superficial carcinoma managed by subcutaneous mastectomy with an elliptical skin excision and axillary dissection through the same approach

Fig. 13.23. Result after immediate reconstruction

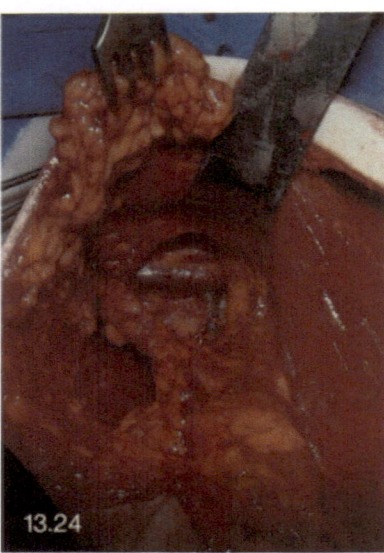

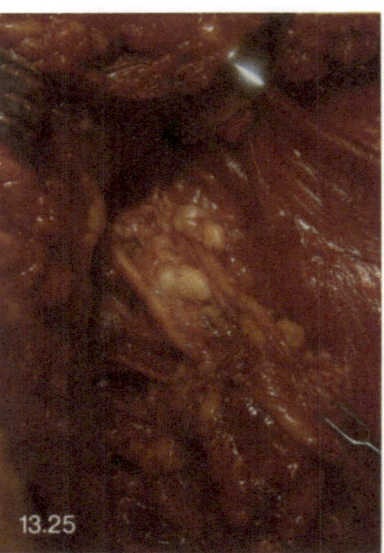

Fig. 13.24. This axilla contains no palpable lymph nodes, so it is necessary only to remove the subaxillary lymph node chain and Rotter's lymph nodes between the pectoralis major and minor muscles for diagnostic purposes

Fig. 13.25. Here there is obvious involvement of the axillary nodes, apparent even on clinical examination, necessitating a radical axillary dissection with skeletization of the veins and removal of all lymph nodes

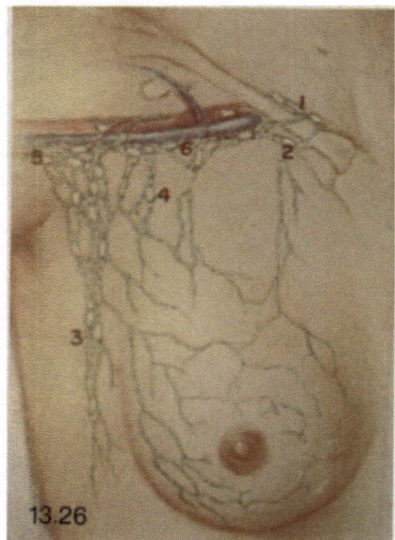

Fig. 13.26. Lymphatic drainage of the mammary tissue. Even when performing the lymph node dissection, the surgeon should be guided by the tumor location and adjust the extent of the resection accordingly

14 Primary Reconstruction

To reduce the risk of recurrence in a woman operated for breast cancer, we believe that the entire mammary gland should be removed by subcutaneous mastectomy, which should include an elliptical skin excision if the tumor is near the skin or removal of the nipple-areola complex if the latter is close to the tumor. A basic principle in all cancer operations is to extirpate the lesion with an adequate margin, which should be approximately twice the tumor diameter. Accordingly, our standard operation for the removal of

a small breast cancer is a simple mastectomy with axillary dissection (Fig. 13.19). Occasionally, when the tumor is in the upper outer quadrant of the breast, it may be possible to preserve the nipple-areola complex (Fig. 13.23). Despite some negative experiences with subcutaneous mastectomy relating to severe capsular contracture, we consistently see results that "cannot be matched by the best reconstruction" (Woods 1986) (Fig. 13.24). Of course patients undergoing a "skin-preserving mastectomy" will require very close oncologic follow-up with particular emphasis placed on palpation of the skin covering the implant.

Fig. 14.1. Appearance following a simple mastectomy with direct intraoperative replantation of the nipple-areola, which was distant from the tumor. This procedure is not recommended due to the difficulty of nipple survival on the thinned skin. It is preferable to bank the nipple-areola in the groin (see Fig. 24.5)

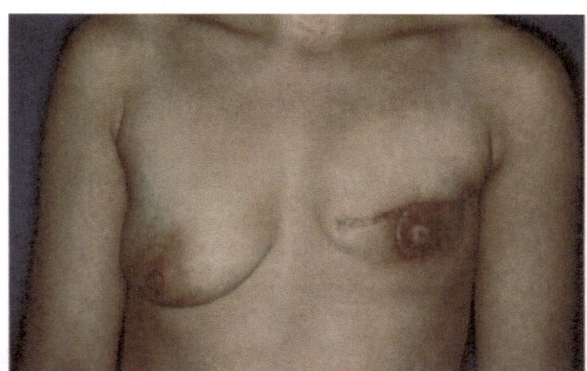

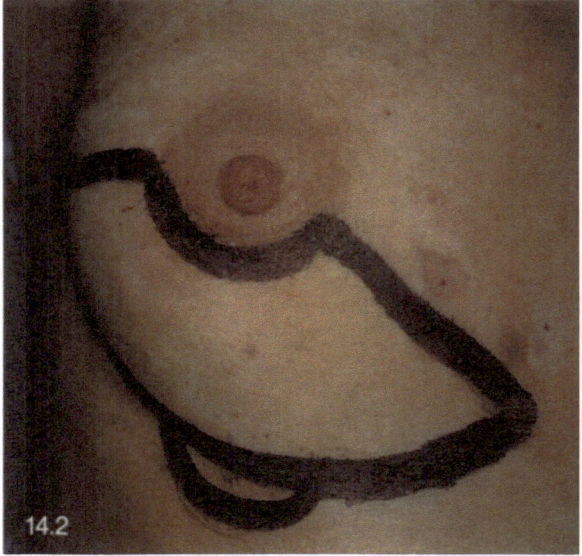
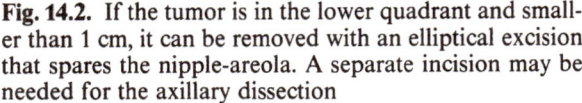

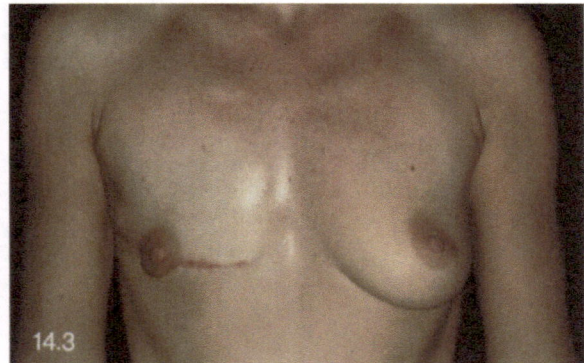

Fig. 14.2. If the tumor is in the lower quadrant and smaller than 1 cm, it can be removed with an elliptical excision that spares the nipple-areola. A separate incision may be needed for the axillary dissection

Fig. 14.3. This immediate postoperative result permits simple reconstruction using an upper abdominal advancement flap (see Fig. 16.2) or a tissue expander (see Fig. 19.3)

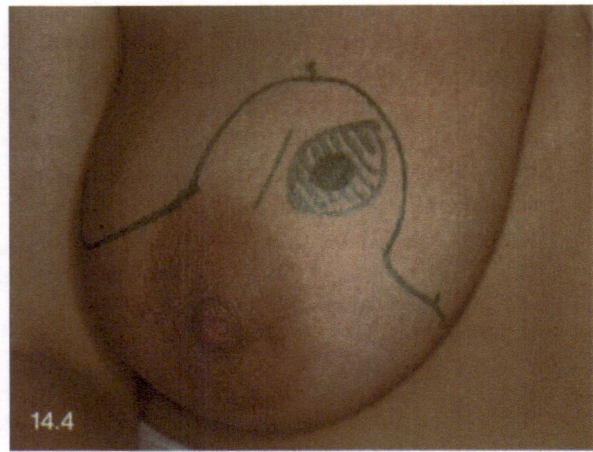

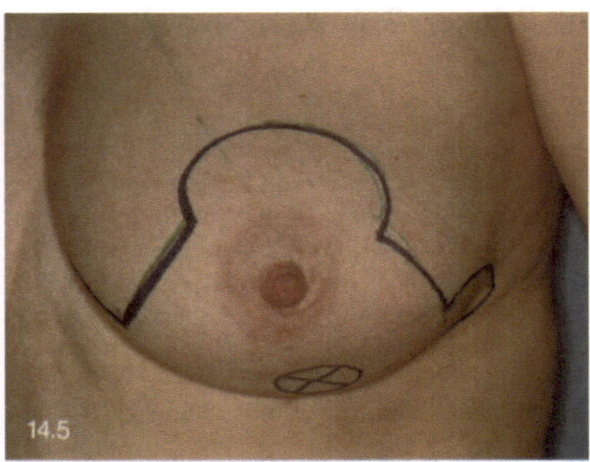

Fig. 14.4. With a small tumor located above the nipple and at least 4 cm from its ducts, the nipple-areola in a ptotic breast can be elevated in the fashion of a masto-pexy. This requires an inferiorly based nipple pedicle (see Fig. 5.2)

Fig. 14.5. A breast with a small, inferiorly located tumor can be removed and immediately reconstructed by a sub-cutaneous reduction mastectomy with a superior nipple pedicle

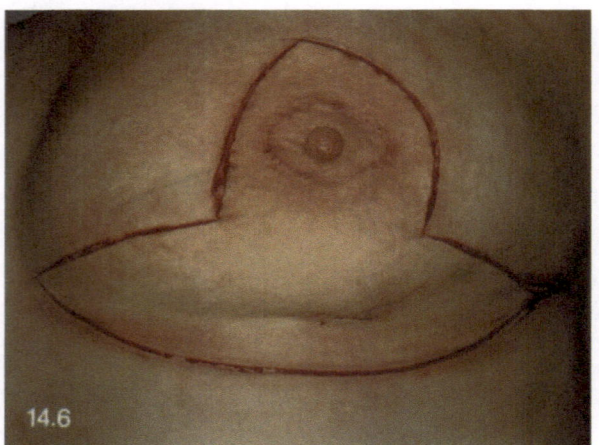

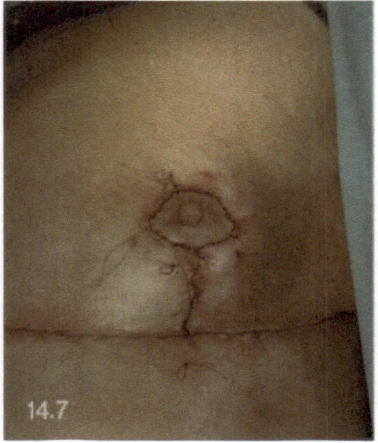

Fig. 14.6. Very small carcinoma ("minimal breast can-cer") at the level of the inframammary crease. In this case the nipple-areola can be based on a superior pedicle, and the remaining skin can be closed in the form of a subcu-taneous reduction mastectomy following axillary dissec-tion

Fig. 14.7. Pleasing postoperative result. Later the left breast can be augmented and the right breast reduced for symmetry

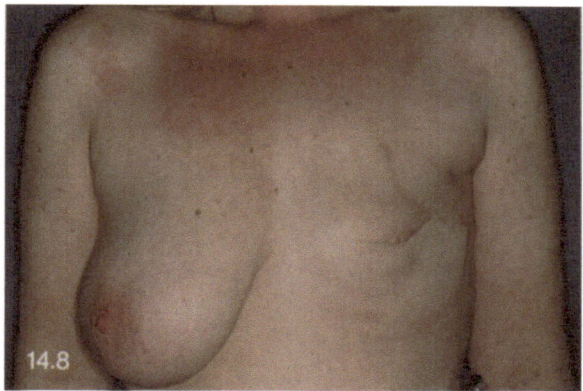

Fig. 14.8. The left breast was ablated for a large intraductal carcinoma, leaving the medial skin intact

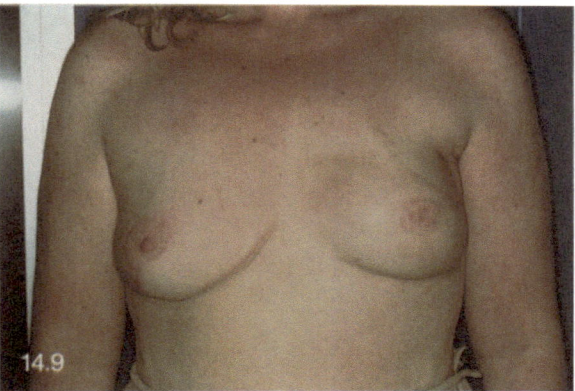

Fig. 14.9. The breast is reconstructed by stretching the residual skin over a prosthesis. The right breast was also reduced, and its nipple-areola was halved to construct a nipple-areola on the left side

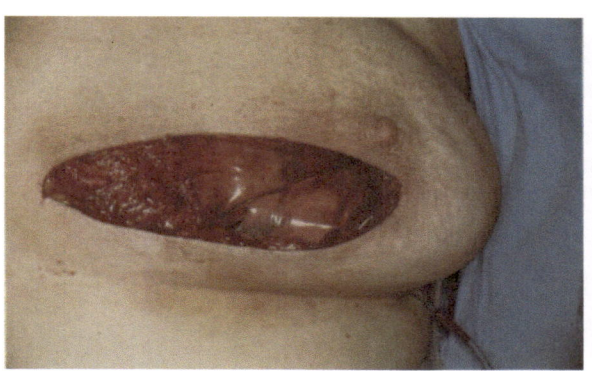

Fig. 14.10. If the tumor was small, far from the nipple, and centrally located in the glandular tissue, implying a low risk of local recurrence, the resected mammary gland can be immediately replaced with a silicone prosthesis. Again, we prefer to place the implant subcutaneously due to a growing dissatisfaction with subpectoral insertions (see Fig. 15.29). Local metastases almost always develop in the skin, so the prosthesis will not obscure pathologic findings

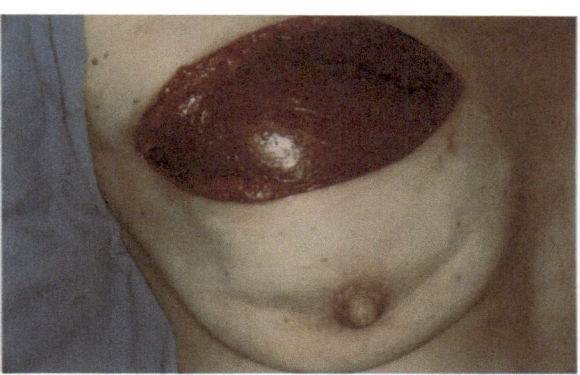

Fig. 14.11. In this case the prosthesis was placed subpectorally due to the precarious blood supply of the skin envelope (it extends upward only as far as the nipple). With a subcutaneous placement, there would have been an exorbitant risk of wound dehiscence

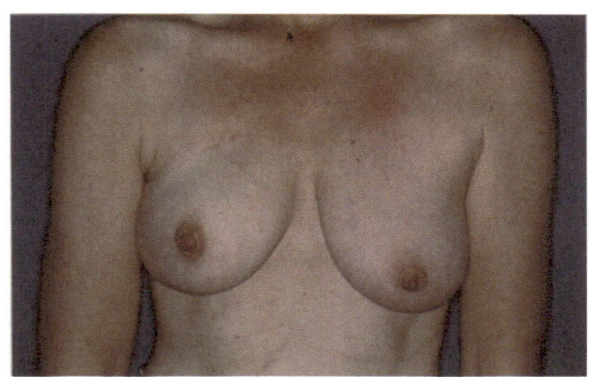

Fig. 14.12. Postoperative result

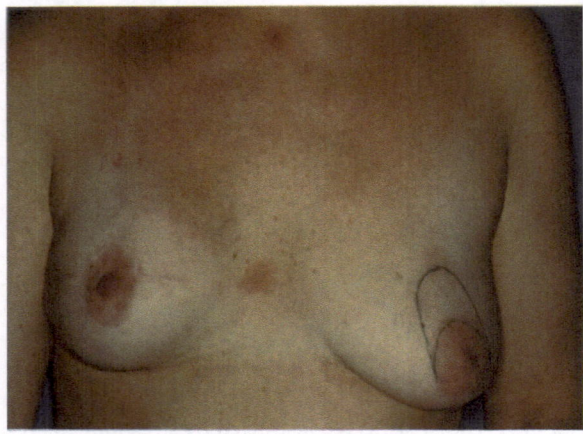

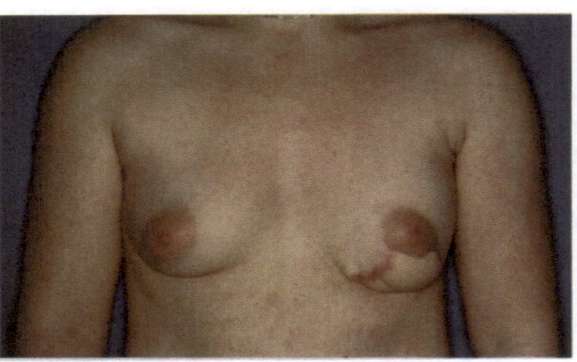

Fig. 14.13. Here as in Fig. 14.2, the excision spares the nipple-areola, which is elevated to the level of the opposite breast. Immediate reconstruction was performed with a bilumen silicone prosthesis

Fig. 14.14. A small carcinoma located near the skin of the inframammary crease was removed by subcutaneous mastectomy with a vertical elliptical skin excision. The defect was repaired with an implant and a thoracoepigastric flap (see Figs. 8.19–8.23)

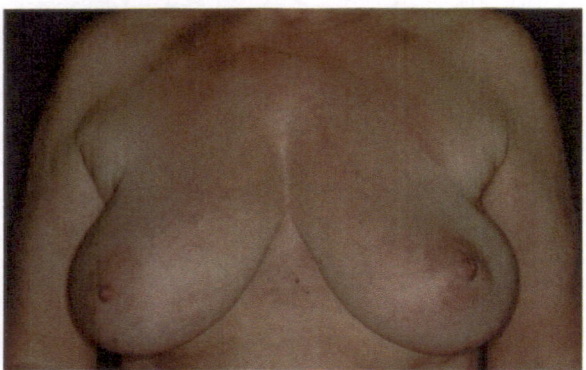

Fig. 14.15. Patient 3 months after removal of a "minimal breast cancer" by subcutaneous mastectomy of the left breast and replacement of the resected glandular tissue by a 650-ml bilumen silicone implant carrying 25 mg of prednisolone

15 Subcutaneous Mastectomy

Indications

Two circumstances have cast doubt on the merits of subcutaneous mastectomy: (1) the 3%–5% of breast tissue that remains, especially beneath the nipple-areola, and (2) the high incidence of capsular contracture, resulting in a poorer aesthetic outcome than simple mastectomy with reconstruction.

We believe that the problem of residual breast tissue is negligible, for in a series of 268 carcinoma patients treated by subcutaneous mastectomy we have observed only two local recurrences of carcinoma and three instances of nipple-areola involvement by an intraductal cancer. Moreover, we find no published quantitative data on local recurrences in the extensive literature on subcutaneous mastectomy, so the percentage must be very low. In any case, even a very small nodule in the skin over the implant is easily detected by palpation, so that a timely referral can be made for additional surgery.

The unsightly aesthetic results of subcutaneous mastectomy ("mastectomy cripple," Olbrisch 1981) date from a period in which double-lumen implants with cortisone were still unknown and the resection was not immediately followed by a skin reduction procedure. Since cortisone has been added to the use of double-lumen implants (Hartley 1976), the incidence of Baker class III and IV capsular contractures has fallen from 54% before 1978 to 24.5%. In most cases a compression capsulotomy can be successfully performed one year after operation. If the closed capsulotomy is not successful, the original implant should be removed and replaced by an implant containing more cortisone (50–100 mg prednisolone) or with a "textured" implant (Lemperle and Exner 1989).

Subcutaneous mastectomy is mainly indicated for benign diseases such as recurrent fibroadenoma phylloides, painful or grade III fibrocystic mastopathy, precancerous disease in the form of ductal or lobular carcinoma in situ, and even for a small, centrally located breast carcinoma. The lesion must be located at least 4 cm from the nipple-areola complex, and there must be no evidence of cutaneous involvement.

Technique

Usually the resection is initiated by a 10-cm inframammary incision, from which the skin is sharply dissected off the gland. If there are already scars from previous biopsies, it may be wise to reopen the scars to ensure adequate blood flow to the nipple-areola. The major cause of nipple necrosis is semicircular scars surrounding the areola. A periareolar incision may be extended laterally as needed to gain access for the glandular resection (see Fig. 11.5).

Subpectoral placement of the prosthesis (see Fig. 14.12), advocated most strongly by gynecologists, is safer than prepectoral placement and carries a lower risk of infection, but the aesthetic result is often marred by an unsightly distortion of the breast during arm movements (Fig. 15.29). For this reason we no longer dissect a subserratopectoral pocket, and we routinely place the implant over the pectoralis muscle, taking meticulous care to preserve the subcutaneous fatty tissue that maintains blood flow to the nipple-areola complex.

Since 1988 we have used "textured" implants covered with polyurethane foam (Replicon) or with a roughened silicone surface (Biocell, Misti, Siltex, Silastic MSI) exclusively for the reconstruction of subcutaneous mastectomies and for the revision of recurrent capsular contractures. In the latter case we emphasize the importance of removing the entire capsule (capsulectomy!) to permit the centripetal ingrowth of connective tissue. The implant should not be manipulated postoperatively, as this might disturb the tissue ingrowth. We have our patients wear an elastic girdle which presses the textured implant down onto the inframammary crease for three weeks after the insertion (Fig. 15.3 b). In a series of 242 implantations, we have observed 13 infections (5.3%) and 40 (16,1%) instances of capsular contracture (Böhling 1989, Rüster 1990). Only in few textured implants could we observe "in growth" of capsular tissue. All implants with pose sizes smaller than 500 mµ caused smooth and detached capsules!

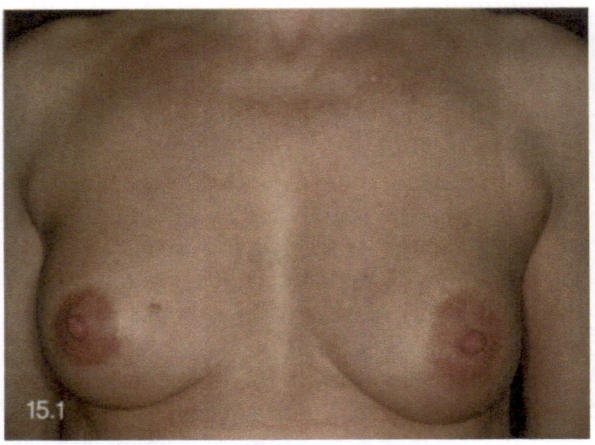

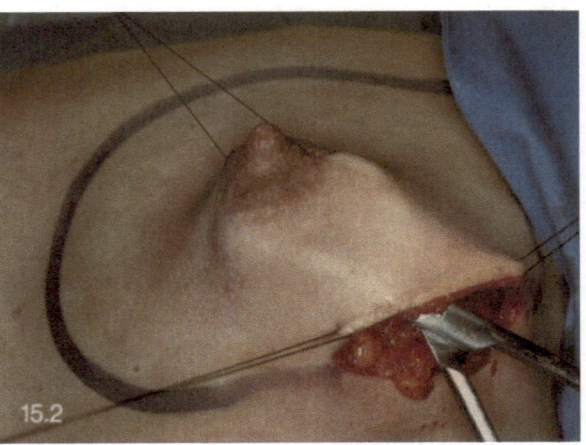

Fig. 15.1. Appearance following subcutaneous mastectomy of the right breast for isolated microcalcifications signifying a lobular carcinoma in situ. *Isolated* microcalcifications do not justify a subcutaneous mastectomy of the opposite breast in all cases

Fig. 15.2. The subcutaneous mastectomy begins with a periareolar or inframammary incision, through which the glandular tissue is dissected from its ligamentous attachments with the skin with a sharp scissors (Castañares), leaving as much subcutaneous fat as possible. Generally an approximately 3-cm button of glandular tissue is left beneath the nipple-areola; the patient must become familiar with the size and shape of this residual tissue

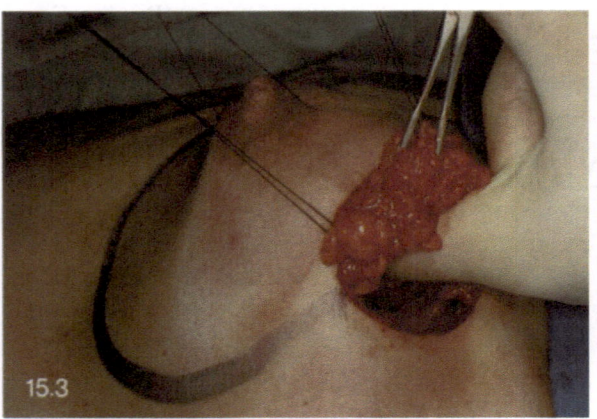

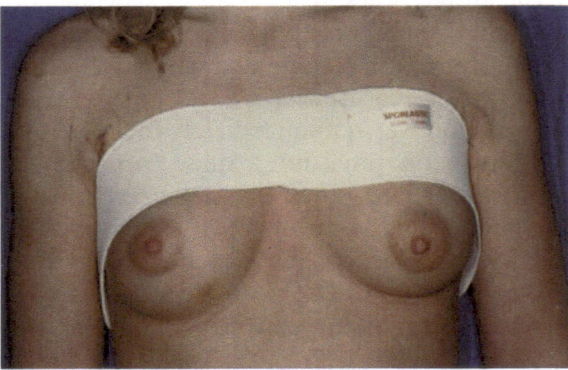

Fig. 15.3. b Postoperatively, an elastic girdle presses the textured implant down into the inframammary crease

Fig. 15.3. a Having been separated from the skin, the gland is now bluntly dissected from the pectoralis fascia. Some peripheral skin adhesions often have to be divided at this time. When the dissection is completed, any remaining breast tissue is identified and removed by everting the breast envelope or inspecting the subcutaneous tissue with a lighted retractor. Finally a suction drain and the appropriate implant are inserted

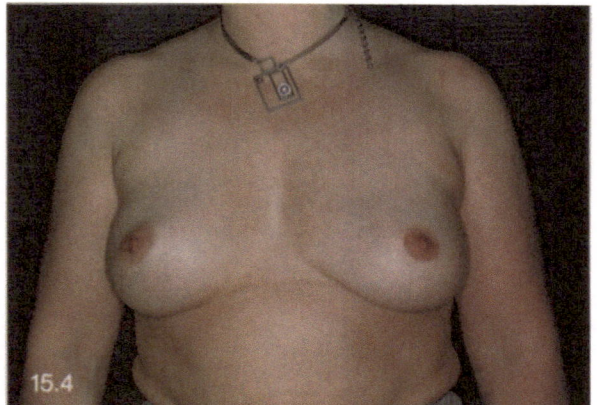

Fig. 15.4. Five years after subcutaneous mastectomy of the right breast for a centrally located minimal breast cancer, axillary dissection, and immediate reconstruction with a silicone prosthesis

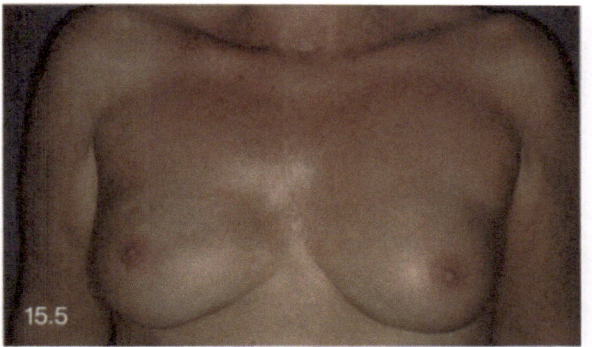

Fig. 15.5. Three years after bilateral subcutaneous mastectomies for an intraductal carcinoma (apparently noninvasive) of the right breast. This is one of two patients who developed a local recurrence of invasive carcinoma after subcutaneous mastectomy

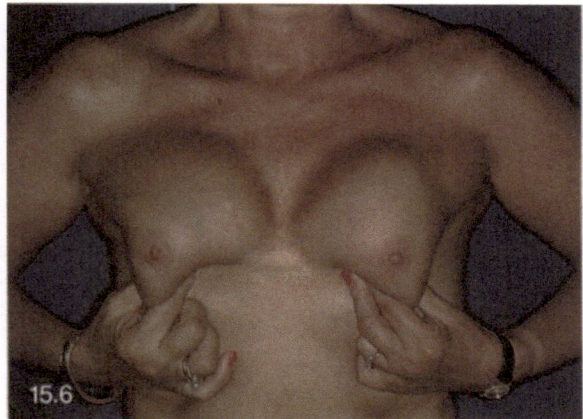

Fig. 15.6. We see this degree of implant mobility and breast pliancy only when the reconstruction has been performed with double-lumen implants carrying 12.5 mg of prednisolone

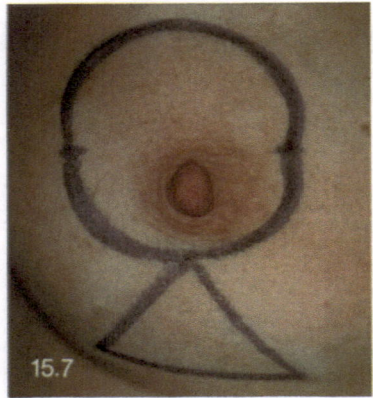

Fig. 15.7. In the mildly ptotic breast, the residual skin envelope can be reduced by a Maillard mastopexy

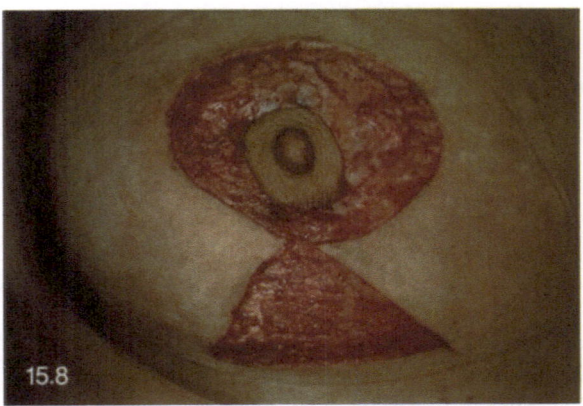

Fig. 15.8. Deepithelization of the outlined areas

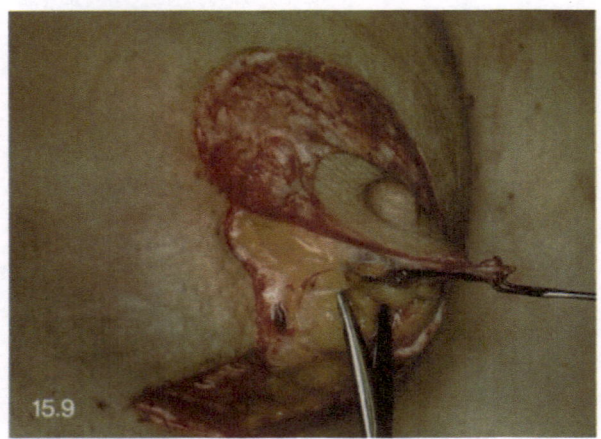

Fig. 15.9. The gland is dissected from the skin envelope with a strong scissors, taking care to preserve the blood supply to the nipple-areola

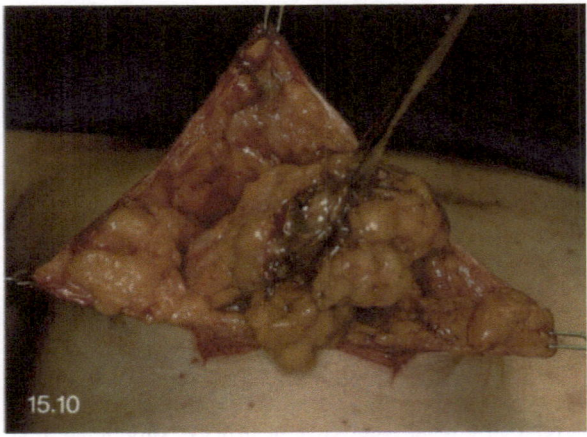

Fig. 15.10. The gland, showing gross cystic changes, is bluntly dissected from the underlying fascia

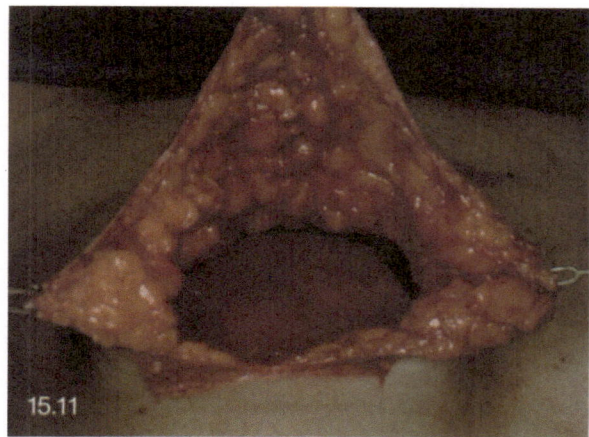

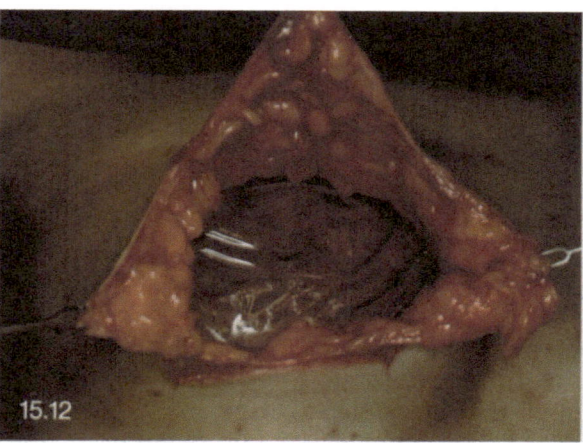

Fig. 15.11. When a simultaneous skin reduction is performed, a large opening is created through which the wound cavity is easily inspected for hemostasis. A lighted retractor is also excellent for this purpose

Fig. 15.12. Prepectoral placement of a double-lumen implant with prednisolone added

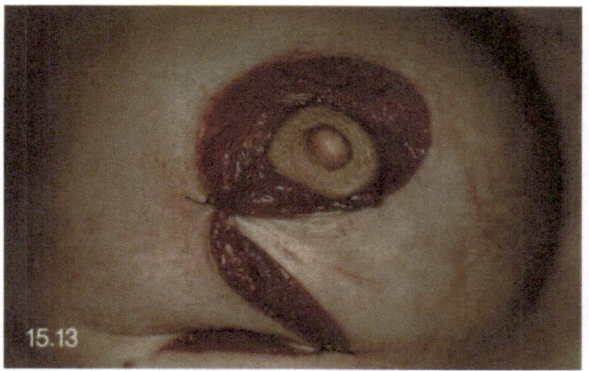

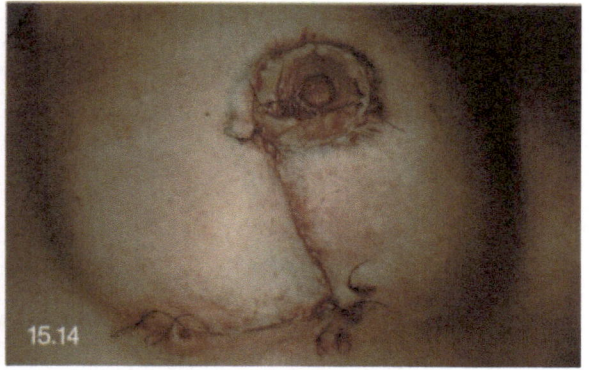

Fig. 15.13. Approximation of the wound edges. The areolar circumference should be at least 12 cm $(d \cdot \pi)$

Fig. 15.14. Intradermal closure

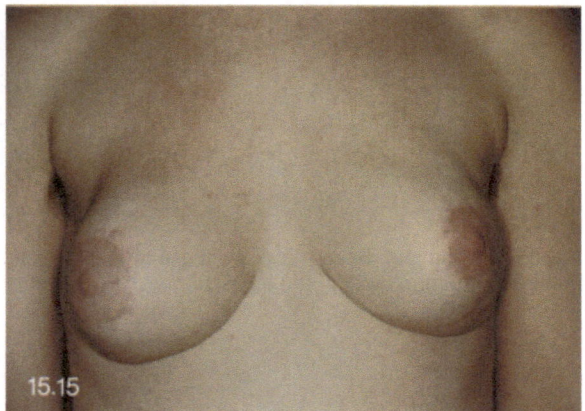

Fig. 15.15. Appearance seven months after subcutaneous mastectomy, Maillard skin reduction, and reconstruction with a bilumen implant

Complications

Subcutaneous mastectomy is always followed by substantial hematoma formation and exudation from the large wound surface, which often has an area of 1/4 me2. Generally this problem is adequately managed by suction catheters, which must be flushed if they become clogged by solid tissues. A more difficult problem is posed by the impending partial or complete necrosis of the nipple-areola complex. The intra- and postoperative administration of dextran 40 and pentoxifylline are an effective prophylaxis against nipple loss but should be discontinued after 8 days. At that time there will be a fairly rapid demarcation of the necrotic areas, which then are surgically removed before the tissues are reclosed over the prosthesis.

Perforation of the skin and exposure of the implant, unless due to a local deficiency of cutaneous blood flow, usually signify a periprosthetic bacterial infection. This complication is managed by instituting suction irrigation with the appropriate antibiotic for 6–10 days and closing the perforation site over the implant.

The major causative organism of infection in the reconstructed breast is the ubiquitous cutaneous bacterium *Staphylococcus epidermidis.* Infections with this organism generally do not become clinically apparent until several weeks after surgery. The reconstructed breast is also vulnerable to *Staphylococcus aureus,* which causes a far more virulent infection that may be associated with true suppuration. Given the many manipulations that are required in a subcutaneous mastectomy, it is entirely possible that swabs, gloves, or the prosthesis itself may seed cutaneous organisms into the surgical cavity, even if a flawless skin prep was carried out. Postoperative washings of the dissected pocket have demonstrated the presence of "nonpathogenic" cutaneous bacteria in 80% (!) of cases (Reinmüller), with most originating from the patient's own skin. The presence of the prosthesis reduces the amount of tissue surface available in the pocket for natural humoral and cellular host defense mechanisms. A fold in the wall of the prosthesis or in the area of the valve can provide a favorable site for bacterial contamination and proliferation. That is why we recommend the intraoperative instillation of approximately 50 ml of a prophylactic antibiotic solution during the first 2 hours.

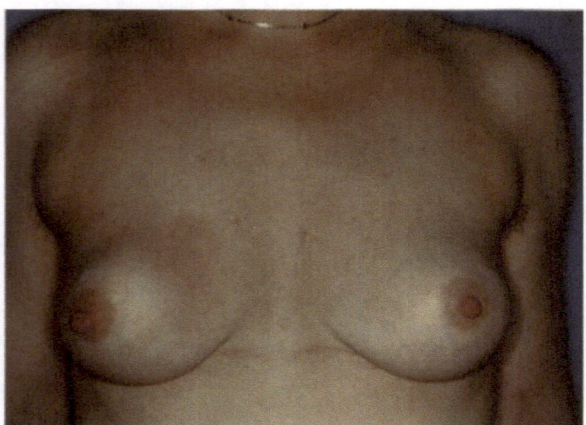

Fig. 15.16. Bilateral Baker class II capsular contracture. With the patient standing, the breasts appear normal

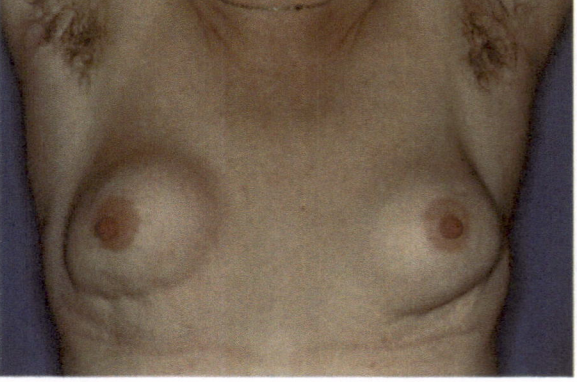

Fig. 15.17. Typical appearance after subcutaneous mastectomy. When the arms are raised, the capsule is drawn upward

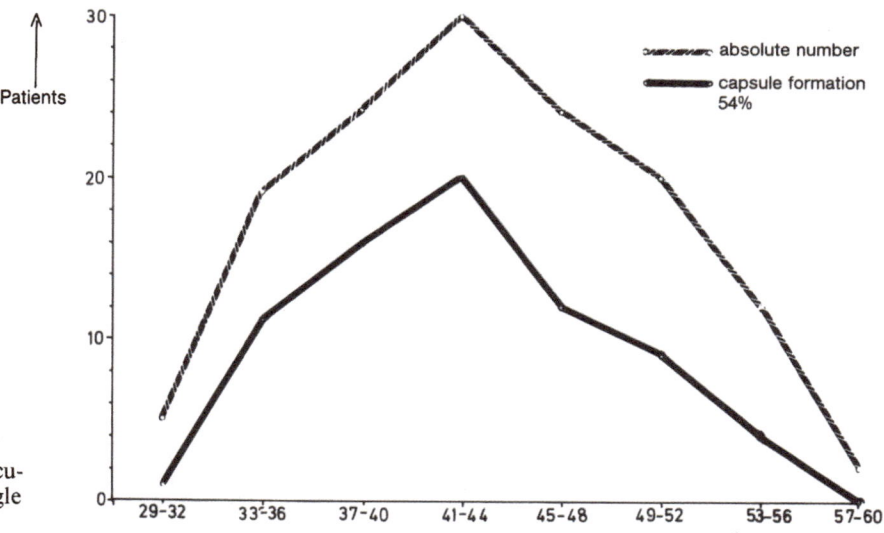

Fig. 15.18. Age distribution of capsular contracture after subcutaneous mastectomy using single lumen implants (1971–1978)

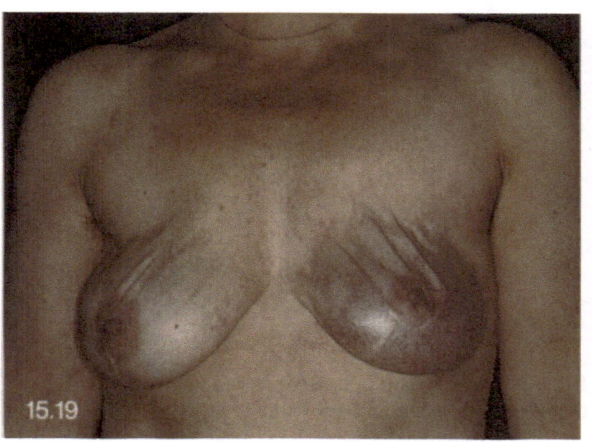

Fig. 15.19. In this patient 20 mg of triamcinolone (Volon-A) was inadvertently instilled on the left side. Within 9 months the skin became extremely thinned – a typical effect of the much stronger-acting corticosteroid. Note the associated systemic effect on the right breast

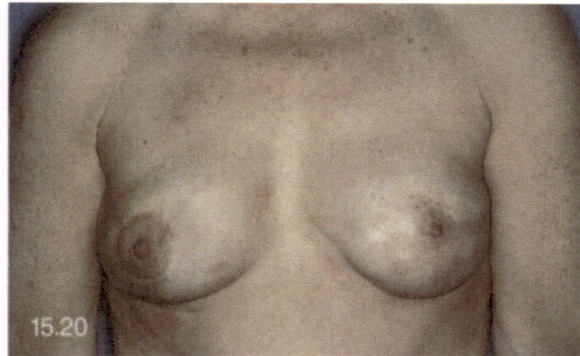

Fig. 15.20. The subcutaneous tissue recovered quickly after removal of the left prosthesis, allowing the reimplantation of a cortisone-free prosthesis 3 months later

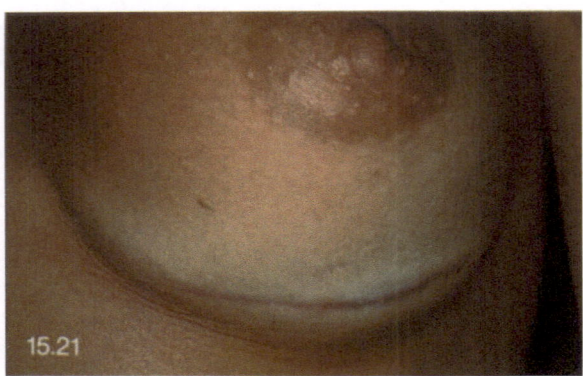

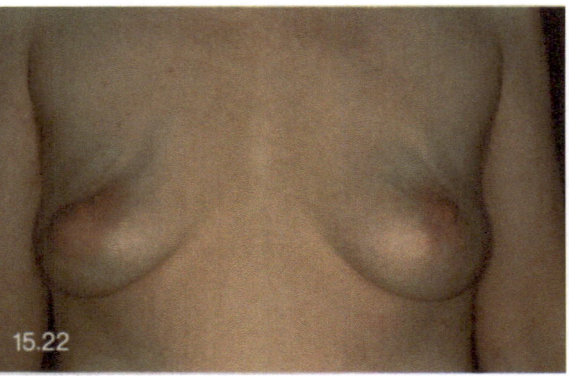

Fig. 15.21. With the current standard dosage of 12.5 mg prednisolone, thinning can sometimes occur in the area of the scar. This may be followed for a period of years, or the thinned area may be excised and doubly closed as an outpatient procedure

Fig. 15.22. Extreme ptosis of both breasts due to thinning of the skin following subcutaneous mastectomy and the instillation of 50 mg prednisolone per side after a capsular contracture (Baker class III) had previously developed with a dose of 12.5 mg. Patients show extremely diverse reactions to the same cortisone doses, so every patient should be aware of the problem of cutaneous thinning

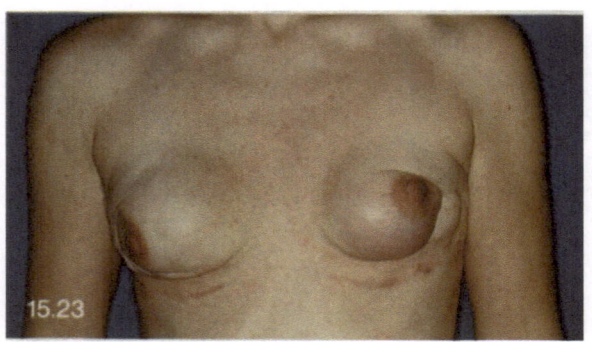

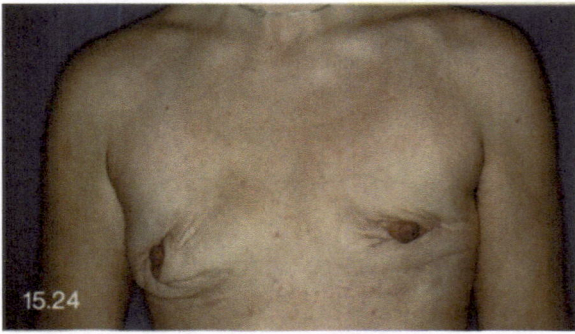

Fig. 15.23. Extreme bilateral capsular contracture after subcutaneous mastectomy

Fig. 15.24. Both implants were removed to allow recovery of the pressure-thinned subcutaneous tissue

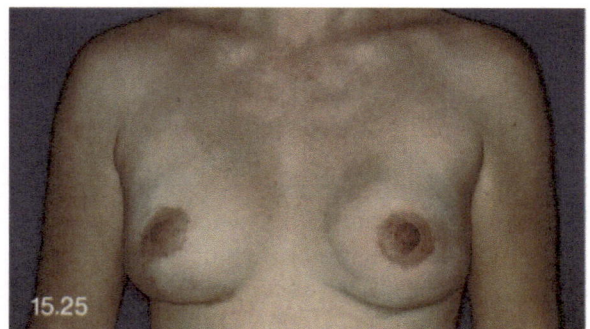

Fig. 15.25. Six months later, following the implantation of two bilumen prostheses carrying 12.5 mg of prednisolone

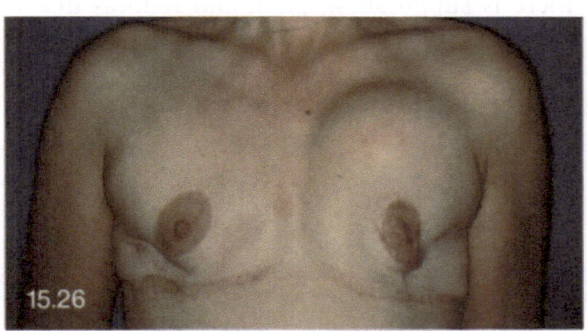

Fig. 15.26. Appearance after subcutaneous mastectomy and breast reconstruction with inflatable implants. The right implant has deflated, while the left implant has been displaced superiorly by scar adhesions

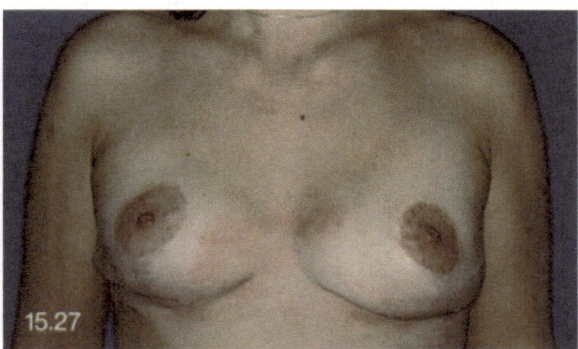

Fig. 15.27. Appearance after the implantation of two bilumen cortisone prostheses

Infected Implant

Various bacteria can cause the formation of mucoid, gelatinous, or even fibrinous deposits in the implant pocket. These are most easily removed by scraping them out with a gynecologic curet.

Capsular contracture, which develops in about 50% of women after subcutaneous mastectomy, is due in part to a genetic predisposition to heavy internal (!) scarring, although a great many cases are caused by low-grade periprosthetic infection with *Staphylococcus epidermidis* (Burkhardt 1986).

Regarding the first cause, we have found that the only effective remedies are the addition of cortisone to bilumen implants and daily implant manipulation. The second cause, infection with *Staphylococcus epidermidis*, rarely leads to perforation; far more commonly the infection is self-limiting but leads to an extreme unilateral capsular contracture. Open capsulotomy should be performed 6–12 months later to allow ample time for the infection to clear.

In all cases it is best to avoid removing an infected prosthesis due to the extreme tendency of the skin to contract following subcutaneous mastectomy, and treatment by suction irrigation (Fig. 15.30) should be attempted.

If there is a recurrence of clinical infection with heavy seroma formation, and especially if there is suppuration, pain, and redness that in-

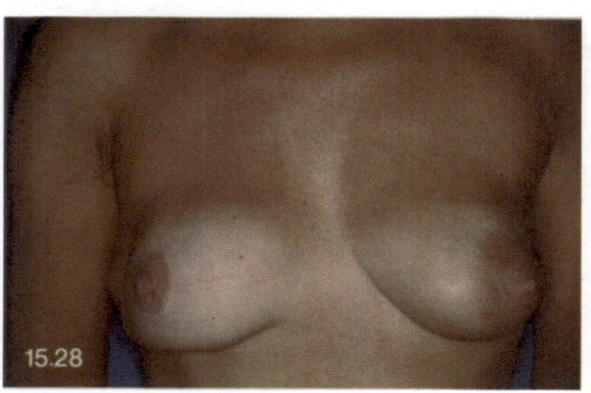

Fig. 15.28. This patient underwent a left subcutaneous mastectomy with the *submuscular* insertion of a bilumen implant

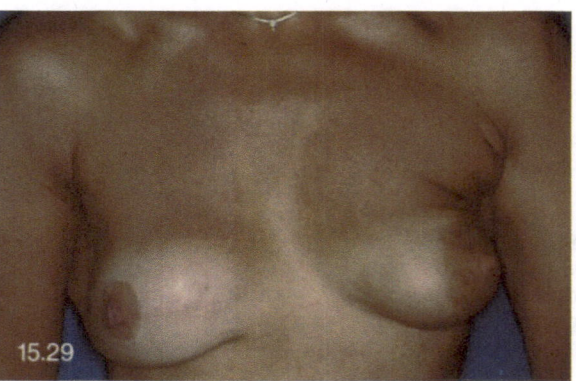

Fig. 15.29. Tensing of the pectoralis major muscle (e. g., during tooth brushing, arm propping, etc.) causes an unsightly distortion of the reconstructed breast

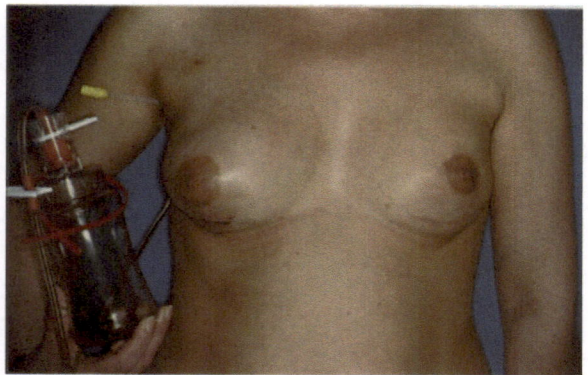

Fig. 15.30. Infection with "nonpathogenic" cutaneous bacteria often presents very early as a persistent increase in the amount of drainage from the suction catheter. In this case we would start the instillation of an antibiotic (gentamycin or cephalothin) even before the fluid is cultured. The antibiotic is instilled by retrograde infusion through the drainage tube and remains in the breast for 3 h, during which time the implant should be well manipulated. If a positive culture is obtained, this regimen is repeated every 6 h for 4–6 days. In this way we have been able to salvage 22 of 31 infected implants (Wolters)

volves the entire breast, and unresponsiveness to systemic antibiotics, an abscess should be suspected, and temporary removal of the prosthesis is indicated.

At the time open capsulotomy is performed, it is wise to obtain a smear for culture study. The presence of more than a teaspoon of fluid around the prosthesis should raise suspicion of infection with *Staphylococcus epidermidis*.

The extreme skin thinning observed formerly (1976-1978) after the use of bilumen silicone implants carrying triamcinolone or prednisolone were due to excessive steroid doses. Today, triamcinolone should be used only in cases of extreme capsular contracture, i. e., in secondary operations. Prednisolone is the primary prophylactic steroid of choice and should be instilled routinely in a dose of 12.5 mg; for secondary procedures the dose should be increased to 50 or 100 mg. In all cases, the subcutaneous tissues should recover their normal thickness within 3-6 months after removal of the prosthesis.

Table 15.1. Incidence of capsular contractures in the "pre-cortisone era" from 1971 to 1975. In 1976 we tested the efficacy of cortisone by instilling 250 mg of prednisolone only into the left double-lumen implant of 10 patients. In all cases the left breast remained soft, although its marked descent in the ensuing years necessitated a change of implants in 8 of the women

Prosthesis-related late complications after subcutaneous mastectomy during the period 1971-1975 (n = 110)		
1. Skin thinning	19.0%	(21)
2. Skin rippling	11.8%	(13)
3. Displacement of prosthesis	5.5%	(6)
4. Rupture of prosthesis	0.9%	(1)
5. Perforation	0.9%	(1)
Total requiring change of implant:	21.8%	(24)

References

Baessler R (1978) Pathologie der Brustdrüse. Springer, Berlin Heidelberg New York

Baral E, Ogenstad S, Wallgren A (1985) The effect of adjuvant radiotherapy on the time of occurrence and prognosis of local recurrence in primary operable breast. Cancer 56: 2779-2782

Berrino P, Campora E, Santi P (1987) Postquadrantectomy breast deformities: Classification and techniques of surgical correction. Plast Reconstr Surg 79: 567-572

Bonadonna G, Rossi A, Valagussa P, Banfi A, Veronesi V (1979) The CMF program for operable breast cancer with positive axillary nodes: up dated analysis on the disease-free interval, size of relapse and drug tolerance. Cancer 39: 2904-2915

Bostwick J, Paletta C (1984) Radiation to the breast: Complications amenable to surgical treatment. Ann Surg 200: 543-553

Clodius L (1977) Secondary arm lymphedema. In: Clodius L (ed) Lymphedema. Thieme, Stuttgart New York

Ellenberg AH, Braun H (1980) A 3½ year experience with double-lumen implants in breast surgery. Plast Reconstr Surg 65: 307-313

Fallowfield LJ, Braum M, Maquire GP (1986) Effects of breast conservation on psychological morbidity associated with diagnosis and treatment of early breast cancer. Br Med J 293: 1331-1334

Ferguson DJ, Sutton HG, Dawson PJ (1985) Delayed hazards of adjuvant radiotherapy for breast cancer. Breast 11: 2-6

Fisher B, Bauer M, Margolese R et al. (1985a) I. Five-year result of randomized clinical trial comparing total mastectomy and segmental mastectomy with or without radiation in the treatment of breast cancer. N Engl J Med 312: 665-673

Fisher B, Redmond C, Fisher ER et al. (1985b) Ten-year results of a randomized clinical trial comparing radical mastectomy and total mastectomy with or without radiation. N Engl J Med 312: 674-681

Fournier D von, Hoeffken W, Junkermann H, Bauer M, Kühn W (1985) Growth rate of primary mammary carcinoma and its metastases. Consequences for early detection and therapy. In: Zander J, Baltzer J (eds) Early breast cancer. Histopathology, diagnosis and treatment. Springer, Berlin Heidelberg New York, pp 73-86

Frank HA, Hale FM, Steer ML (1976) Preoperativ localization of nonpalpable breast lesions demonstrated by mammography. N Engl J Med 295: 259-260

Freeman BS (1962) Subcutaneous mastectomy for benign lesions with immediate or delayed prosthetic replacement. Plast Reconstr Surg 30: 676-682

Frischbier HJ (1986) Empfehlungen der Dt. Gesellschaft für Senologie zur Indikation und Technik der Radiotherapie im Rahmen der brusterhaltenden Behandlung des Mammacarcinoms, Hamburg

Halverson JD, Hori-Robaina JM (1974) Cystosarcoma phylloides of the breast. Am Surg 40: 295-301

Harder F, Laffer U, Walther E (1989) Behandlung des kleinen Mammacarcinoms nach den Richtlinien der Basler Studie. In: Bohmert H (Hrsg) Brustkrebs: Organerhaltung oder Rekonstruktion. Thieme, Stuttgart, S 104

Harris JR, Hellman S, Silen W (1983) Conservative management of breast cancer. Lippincott, Philadelphia

Hartley JH (1976) Specific applications of double lumen prosthesis. Clin Plast Surg 3: 247-263

Herrmann RE, Esselstyn CB, Crile G Jr (1985) Results of conservative operations for breast cancer. Arch Surg 1985: 746-751

Kindermann G, Genz T (1985) A comparison between the results of simple mastectomy and tumorectomy for breast cancer: the problem of local recurrence. Arch Gynecol 237: 67-73

Kubli F (1988) Lokalrezidive nach brusterhaltender Therapie. In: Bohmert H (Hrsg) Brustkrebs: Organerhaltung oder Rekonstruktion. Thieme, Stuttgart

Kusche M, Scharl A, Reusch K, Bolte A (1987) Therapie und Prognose des inflammatorischen Mammacarcinoms. Tumor Diagnostik Therapie 8: 108–114

Lemperle G (1985) Radikal operieren oder die Brust erhalten? Selecta-Forum über das Mammacarcinom. Selecta 46: 4102–4104

Lemperle G, Exner K (1989) Skin-preserving mastectomy in early breast cancer. In: Bohmert H, Leis HP, Jackson IT (eds) Breast cancer – conservative and reconstructive surgery. Thieme, Stuttgart, pp 212–219

Martin JK, van Heerden JA, Taylor WF, Gaffey TA (1986) Is modified radical mastectomy really equivalent to radical mastectomy in treatment of carcinoma of the breast? Cancer 57: 510–518

Mühlbauer W (1978) Zur Problematik der subcutanen Mastektomie. Zentralbl Chir 103: 781–789

Olbrisch RR (1981) Gibt es noch Indikationen zur subcutanen Mastektomie? Chirurg 52: 467

Patey DH, Dyson WH (1948) The prognosis of carcinoma of the breast in relation to the type of operation performed. Br J Cancer 2: 7–13

Rice CO, Strickler JH (1951) Adenomammectomy for benign lesions. Surg Gynecol Obstet 93: 759

Rigg BM (1986) A continuous breast irrigation system. Plast Reconstr Surg 78: 102–103

Rosen PP (1980) Axillary lymph node metastases in patients with occult noninvasive breast carcinoma. Cancer 46: 1298

Spahn I (1986) Brustrekonstruktion nach Ablatio mammae und ihre Komplikationen. Thesis, Frankfurt

Spitalny HH, Lemperle G (1984) Wirkung und Komplikationen doppellumiger Silikonprothesen mit Cortisonfüllung nach subcutaner Mastektomie. In: Kubli F, Fournier D von (Hrsg) Neue Konzepte der Diagnostik und Therapie des Mammacarcinoms. Springer, Berlin Heidelberg New York Tokyo, S 96–193

Strömbeck JO (1982) Subcutaneous mastectomy has to be a mastectomy. In: Bohmert H (ed) Breast cancer and breast reconstruction. Thieme, Stuttgart New York, pp 70–74

Thomsen K (1987) Wandel in der Therapie des operablen Mammakarzinoms. Fortschr Med 105: 425–428

Tinnemans JGM, Wobbes T, van der Sluis RF, Lubbers EYC, de Boer HHM (1986) Multicentricity in nonpalpable breast carcinoma and its implications for treatment. Am J Surg 151: 334–338

Veronesi U, Banti A, Del Vecchio M et al. (1986) Comparison of Halsted mastectomy with quadrantectomy, axillary dissection and radiotherapy in early breast cancer: long-term results. Eur J Cancer Clin Oncol 22: 1085–1089

Part E

Breast Reconstruction

16 Abdominal Advancement Flap

The first postmastectomy breast reconstructions with silicone prostheses were described by Lewis (1971) and Snyderman (1971), who used the gel implants commercially available since 1962 and simply inserted them beneath the skin. This technique resulted in hemispherical, unnatural "brassiere" breasts which, while giving the patient security, were not aesthetically appealing. A very important feature of the female breast, besides its volume and nipple-areola complex, is the inframammary crease, which provides for a natural ptosis. In 1973, when the first women with transverse mastectomy scars asked about reconstruction, we began to fix the inframammary crease separately to the chest wall with interrupted sutures. All the skin of the ipsilateral upper abdomen must be undermined from the operative scar in order to mobilize sufficient skin (about a hand's width) to cover the implant (Höhler and Lemperle 1975; Spitalny and Lemperle 1978).

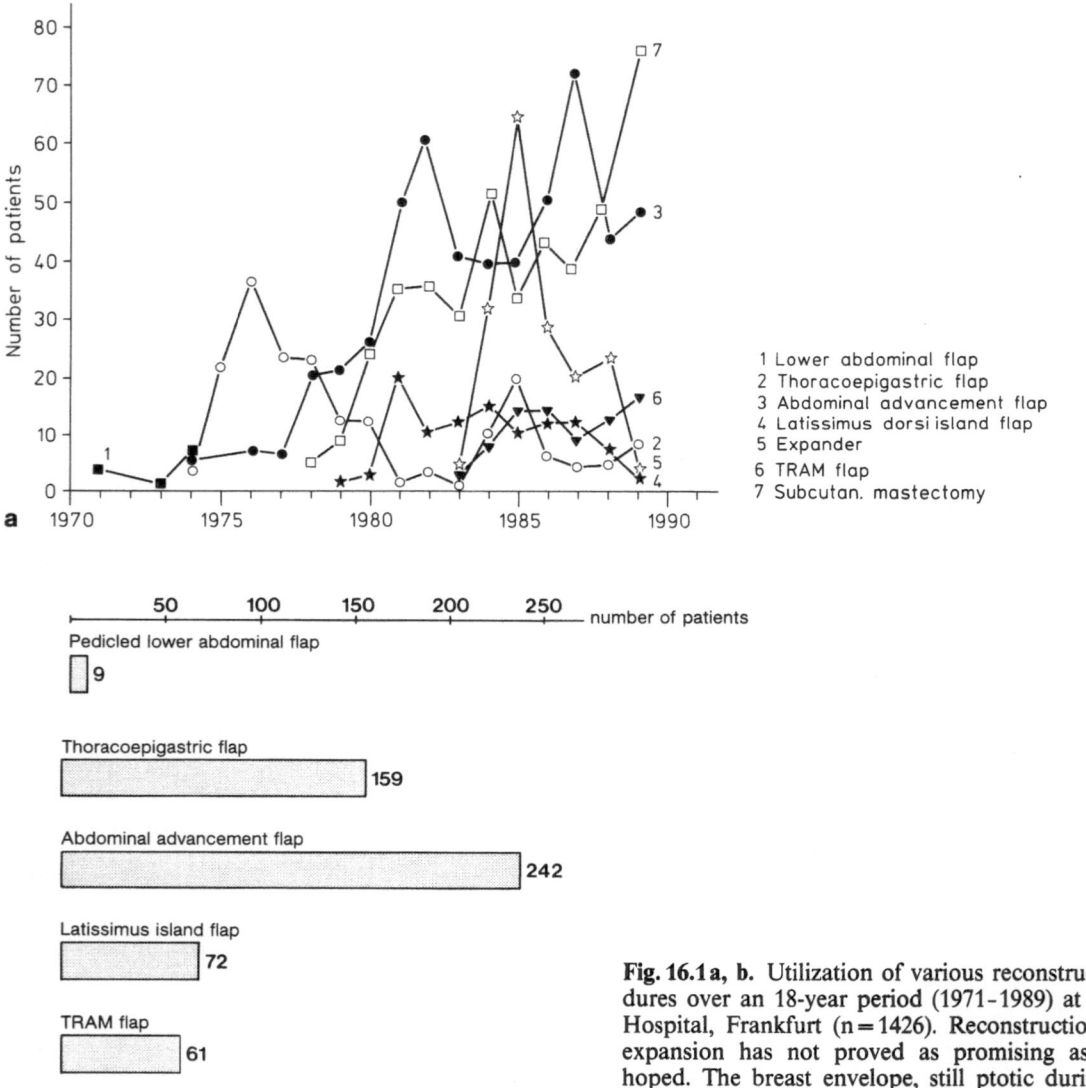

Fig. 16.1a, b. Utilization of various reconstructive procedures over an 18-year period (1971–1989) at St. Markus Hospital, Frankfurt (n = 1426). Reconstruction by tissue expansion has not proved as promising as was once hoped. The breast envelope, still ptotic during the first week, shrinks very rapidly in most patients so that the result at 4 weeks is usually no better than that obtained with upper abdominal skin advancement (see Table 16.1)

Indications

Virtually any patient with a transverse mastectomy scar is a candidate for this advancement procedure. Preferably, the subcutaneous tissue should form a sufficiently thick layer to allow prepectoral placement of the implant. On the irradiated chest wall, we strongly recommend a subpectoral placement in which the inferior and medial origins of the pectoralis major muscle are released from the fifth rib and sternum.

Technique

Reconstruction by upper abdominal skin advancement is performed an average of 6–12 months after mastectomy. This allows sufficient time for the completion of chemotherapy, the subsidence of any acute radiation effects, and the regression of scars. The patient's own brassiere can be used to select the appropriate implant size prior to operation (Fig. 16.4). This can be done in all women who will not undergo a subsequent contralateral reduction.

It is then decided whether the implant will be placed above or below the pectoralis major muscle. We favor subpectoral placement only in patients with an irradiated chest wall or thin subcutaneous fat. Otherwise we prefer the prepectoral implantation, which affords a more natural appearance. The subpectoral position often leads to unsightly movements of the breast when the patient brushes her teeth, leans upon her arm, or performs other acts involving contraction of the pectoralis major. In many cases we have even had to move an initially subpectoral implant to the prepectoral position.

After excision of the external scar, the pocket for the prosthesis, either above or below the pectoralis major, is sharply dissected inferiorly and medially. The skin of the upper abdomen is then separated from the aponeurosis by blunt finger dissection until the umbilicus and iliac crest are palpated (Fig. 16.8). Medial to the rectus abdominis muscle, care is taken to preserve the perforating vessels from the superior epigastric artery as in the thoracoepigastric flap procedure (Bohmert 1982).

When the pocket for the prosthesis has been developed far enough laterally and superiorly and a "second look" has been taken to exclude local recurrence in the chest wall, subcutaneous tissue or axilla, fixation of the new inframammary crease is begun. For this a line is drawn with gentian violet along the sixth rib at the level of the contralateral inframammary crease, i.e., about two fingerwidths below the origin of the pectoralis major, and several fixation sutures are placed between the intercostal muscles and subcutaneous tissue (Fig. 16.9). When these sutures are tied, proceeding medially to laterally, it is recommended that the patient be raised to an upright position to relieve stress on the suture line. For the next 8 days the patient should also sleep in a propped position and bend slightly forward when walking.

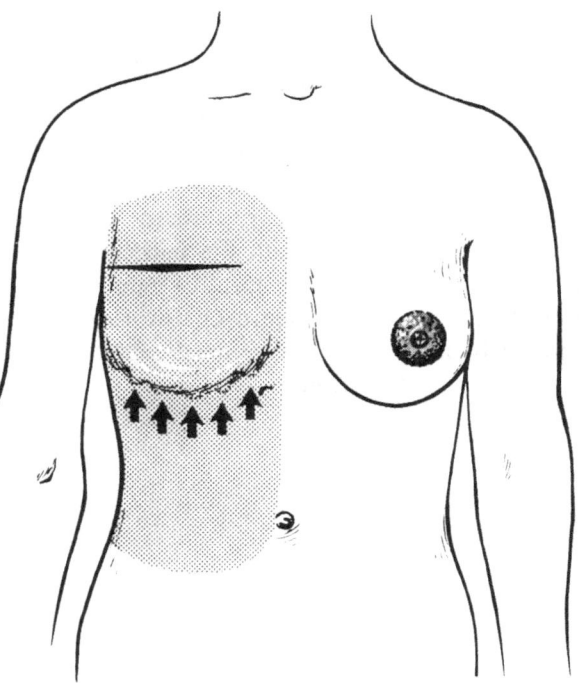

Fig. 16.2. Upper abdominal advancement flap: An incision is made on the existing scar, and the upper abdominal skin is undermined as far as the midline and iliac crest. The undermined tissues are advanced superiorly and secured along the sixth rib with interrupted sutures to create a new inframammary crease

A new incision at the level of the proposed inframammary crease, as described by Pennisi
(1977), Bohmert (1982), and Ryan (1982), is recommended when the mastectomy scar is inconspicuous (i. e., requires no improvement) and the
prosthesis is placed submuscularly. This second
incision is also recommended in obese women,
as it allows the simultaneous selective trimming
of subcutaneous fat so that there is less circulatory impairment by the direct fixation of the corium to the chest wall.

Complications

Wound healing problems in the area of the transverse scar are most common in patients who
have received radiation to the chest wall. Wound
healing can also be compromised by the placement of too many sutures on the new inframammary crease, causing impairment of blood flow
above the suture line. Six sutures spaced at 2-cm
intervals should be enough! The height of the inframammary crease cannot always be accurately
defined, because residual tension in the upper
abdominal skin may pull the new crease inferiorly in the ensuing weeks, or extreme capsular contracture may draw the crease upward. After the
contralateral inframammary crease has been
marked preoperatively with the patient in a sitting position, it may be helpful to mark the proposed inframammary crease on the ribs percu-
taneously using a thin-gauge needle on a syringe
containing gentian violet.

Individual sutures may pull loose, resulting in
a bulge on the inframammary line. If the implant
is still mobile, these sites can be reattached to the
chest wall with a buried mattress suture on a
large needle (Fig. 16.11) as an outpatient procedure.

The danger of local recurrence or regional metastasis is the same as in patients who do not undergo reconstruction. Of 425 patients reconstructed with an upper abdominal advancement
or thoracoepigastric flap between 1973 and 1985,
12 (2.8%) have developed a recurrence in the
skin over the prosthesis necessitating a skin excision, and 4 of these have had to have their prosthesis removed (Spahn 1987).

In our view, the upper abdominal advancement flap provides the simplest and safest means
of constructing an aesthetically pleasing breast
shape in the mastectomized patient. Reconstruction with a tissue expander or with a musculocutaneous flap from the back or lower abdomen is indicated only in women with very tight
skin or an irradiated chest wall (Table 16.1).

Table 16.1. Indications for breast reconstruction procedures

Abdominal advancement flap	Tissue expansion	Latissimus or TRAM flap
Transverse mastectomy scar with no apparent radiation fibrosis	1. Immediate reconstruction 2. Tight, nonirradiated skin	1. Irradiated chest wall 2. Obesity

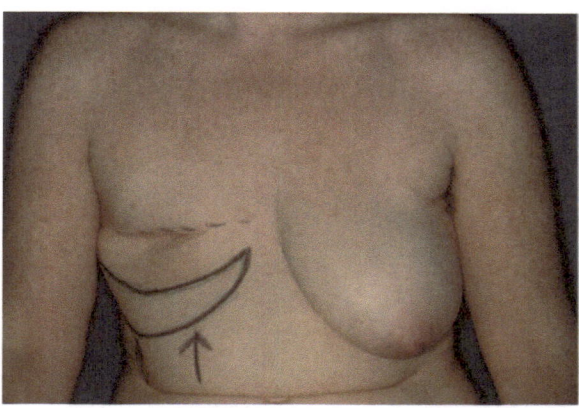

Fig. 16.3. The skin marking are drawn with the patient in a sitting position. Particular care is taken to mark the height of the contralateral inframammary fold, as it will guide the reconstruction. Approximately 6 cm of skin advancement is necessary in this patient

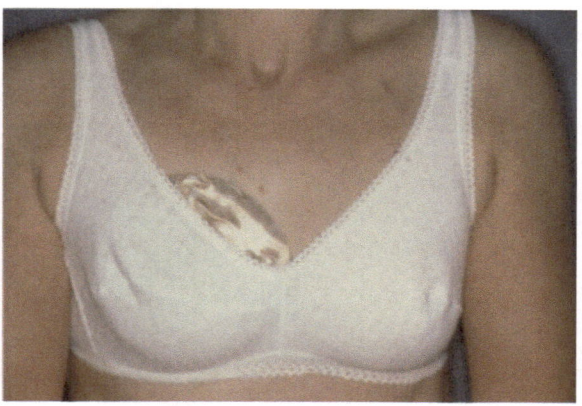

Fig. 16.4. The correct implant size is often difficult to determine on the operating table. We solve this problem by having the patient fit prostheses of different sizes into her brassiere preoperatively to see which she likes best. For the upper abdominal flap procedure, allowance must be made for the contribution of the advanced skin

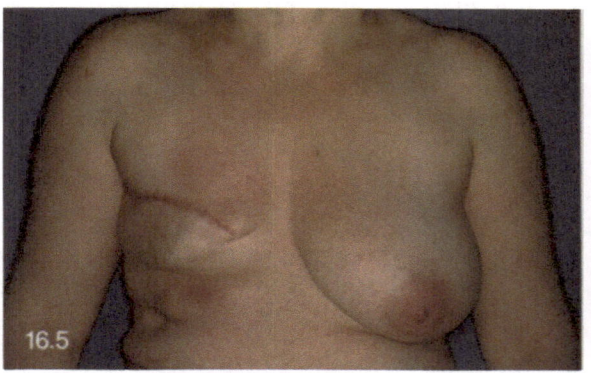

Fig. 16.5. If the residual skin envelope after the first operation is sufficient for a small breast, the envelope can simply be loosened and the implant inserted without altering the inframammary crease. The wound is closed with simple interrupted sutures and an intradermal suture line

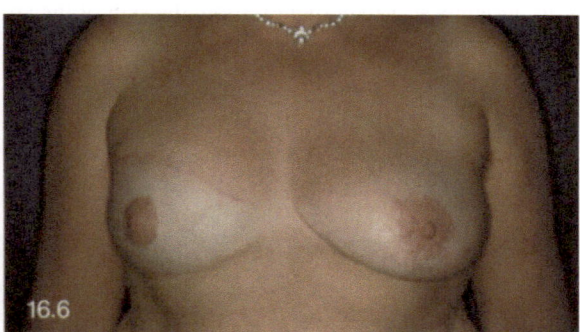

Fig. 16.6. Postoperative result

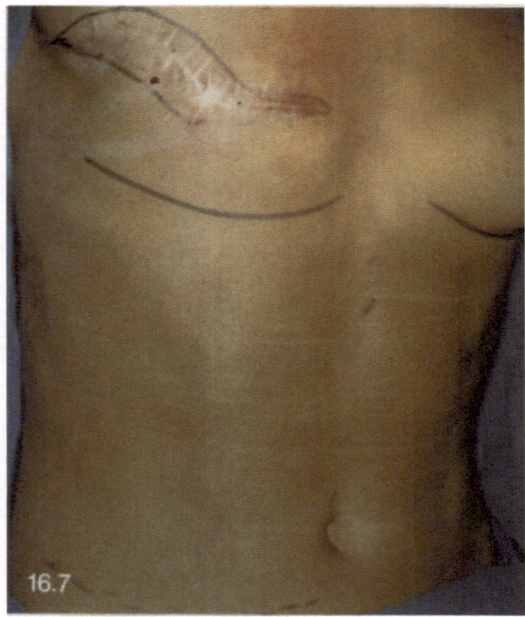

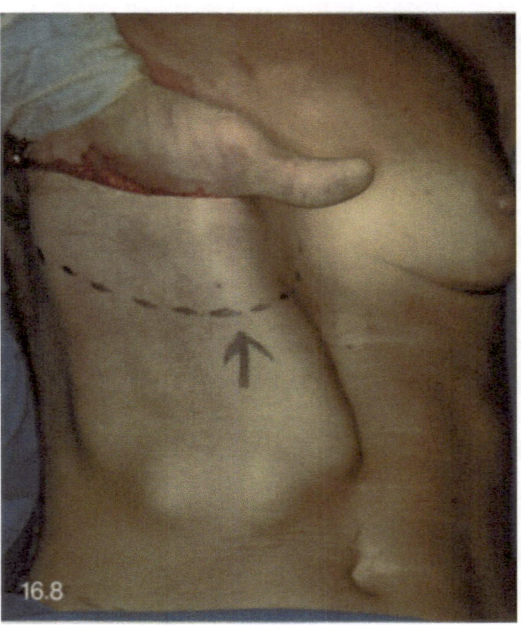

Fig. 16.7. If the skin over the chest wall is tight and there is an unsightly scar requiring excision, the skin of the entire upper abdomen can be mobilized and advanced superiorly

Fig. 16.8. Blunt dissection of the advancement flap rarely causes bleeding, because the intima and media of the torn vessels retract into the adventitia, stopping the extravasation of blood. Thus, it is rarely necessary to insert a suction drain at the level of the umbilicus

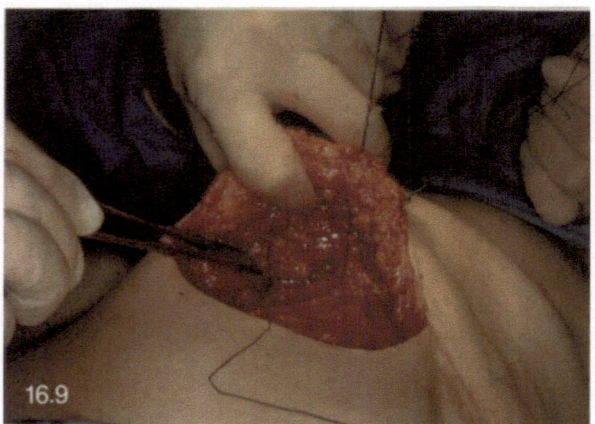

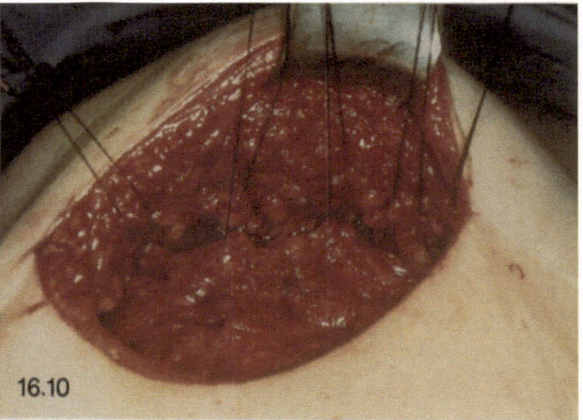

Fig. 16.9. The skin having been mobilized, markings are made at the level of the contralateral inframammary crease, and the skin is brought up and fixed to the intercostal muscle between the fifth and sixth ribs with 6–8 simple interrupted sutures. These stitches should be placed too high rather than too low, for the tension of the advanced skin and the cortisone effect of the implant tend to cause descent of the inframammary crease

Fig. 16.10. We still prefer silk sutures for the fixation of the inframammary crease, our rationale being that absorbable threads might loosen too early, while the ends of monofilament threads might damage the delicate implant shell

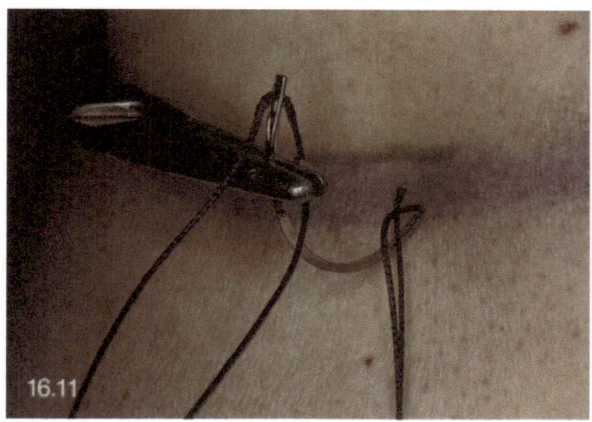

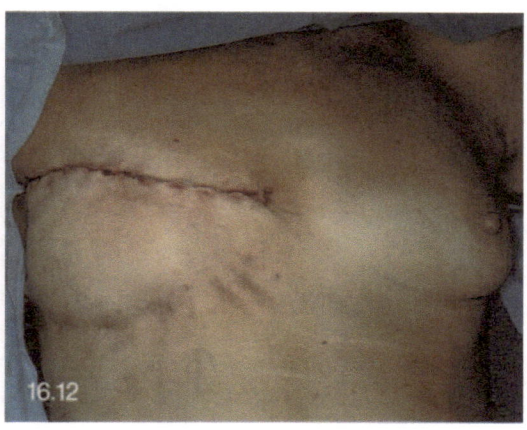

Fig. 16.11. If the subcutaneous tissue is so loose that the sutures tear out, the cutis may be fixed to the intercostal muscles using all-layer sutures

Fig. 16.12. At the end of the operation the patient is raised to a semi-sitting position and should try to maintain a somewhat upright position for the next week to reduce tension on the inframammary sutures. The irregularities in the recreated inframammary fold generally soften and disappear completely in 2–6 months (see Fig. 19.11)

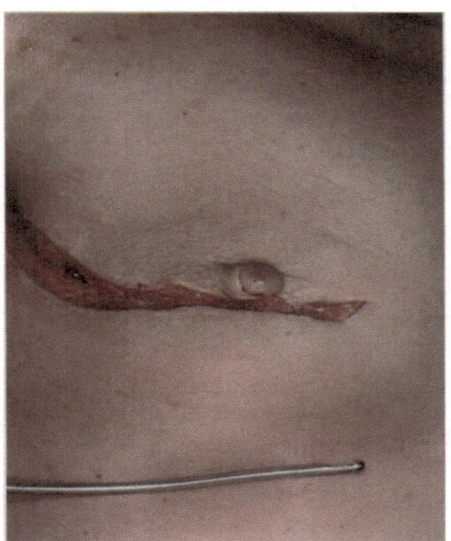

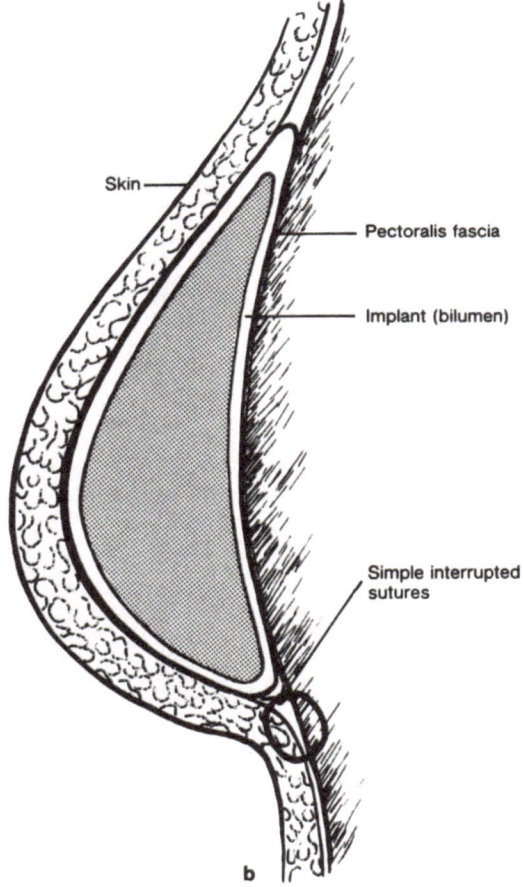

Fig. 16.13 a. In obese patients the future inframammary crease should be thinned out by suction lipectomy before suturing it to the 6th intercostal space

Fig. 16.13 b. Cross-sectional view of the implanted bilumen prosthesis carrying 12.5 mg of prednisolone. An additional advantage of this type of implant is that, if the shell is damaged, there is no gel leakage into tissues (from Spitalny et al. 1981)

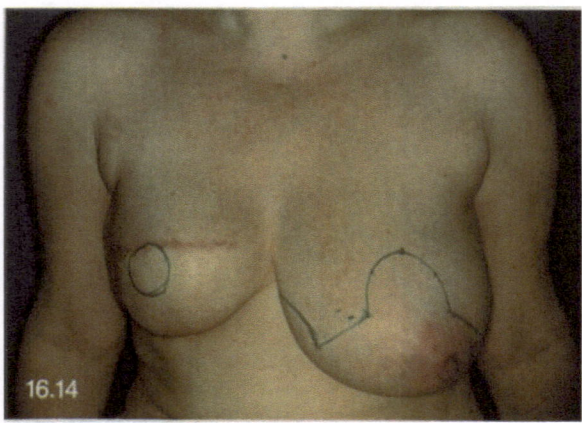

Fig. 16.14. The second stage of the reconstruction, involving reduction or symmetrization of the opposite breast and nipple-areola reconstruction, is performed about 3 months later

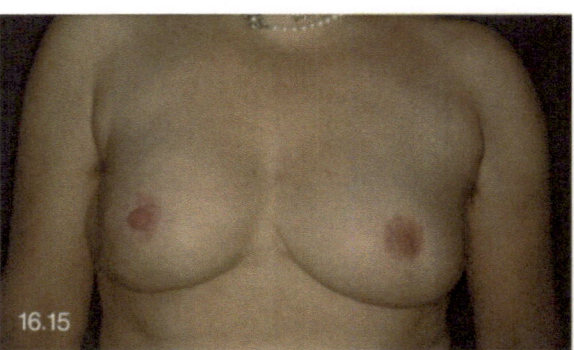

Fig. 16.15. The nipple has been reconstructed from half of the opposite nipple, and the areola from a concentric circle from the opposite areola

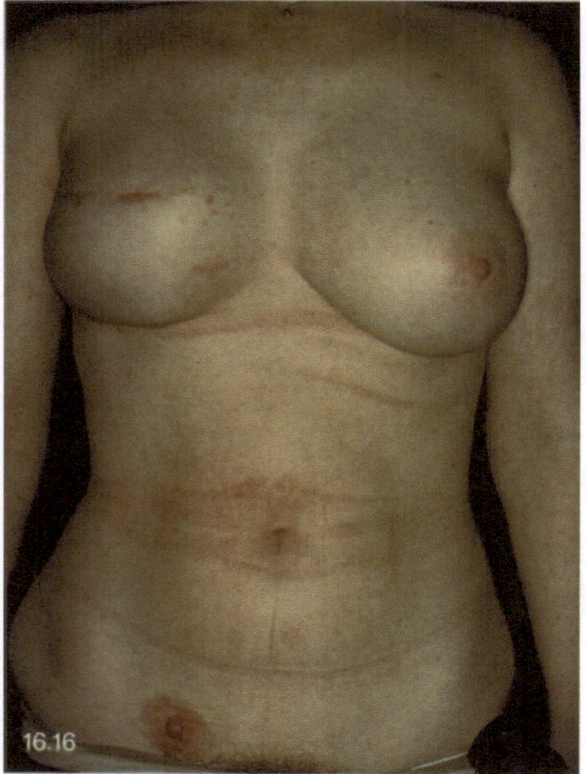

Fig. 16.16. In this young patient the nipple-areola was removed at primary operation and banked in the lower abdomen

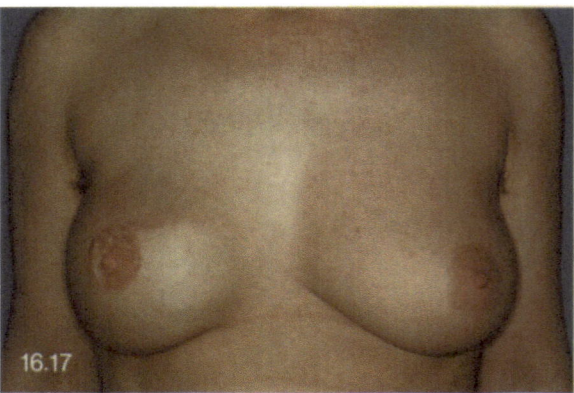

Fig. 16.17. Appearance after replantation of the banked nipple-areola. Note the cortisone effect in the right breast. The upper abdominal flap advancement performed in this patient was documented on film (Spitalny and Lemperle 1978)

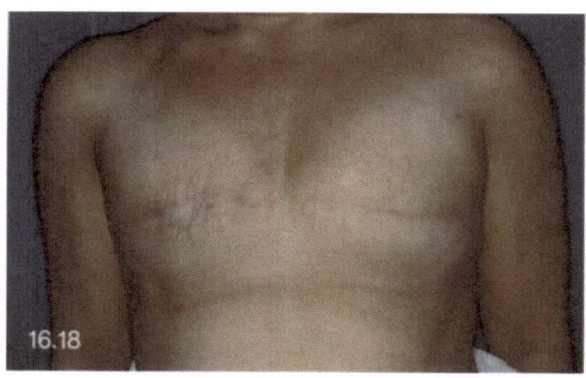

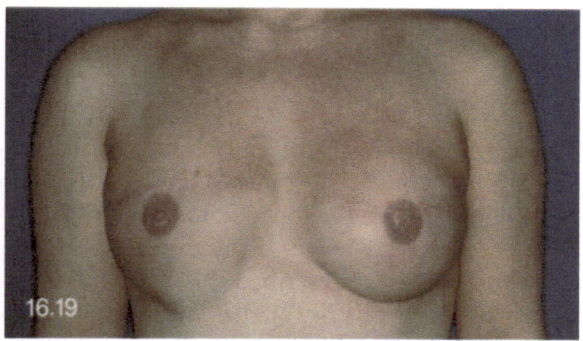

Fig. 16.18. Appearance 5 years after bilateral mastectomy. After excision of the scars, upper abdominal skin advancements were performed in the same sitting, and 280-ml silicone prostheses were inserted

Fig. 16.19. Three months later, after the prostheses have settled into their definitive positions, the nipple-areola complexes are reconstructed using local flaps and areolar tattooing. Two sutures that have pulled loose in the right inframammary crease can be replaced with percutaneous threads (see Fig. 16.11)

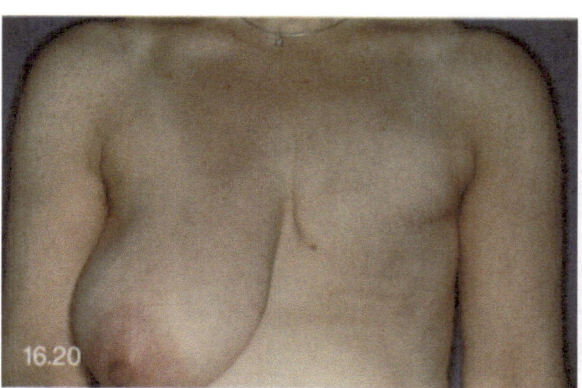

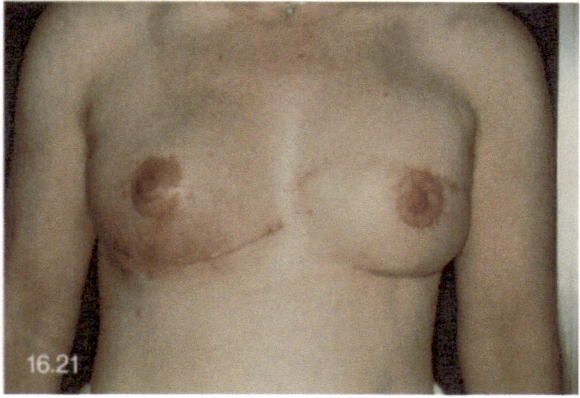

Fig. 16.20. In this case reduction of the healthy breast alone would provide an effective static improvement

Fig. 16.21. Appearance following reconstruction of the left breast with an abdominal advancement flap and a 280-ml silicone implant, right reduction mammoplasty, and nipple halving. The positive effect of the reconstruction on the patient's psychological state is easily appreciated

17 Thoracoepigastric Flap

In patients with a vertical or oblique scar following a Rotter or Halsted mastectomy, a flap can be fashioned from the loose skin of the upper abdomen to give coverage of the excisional defect. Tai and Hasegawa described this "transverse abdominal flap" in 1974 for the coverage of chest-wall recurrences, while in 1975 Brown et al. investigated the axial pattern of vascular distribution in the flap. Bohmert inaugurated the use of the flap for breast reconstruction in 1974 and later used selective angiography to show that the axial vascular supply from a lateral branch of the superior epigastric artery provides optimum circulation when the length-width ratio of the flap

is 2:1. The superior edge of the flap lies on the original inframammary crease, while the inferior edge is parallel to the superior edge and 8–10 cm below it. The average flap length is 20 cm and should not transgress the midaxillary line.

For closure of the large donor site, the skin must be undermined as far as the umbilicus and iliac crest, as in the upper abdominal skin advancement, and is fixed at the level of the proposed inframammary crease with absorbable interrupted sutures. Again, the patient should avoid recumbency and walk in a slightly stooped posture for 8 days to decrease suture line tension.

The true inframammary crease is not restored in the initial operation but generally is effaced and must be created at a second operation 3 months later by a vertical elliptical excision and defatting of the flap base.

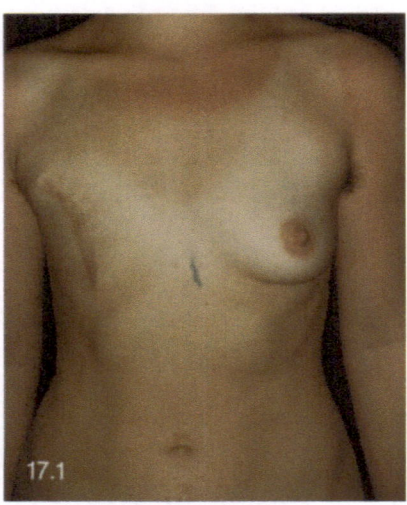 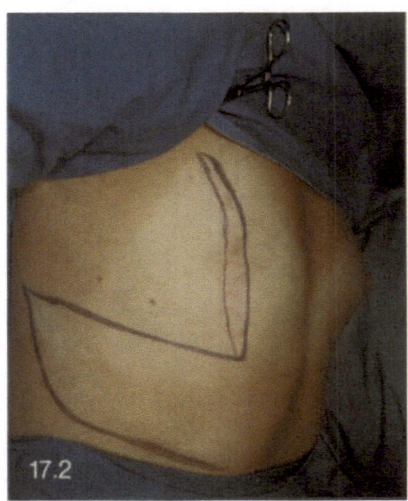

Fig. 17.1. With a vertical scar following a Halsted radical mastectomy, additional skin must be recruited for the breast reconstruction. Here a thoracoepigastric flap has been selected for that purpose

Fig. 17.2. The thoracoepigastric flap is supplied by perforating vessels from the superior epigastric artery. The flap may be extended to the midaxillary line

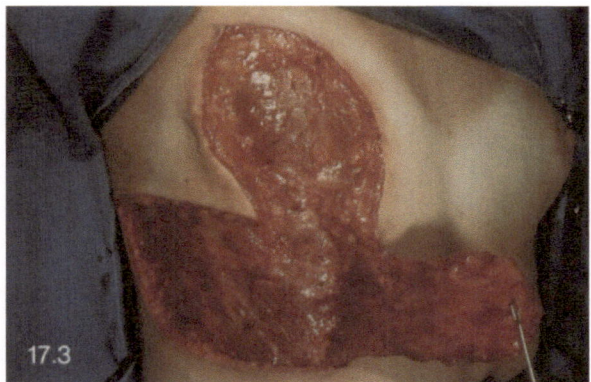

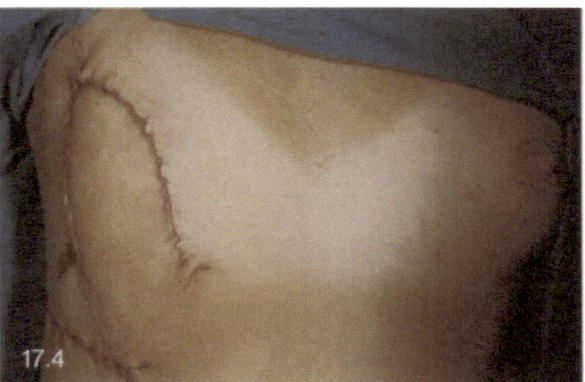

Fig. 17.3. While raising the fasciocutaneous flap, the surgeon must be careful not to damage any blood vessels above the fascia. It is important that the flap be cleanly dissected in the fascial plane. Undermining of the final, proximal third of the flap is done bluntly to preserve the perforating vessels. As in the upper abdominal skin advancement (see Fig. 16.8), the inferior wound margin must be undermined and advanced superiorly

Fig. 17.4. The thoracoepigastric flap is transposed and fixed with simple interrupted sutures for the subcutis and an intradermal suture line

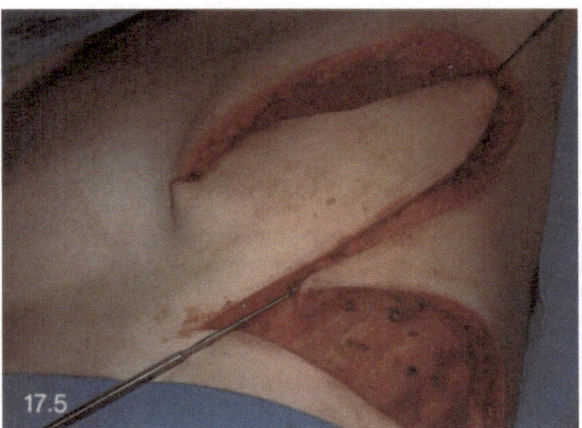

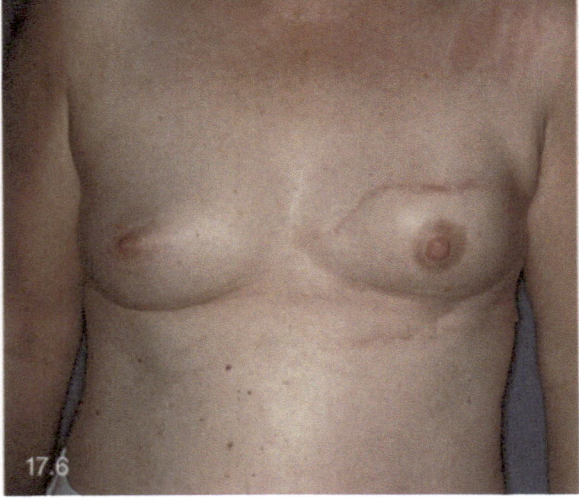

Fig. 17.5. If the skin is sufficiently loose and the opposite breast is not too large, a silicone implant may be inserted right away

Fig. 17.6. Three months later an acceptable inframammary crease is fashioned and the nipple-areola complex is reconstructed, here by halving the opposite nipple and tattooing the areola

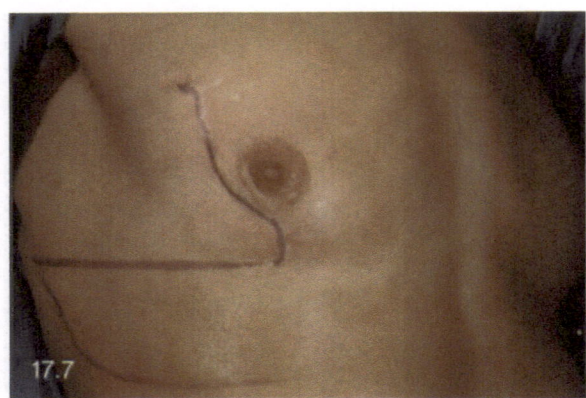

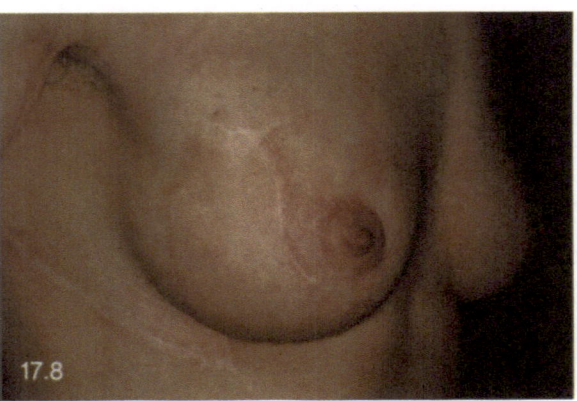

Fig. 17.7. If the nipple-areola complex was not removed at mastectomy, it is sufficient to replace the resected skin

Fig. 17.8. Ideal postoperative result after replacement of the missing skin. This procedure was recently publicized by Holmström (1988) as the "thoracolateral flap"

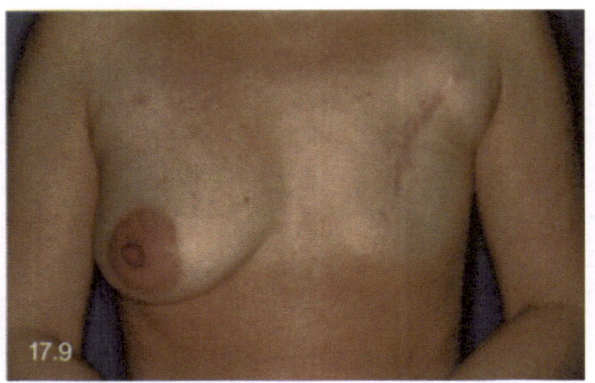

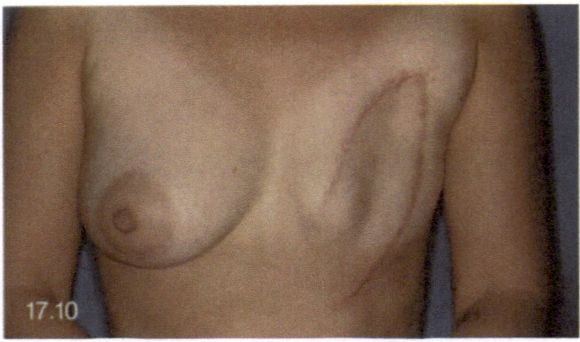

Fig. 17.9. Vertical scar 3 years after mastectomy in a 28-year-old woman

Fig. 17.10. The transposed thoracoepigastric flap has healed well, and the breast can now be reconstructed with a 230-ml silicone implant (see Fig. 2.1)

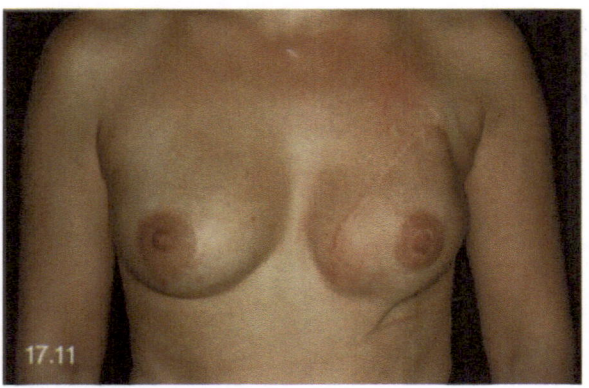

Fig. 17.11. Three months later the nipple and areola were reconstructed by concentric halving of the right nipple-areola complex. A Z-plasty could additionally be performed to correct the inframammary crease

Complications

Tip necrosis can be a problem at the distal end of the flap and at the point of skin left on the lateral side of the inframammary line. We have found that this necrosis is preventable by the postoperative infusion of Rheomacrodex and Trental. If demarcation still occurs – necrosis of the subcutaneous fatty tissue is generally much more ex-

tensive than necrosis of the dermis (!) – the necrotic area is excised after 14 days and the defect closed by secondary suture after first flushing the periprosthetic area with antibiotic solution.

If it is found at operation that the flap circulation is less than optimum, insertion of the prosthesis should be delayed until a later sitting due to the pressure exerted by the implant on the flap and its nutrient vessels.

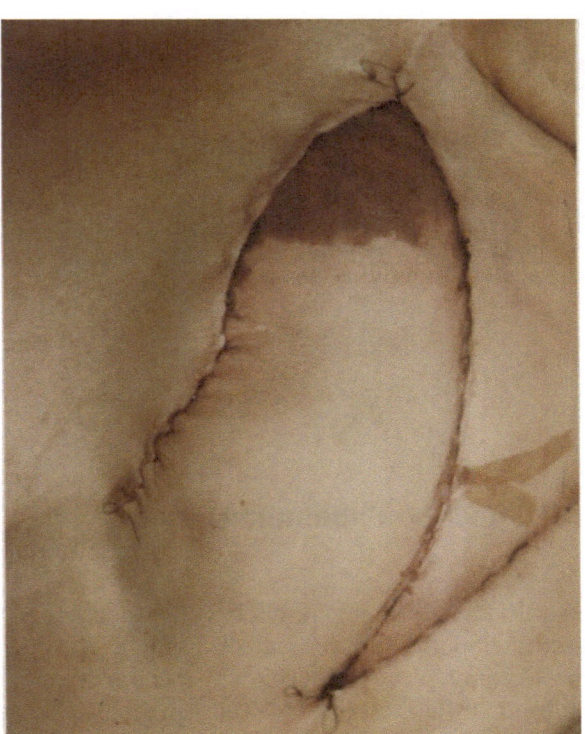

Fig. 17.12. Complications such as tip necrosis and wound dehiscence are most common in obese patients and when proper attention is not given to the median perforating vessels. Otherwise the thoracoepigastric flap is absolutely reliable. The necrosis shown here might have been prevented by direct postoperative infusions of 2 x 250 ml dextran 40 with 2 x 150 mg pentoxifylline

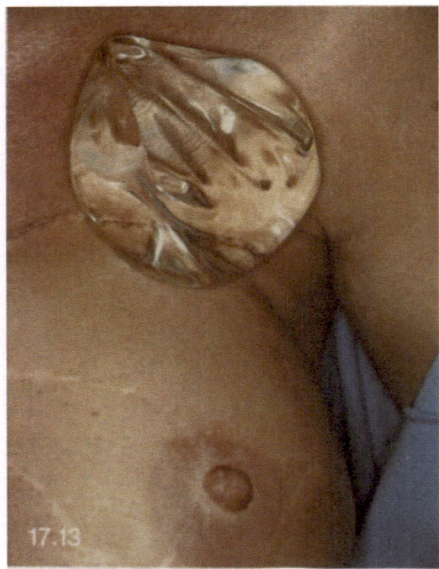

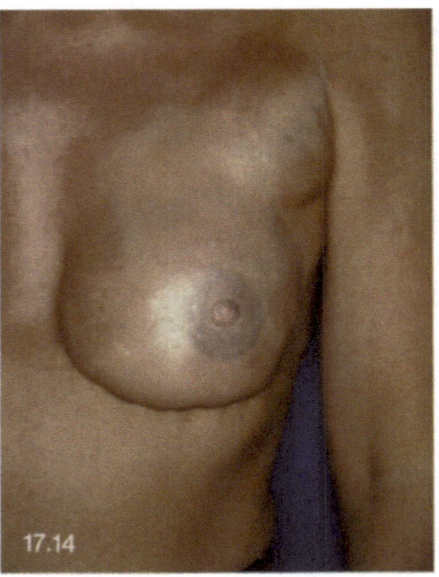

Fig. 17.13. A conspicuous infraclavicular hollow following a Halsted mastectomy with radical removal of the pectoralis muscle can be augmented by the insertion of a low-profile 60-ml silicone implant

Fig. 17.14. A constricting capsule has formed around the infraclavicular implant. At 6 months the capsule can be manually ruptured to relieve the contracture and give better correction of the contour defect

18 Upper Midabdominal Flap

Shortly after Bohmert publicized his thoracoepigastric flap for the vertical or oblique Halsted mastectomy scar, we developed the upper mid-abdominal flap (Höhler 1977) for patients with a transverse simple mastectomy scar. The main advantages of this flap are its excellent medial blood supply by perforating vessels, and that its swing point lies at the site where the most skin is needed. This provides for an optimum breast shape that is further underscored by the "wasp waist" created by the transfer.

The main disadvantage of this flap is the residual upper abdominal scar, which may remain conspicuous in patients who are prone to hypertrophic scarring (Fig. 18.4). Therefore we use this flap only in patients with radiation-damaged skin who are not good candidates for an upper abdominal advancement flap.

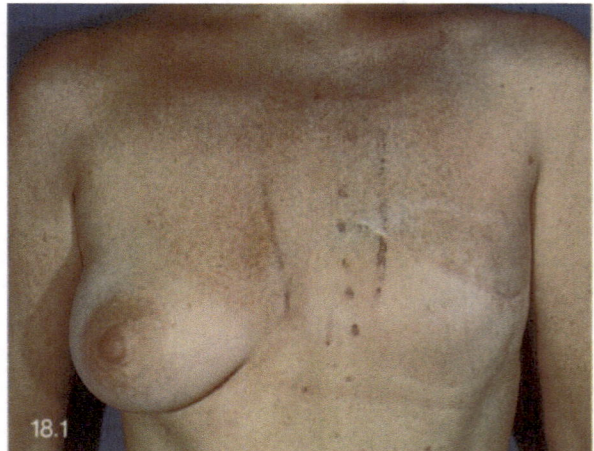

Fig. 18.1. The well-perfused vertical epigastric flap is excellently suited for the mastectomy patient who is bothered by excess upper abdominal subcutaneous tissue

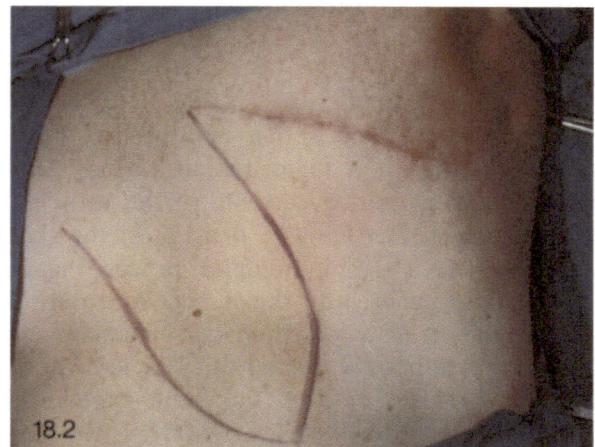

Fig. 18.2. The fasciocutaneous flap is dissected inferiorly to the umbilicus and superiorly to the xyphoid, where it receives an adequate blood supply from perforating vessels

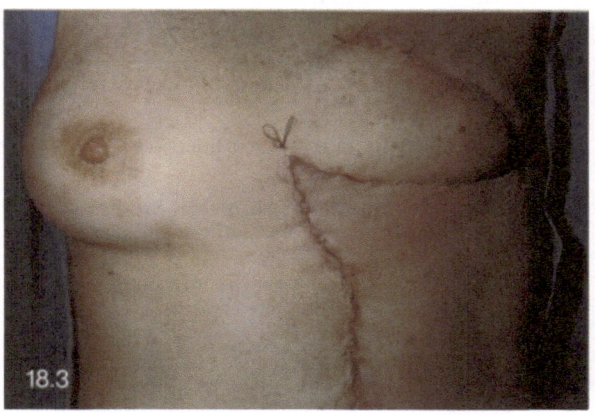

Fig. 18.3. The flap is swung up into the mastectomy scar. Note that this flap, unlike the thoracoepigastric flap, transposes in a manner favorable for creating an inframammary sulcus

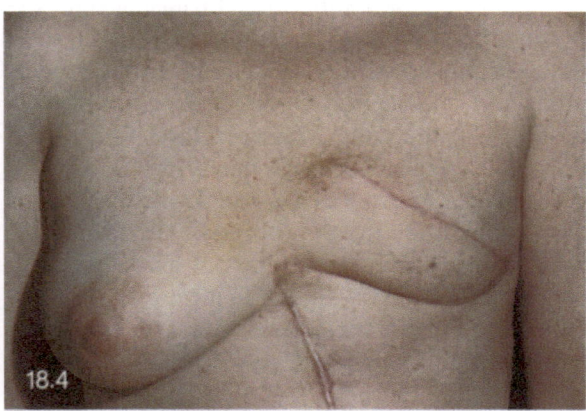

Fig. 18.4. Because the scar at the donor site in the upper abdomen runs across skin lines, hypertrophic scarring is likely

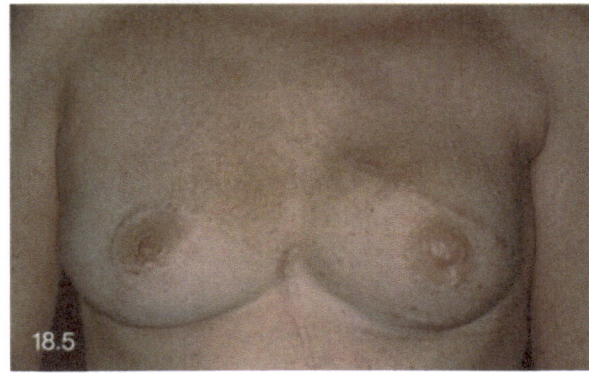

Fig. 18.5. Eight months after insertion of a 280-ml implant and 6 months after left nipple-areola reconstruction by halving the opposite nipple-areola

19 Tissue Expanders

A basic disadvantage of swinging flaps, island flaps, and free flaps is that they often do not match the thickness, pigmentation, texture, sensation, or hair-bearing capacity of the recipient area. On the other hand, expansion of the skin and soft tissues is a physiological process that is seen in pregnancy, growth, obesity, and during the formation of a hematoma or subcutaneous tumor. These natural tissue responses led Radovan, in 1976, to develop the tissue-expanding prosthesis, a device that has become widely utilized in plastic surgery (Lampe et al. 1985) and especially in postmastectomy reconstructions (Radovan 1982; Argenta 1984; Olbrisch et al. 1987).

Following successful clinical trials, several experimental studies were published showing that tissue expansion stimulates activity in the epidermis while causing mitotic the destruction of elastic fibers in the cutis. The vascularization of the fibrous capsule increases markedly under the pressure of the expander, while the subcutaneous tissue becomes greatly thinned. However, our own experimental studies and our clinical experience since 1983 have shown that permanent loosening of the skin is not achieved with tissue expansion. Since we cannot confirm the hypothesis of skin growth over the expander, we continue to prefer upper abdominal skin advancement for secondary reconstruction of the female breast (Table 19.1). We have found that even when a fully inflated expander is left in place for 6 months and then exchanged for a prosthesis half its volume, the initially loose skin contracts markedly within 2 weeks while the atrophied subcutaneous tissue largely regenerates within another 4 weeks.

Following subpectoral tissue expansion, the stretched pectoralis muscle will contract and mold to the smaller permanent prosthesis within hours, holding it firmly against the chest wall.

Table 19.1. Tissue expanders

Advantages	Disadvantages
Ideal for primary reconstruction	Require two operations
Ideal in patients with tight epigastric skin	Cost-intensive
Gradual "growth" of the breast is often more acceptable than rapid stretching	Displacement during inflation, leading to uncertainty in the position of the inframammary crease
	Skin still tends to contract!

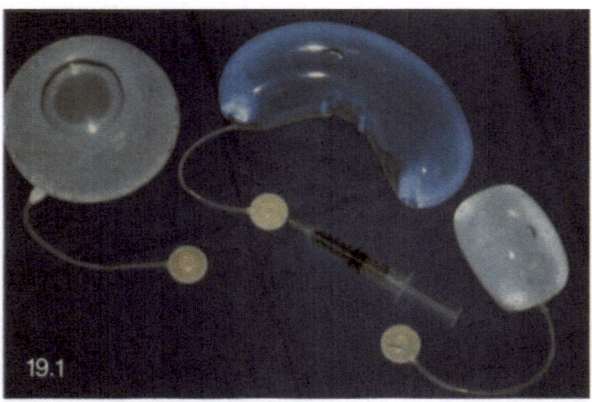

Fig. 19.1a. Various types of tissue expander that can be used for breast reconstruction. These implants can be inflated to twice the designated volume without rupturing

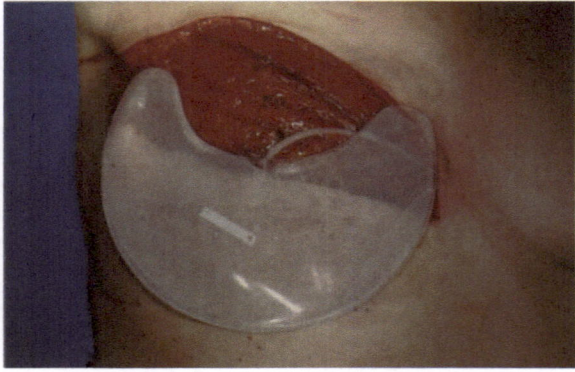

Fig. 19.1b. At present the croissant-shaped expander is our favorite implant since there is never any need to expand the skin of the two upper quadrants

Indications

Tissue expansion is also indicated for (1) primary reconstructions following simple mastectomy, in which the expander is placed pre- or subpectorally depending on the circulatory status of the residual skin (Figs. 19.3, 19.4); (2) patients with tight thoracic and upper abdominal skin that has not been irradiated; and (3) patients who require a relatively large breast that cannot be adequately fashioned by a simple upper abdominal skin advancement.

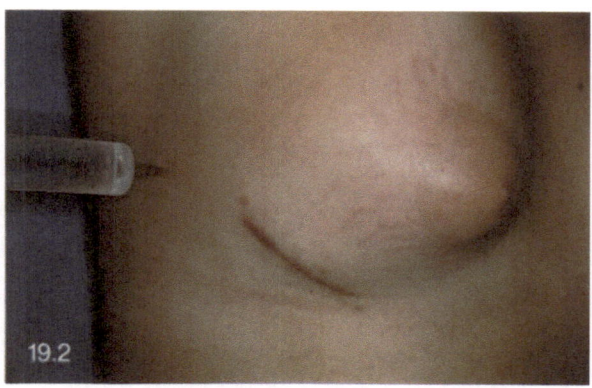

Fig. 19.2. Filling of the tissue expander through the subcutaneously placed valve should be done as rapidly as possible after operation, i. e., at 2-day intervals. Here expansion is being employed for unilateral mammary hyperplasia

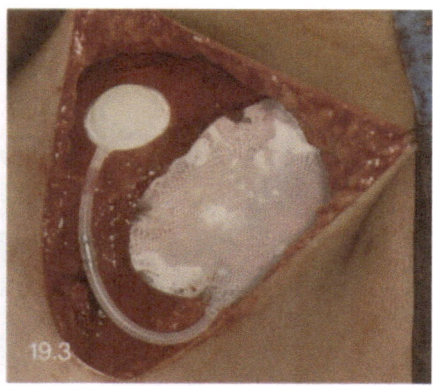

Fig. 19.3. The tissue expander may be placed subcutaneously or, as shown here, in a submuscular pocket. The latter placement is especially well suited for primary reconstructions

Fig. 19.4. This patient has undergone a mastectomy that spared the nipple-areola. While she is still on the operating table, a subserratopectoral pocket is dissected for insertion of the tissue expander. The valve should be placed as close to the expander as possible so that a long tunnel will not have to be opened during later replacement. At operation the implant is already inflated to its maximum safe size. When the large expander is later exchanged for a smaller silicone prosthesis, the stretched pectoral muscle will quickly assume the shortest shape, causing the oversized pocket to contract around the new implant

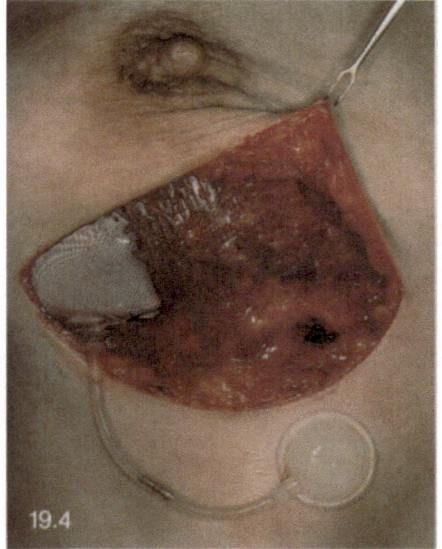

Technique

Expansion of the thoracic skin can be accomplished with a round or kidney-shaped (Scheflan, Fig. 19.13) tissue expander. The implant is inserted through the old mastectomy scar and may be placed pre- or subpectorally depending on the thickness and mobility of the subcutaneous tissue. With an irradiated chest wall, subpectoral placement is indicated to avoid wound healing problems. In this case, the pocket should extend 2 fingerwidths below the prospective inframammary line, and the expander should be placed as low as possible so that there will be sufficient skin in that area for the later creation of an inframammary crease.

The tissue expander is filled with physiological saline as rapidly as possible, the fluid being in-

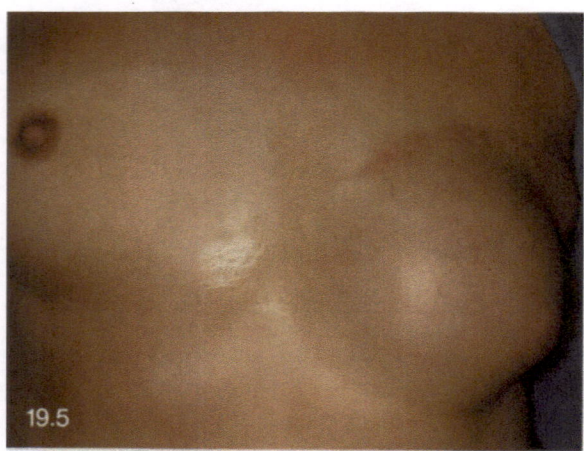

Fig. 19.5. It is very important that the expander be positioned as low as possible. The inferior edge of the expander should be at least 2 fingerwidths below the inframammary line

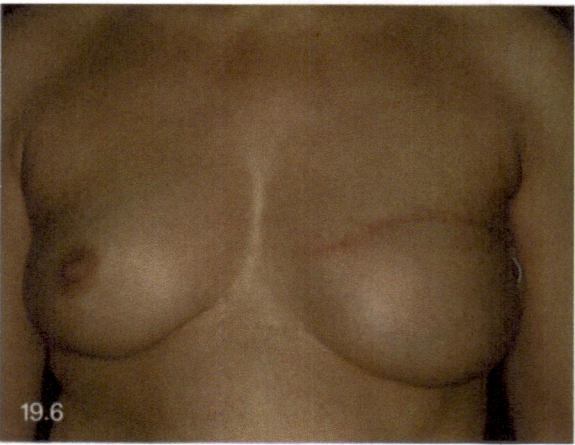

Fig. 19.6. A low initial placement of the expander ensures that, when the permanent prosthesis is inserted (bilumen silicone implant with cortisone), there will be skin available for refixation of the inframammary crease, if such is required

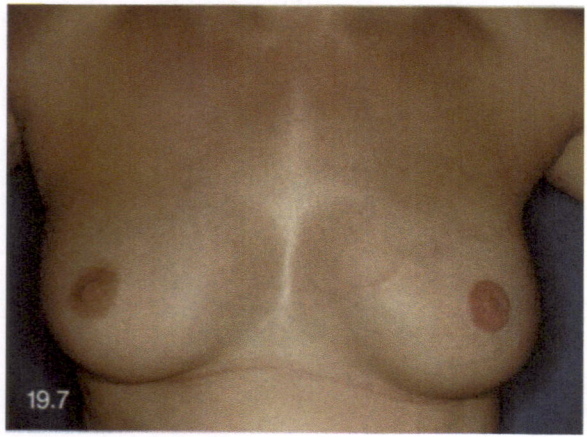

Fig. 19.7. Appearance after nipple-areola reconstruction from local rotating flaps and inner thigh skin

stilled through the subcutaneously placed fill valve using a special syringe with a detachable needle (20–26 gauge) or a small stopcock. As soon as the implant has been placed, it is inflated to the extent that the cutaneous circulation will tolerate. Additional insufflations may be performed on the second, fourth, and sixth postoperative days and so on until, by 4 weeks, the expander usually has been inflated to twice the volume of the permanent prosthesis. An additional 2 months should then elapse before the definitive prosthesis is inserted.

Rather than use a standard calculation to select the prosthesis, we find it more reliable to withdraw fluid from the expander preoperatively until, in the patient's estimation, a satisfactory volume is achieved.

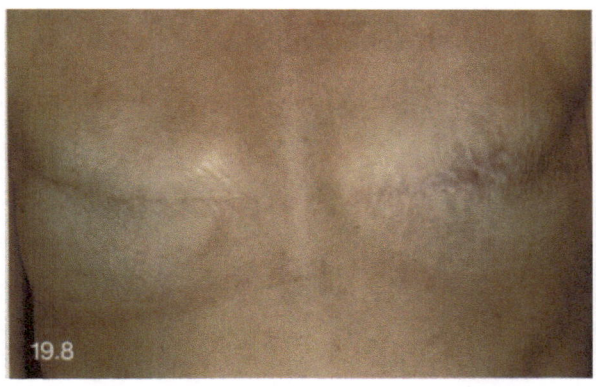

Fig. 19.8. Appearance 10 years after bilateral mastectomy

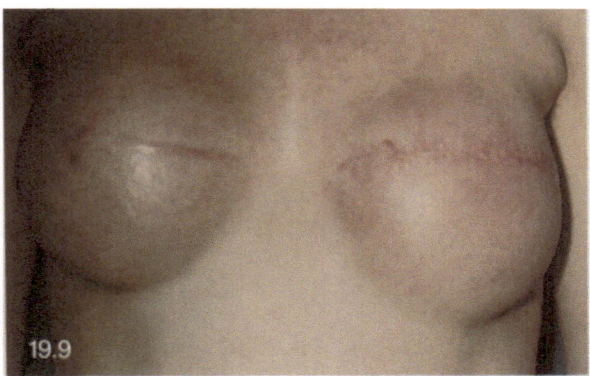

Fig. 19.9. Two tissue expanders were inserted, and each was inflated to 600 ml

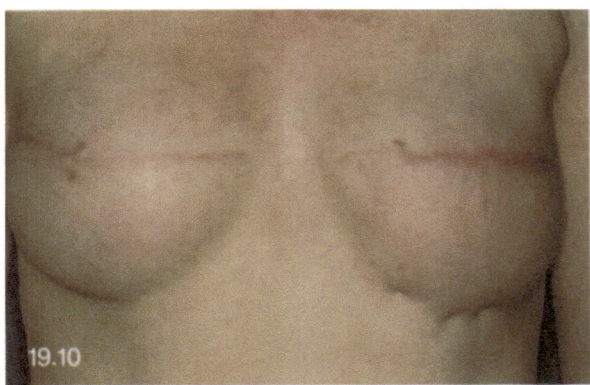

Fig. 19.10. Three months later the expanders were exchanged for bilumen silicone implants with cortisone, at which time the left inframammary crease was raised and secured with five loop sutures

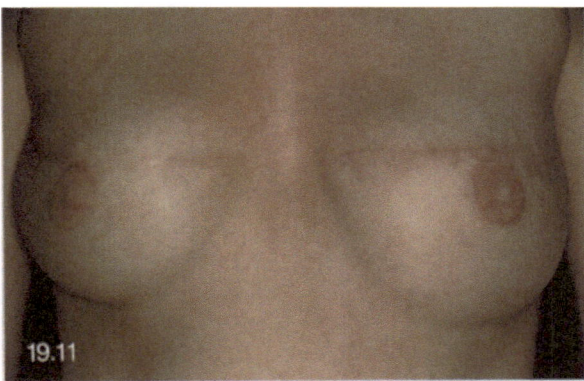

Fig. 19.11. Postoperative result 3 months after bilateral nipple-areola reconstruction with local flaps and inner thigh skin

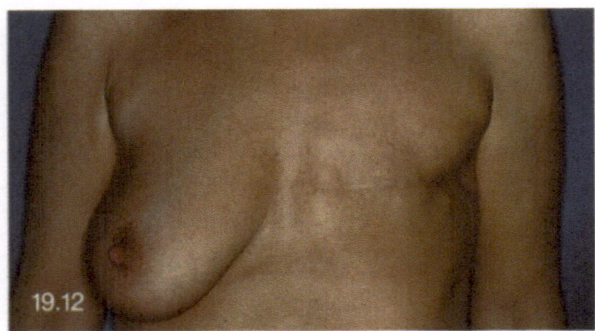

Fig. 19.12. Appearance of a 28-year-old woman after left mastectomy

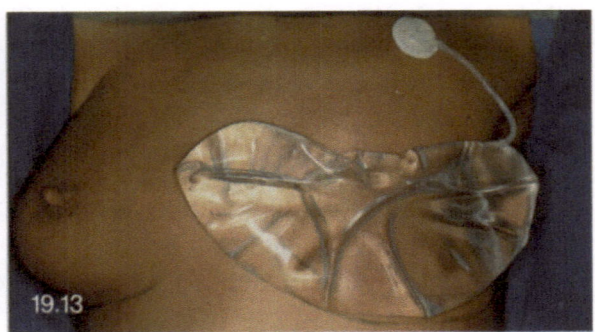

Fig. 19.13. Since the greatest projection, and thus the most skin, is needed in the lower third of the reconstructed breast, a kidney-shaped tissue expander can be advantageous (Scheflan, personal communication). This 600-ml reniform expander is inserted at the level of the lower breast half and is inflated to 800 ml

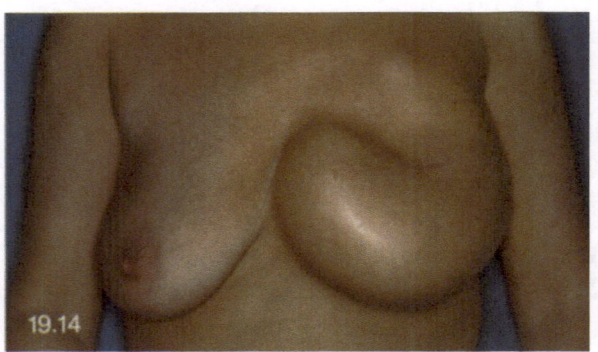

Fig. 19.14. Appearance after expansion to 800 ml

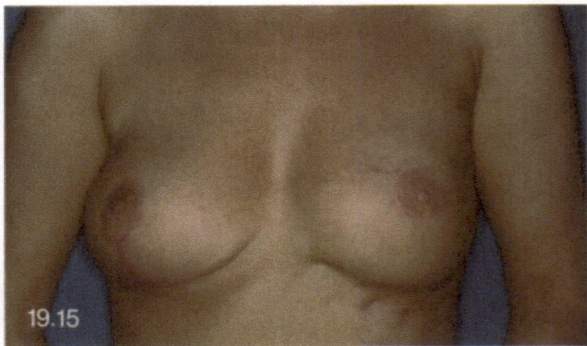

Fig. 19.15. Appearance 3 months after replacement of the expander with a 450-ml prosthesis, nipple-areola reconstruction, and right mastopexy

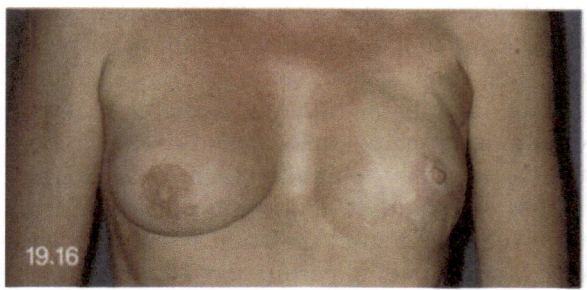

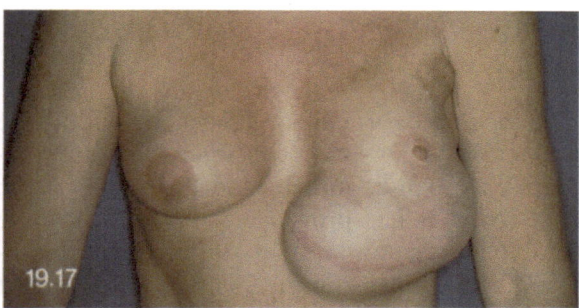

Fig. 19.16. Fifteen years after breast reconstruction with a pedicled lower abdominal flap (see Fig. 21.2) there is almost complete effacement of the inframammary crease on the left side

Fig. 19.17. To obtain more skin, a kidney-shaped tissue expander is inserted into this area and inflated to 450 ml

Fig. 19.18. Three months later the expander was removed, a new inframammary crease was created, and the areola was tattooed. A skin strip measuring 15x2 cm is all that remains of the skin area previously expanded to 30x12 cm

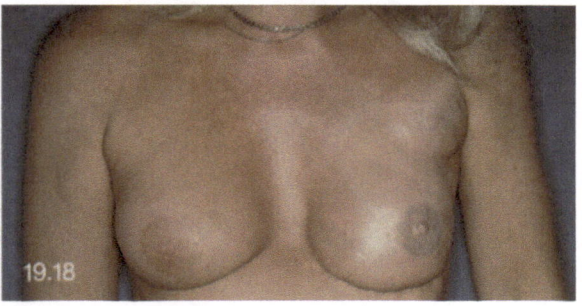

Complications

The incidence of infection associated with tissue expansion for breast reconstruction is approximately as high as in subcutaneous mastectomy: 10%–20%! It has proved beneficial to institute antibiotic irrigation through the suction drain intraoperatively, leaving the solution in the breast for 3 hours. If drainage persists for 4–6 days, one should consider the possibility of infection with *Staphylococcus epidermidis,* which often cannot be detected initially. If there is clinical suspicion of infection, irrigation with approximately 100 ml of antibiotic solution should be started at once and repeated 3 times daily for 1 week, each time leaving the solution for 3 hours. Occasionally this will require withdrawing some fluid from the expander. Partial deflation is likewise indicated for impending perforation. However, as infection is frequently present in these cases, removal of the implant is often required.

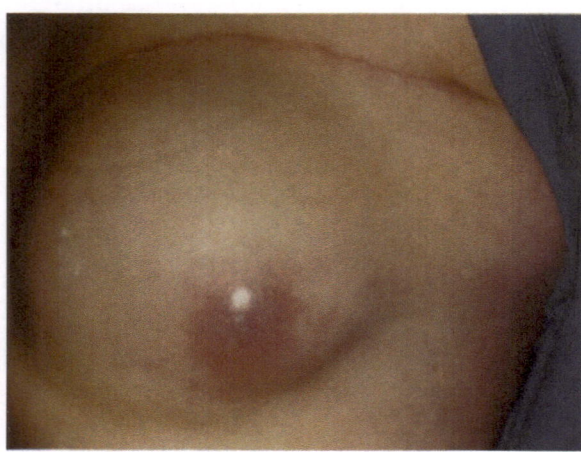

Fig. 19.19. Impending perforation due to too-rapid expansion (see Fig. 19.5) is managed either by withdrawing fluid through the valve *(right edge of photo)* or by exchanging the implant as soon as possible. If the cause is infection with nonpathogenic organisms, treatment by suction-irrigation is advised (see Fig. 15.18)

20 Latissimus Island Flap

Indications

The latissimus dorsi musculocutaneous flap was described by Olivari in 1976 for the coverage of large radiation ulcers of the chest wall, having been originated by Tansini in 1906 for the coverage of extensive mastectomy defects and subsequently forgotten. Bostwick (1978) adopted Olivari's idea and developed a latissimus island flap for breast reconstruction (Fig. 20.3). Copiously perfused and therefore reliable, the latissimus island flap can generally be cut to the same size as the resected specimen and has enough bulk to replace a small breast volume even without a silicone implant. With a vertical mastectomy scar, a transverse elliptical skin island is cut over the central to inferior portion of the latissimus dorsi muscle. With an oblique scar, the skin island is designed obliquely over the center of the muscle, and with a transverse scar the island is placed more vertically over the lateral border of the muscle. The range of the skin island can be extended by releasing the latissimus dorsi at its humeral insertion. Reattached to the lateral end of the clavicle, the muscle can then augment a deficient anterior axillary fold in cases where the pectoralis major has been removed. The ideal indication for this flap is the irradiated chest wall where fibrosis of the subcutaneous tissue greatly restricts skin mobility in the irradiated area. In these cases implantation of the latissimus dorsi, which is richly supplied by the thoracodorsal artery, often leads to improvement of radiation damage through marginal capillarization.

Technique

The operation is usually performed in the lateral decubitus position. The use of two teams can greatly accelerate the technical phase of the procedure and can reduce the total operating time to about 2 hours. This requires comprehensive preparations that include the accurate pre-

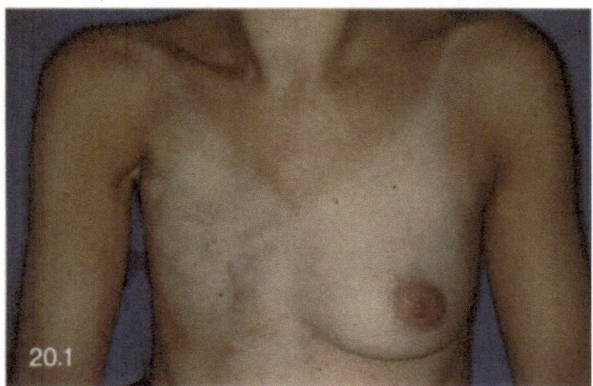

Fig. 20.1. Status following radical mastectomy of the right breast with removal of the pectoralis major muscle and subsequent irradiation of the chest wall

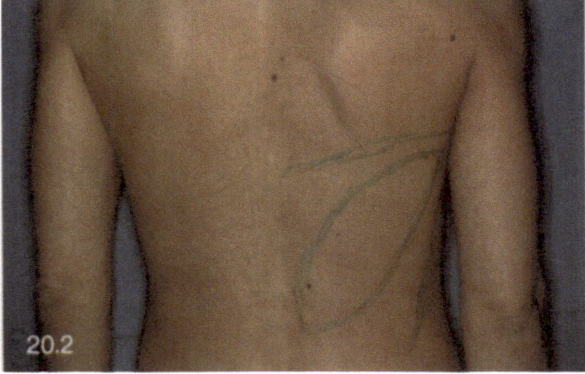

Fig. 20.2. After latissimus dorsi muscle function has been tested by having the patient put her right hand on her hip and press downward, the necessary island is outlined on the skin. The island should always be oriented at right angles to the scar on the anterior chest wall. Thus, a vertical skin island is needed for a transverse scar, while a more transverse island is needed for a vertical scar

marking of the inframammary line and all concavities to ensure the correct placement of the muscle flap. In calculating the replacement volume, it should be considered that two-thirds of the latissimus dorsi volume will be lost to atrophy in the ensuing 6 months.

With an oblique mastectomy scar that is inconspicuous and needs no correction, we recommend placing the flap transversely at the level of the inframammary crease whenever possible (Fig. 20.18) since the greatest projection is desired in that area.

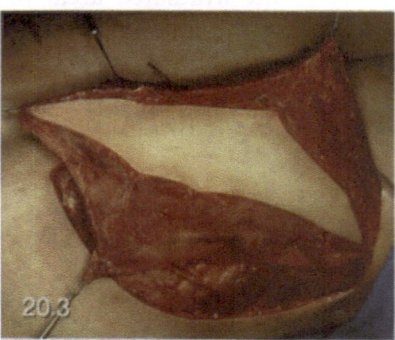

Fig. 20.3. The latissimus dorsi muscle is completely released from its origins on the spine, and the skin island is fixed to the muscle with catgut sutures so it will not slip when the flap is pulled through

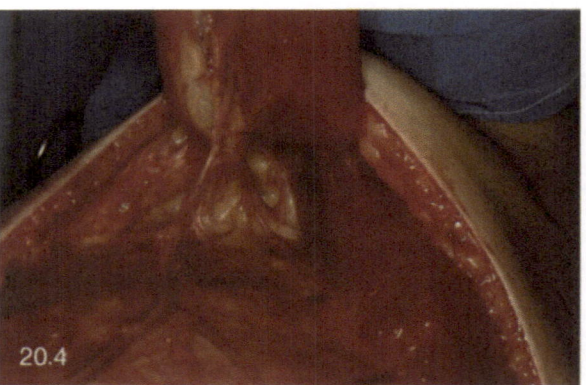

Fig. 20.4. The major vessel supplying the latissimus dorsi muscle, the thoracodorsal artery, should be sought during the dissection and positively identified

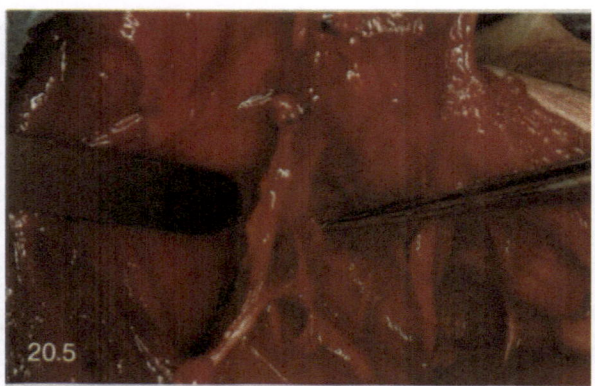

Fig. 20.5. If the thoracodorsal artery was ligated during the axillary lymph node dissection, it is necessary to preserve the serratus arcade

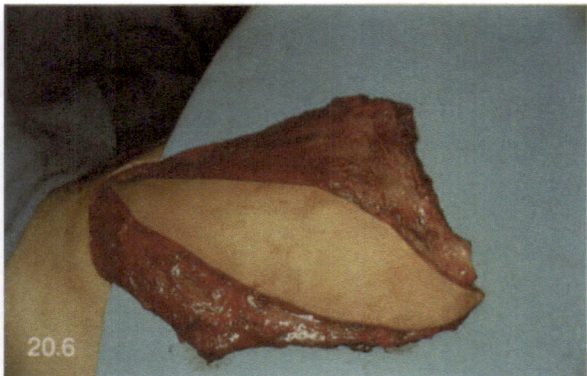

Fig. 20.6. The latissimus island flap has been pulled through the tunnel in the axillary skin and is ready for insertion into the defect

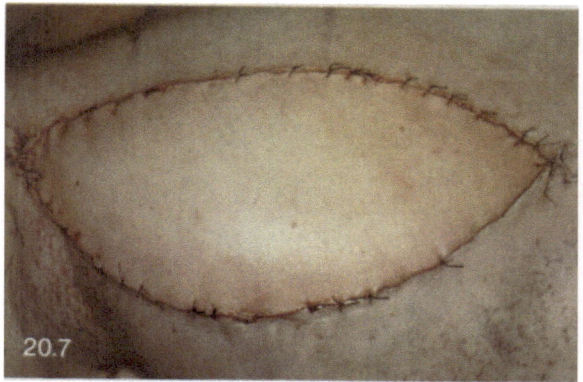

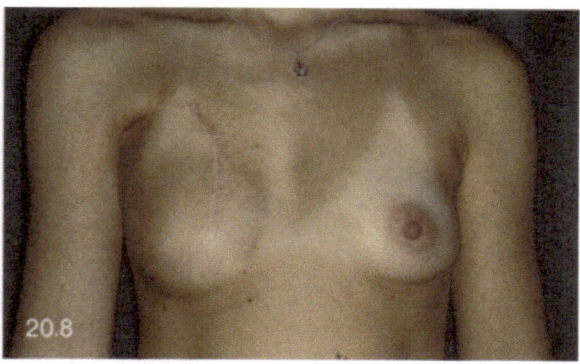

Fig. 20.7. The free ends of the latissimus dorsi muscle have been fixed parasternally and below the inframammary crease with absorbable sutures, a silicone implant has been inserted, and the skin island has been sutured into place

Fig. 20.8. Postoperative appearance prior to nipple-areola reconstruction (see Fig. 20.1). The hollow on the anterior axillary line could be augmented by releasing the latissimus from the humerus and reattaching it to the coracoid

Fig. 20.9. The scar of the donor defect at 10 days (see also Fig. 20.2)

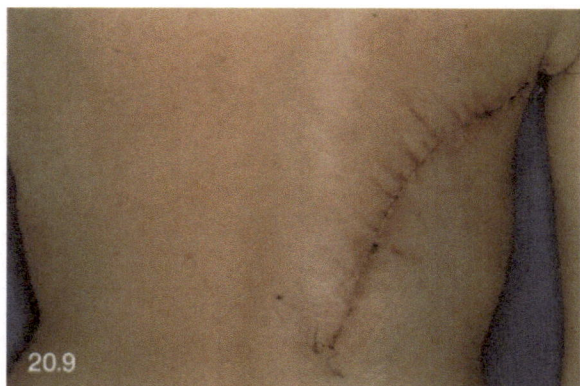

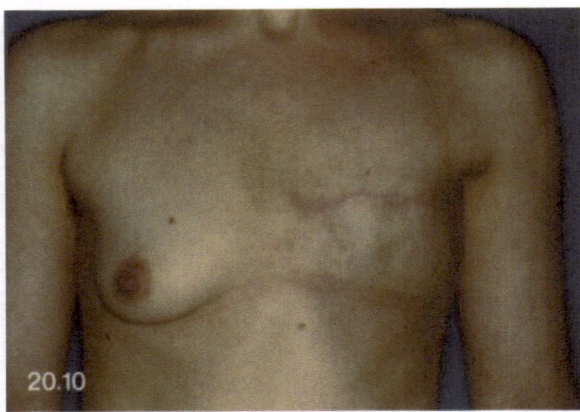

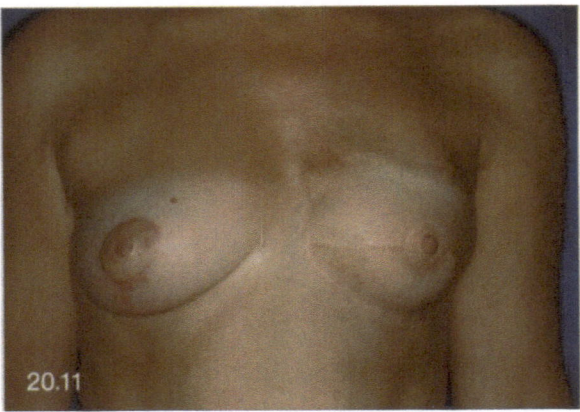

Fig. 20.10. Left radical mastectomy with removal of the pectoralis major muscle

Fig. 20.11. For coverage of a horizontal defect, the skin island on the flap should be cut vertically and placed at the level of the inframammary crease (!) and then underlaid with a 150 ml implant

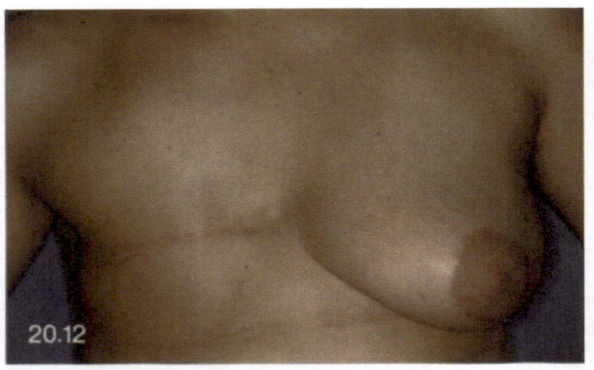

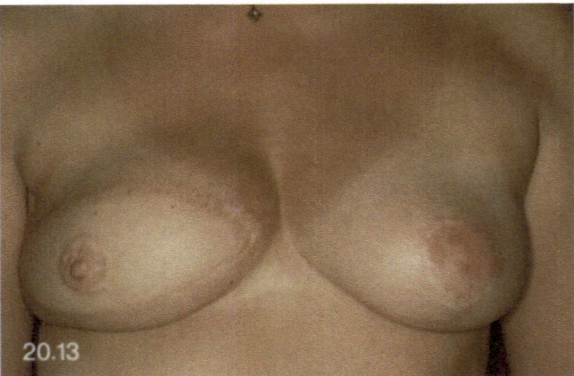

Fig. 20.12. Young patient with a right transverse mastectomy scar. The chest wall was subsequently irradiated, so an upper abdominal advancement flap cannot be used

Fig. 20.13. Appearance after transfer of a vertical-island latissimus dorsi flap and nipple-areola reconstruction with local flaps and a concentric areolar graft

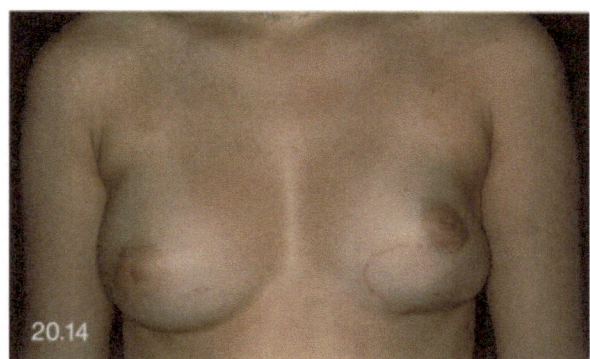

Fig. 20.14. Sixteen-year-old girl with a fourth recurrence of *cystadenoma* phyllodes in the left breast

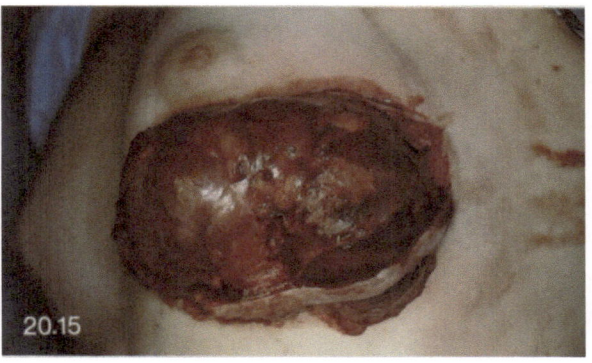

Fig. 20.15. A large skin ellipse is excised together with the underlying pectoralis muscle. Histologic examination again showed no evidence of invasive disease

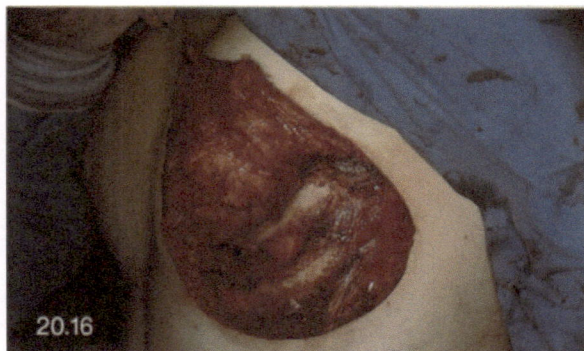

Fig. 20.16. Intrapleural palpation revealed a small metastasis from the *cystosarcoma* phyllodes in the sixth intercostal space, so a partial resection of the fifth through seventh ribs was performed

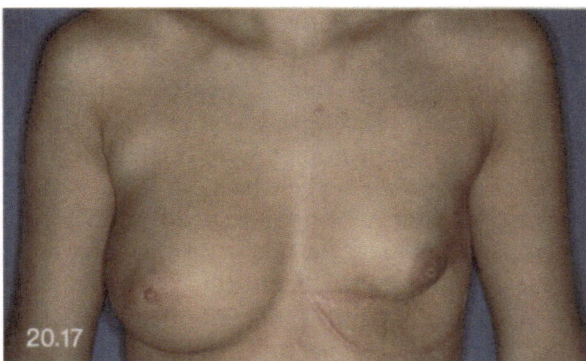

Fig. 20.17. Six months after coverage of the defect with a latissimus island flap

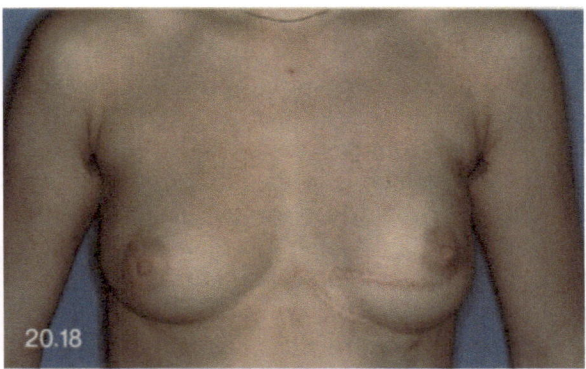

Fig. 20.18. Two years after the fifth operation (bilumen silicone implant) there was no local recurrence. Three months later an overwhelming pulmonary metastasis ensued, leading to the patient's death at 19 years of age

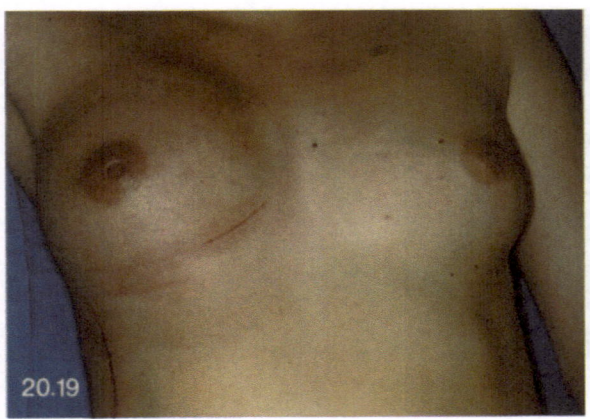

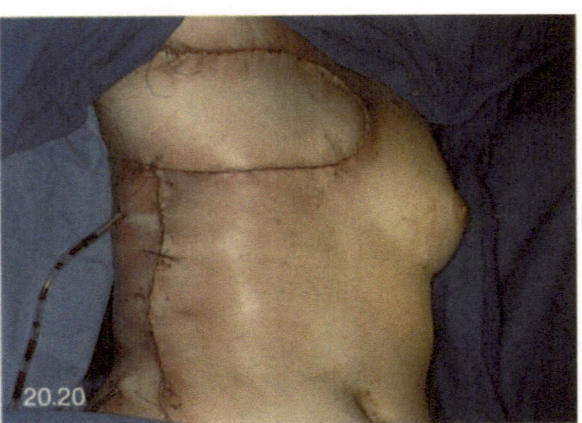

Fig. 20.19. Inflammatory carcinoma of the right breast, which was widely excised following preoperative irradiation

Fig. 20.20. The excisional defect is covered with a pedicled latissimus dorsi flap extending to the iliac crest

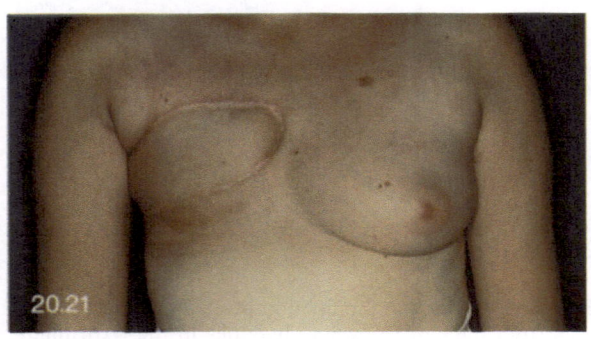

Fig. 20.21. At 3 years postoperatively the patient is still free of disease

Complications

In the rare cases where the thoracodorsal artery has been ligated during the primary axillary dissection, the latissimus dorsi muscle is nourished by an arcade from the serratus muscle. An essential first step, then, is to identify the thoracodorsal artery and, if it is disrupted, to preserve the serratus arcade. Among 72 latissimus island flaps, we have seen three with a pronounced serratus arcade.

Although tip necrosis is a common problem in flap procedures, we have not encountered it in any of our latissimus island flaps, nor have we seen any instances of infection. In three cases we have had muscle sutures tear loose from the sternum or clavicle, and once a suture tore loose from the pectoralis major stump. These resulted in permanent but relatively inconspicuous concavities.

Twenty-eight of our patients required a symmetrization procedure and nipple-areolar reconstruction. Some women were bothered by the bulge of the muscle pedicle beneath the axilla.

The reason we have not adopted the latissimus island flap routinely for breast reconstructions is that it does not match the texture, pigmentation, or subcutaneous tissue of the recipient area. Sometimes the flap has a "patch" appearance, and it feels harder than an unconstricted silicone implant. Additionally, the flap adds an extra scar to the breast, and this can be objectionable in patients who are prone to hypertrophic scarring.

21 Lower Transverse Rectus Abdominis Muscle Flap (TRAM Flap)

Indications

In 1982, Hartrampf and coworkers described a lower abdominal musculocutaneous flap for breast reconstructions that has become widely utilized. Its major advantage is that it eliminates the need for a silicone implant, since almost every woman has lower abdominal subcutaneous fat in sufficient quantity for the reconstruction of a breast. Based on the superior epigastric artery, two-thirds of the entire rectus abdominis muscle is removed from the rectus sheath and transposed to the defect in the contralateral breast together with a large island of skin and subcutaneous tissue. This flap is not as reliable as the latissimus island flap in terms of its susceptibility to tip necrosis or even partial necrosis. However, there is often a temptation to elevate more subcutaneous and skin than the blood supply will support. Understandably, the contralateral third of the transverse abdominal ellipse must be discarded.

Anatomic studies have shown that the most important perforating vessels supplying the skin of the flap are located in the periumbilical area. Therefore the upper incision is placed 5 cm above the umbilicus and the lower incision 5 cm above the pubic hairline; the umbilicus itself is excised.

Technique of the Unilateral TRAM Flap

Dissection of the skin island proceeds from the lateral side, incising the skin down to the fascia along the lateral rectus border on the contralateral side and then elevating the subcutaneous tissue as far as the linea alba. The rectus fascia is incised along a line 2 cm lateral to the linea alba, and the rectus abdominis muscle is undermined with the hand to its lateral border and elevated. The inferior epigastric artery is identified at its

entry into the inferior portion of the rectus, and the medial two-thirds of the muscle belly is elevated past the intersectiones tendinea to the costal margin, taking with it a 4-cm-wide strip of rectus fascia.

While the inferior portions of the rectus abdominis muscle are denervated during the dissection, the most superior segment, supplied by the eighth intercostal nerve, often retains its innervation and is still contractile after surgery. This can cause tension to be exerted on the transposed flap, leading to an unsightly muscle bulge in the epigastrium. It is best, therefore, to identify the muscular branch of the eighth intercostal nerve and transect it at the lateral border of the rectus over the eighth rib.

The lateral third of the rectus muscle does not contain superior epigastric vessels but is supplied by branches from the inferior epigastric artery. Since intercostal nerve ingrowth from the lateral side will continue to provide tonus, the lateral third of the muscle should be left with the closed rectus sheath, to which it is fixed with permanent sutures. As this displaces the umbilicus about 2 cm from the midline, the umbilicus should be recentered by narrowing the anterior layer of the contralateral rectus sheath by about 4 cm (i. e., an equal amount) using nonabsorbable sutures.

After the skin of the upper abdoman has been elevated to the costal margins as in a flap advancement procedure, a tunnel is created for passing the rectus flap to the defect over the contralateral chest wall formed by excision of the mastectomy scar. The subcutaneous tissue, fascia, and muscle stump are fixed to one another with several interrupted sutures to protect the delicate blood vessels from sheer tension during delivery of the flap. If the weight of the resected breast is known from the operating report or pathology findings, the TRAM flap can be weighed on a sterile spring scale and trimmed accordingly.

After the rectus abdominis flap with the fascial strip and triangular skin island has been delivered to the chest, its distal end is fixed to the clavicle or the pectoralis major stump with heavy absorbable sutures. The skin island is deepithelialized according to the size and shape of the defect, and its edges are tucked beneath the breast skin. The defect left by excision of the umbilicus is closed vertically, and the wound edges are closed with intradermal sutures. Suction catheters are placed as for an abdominoplasty.

Technique of the Bilateral TRAM Flap

A much safer method is to use both rectus muscles and raise a full-size TRAM flap based on two pedicles. Hartrampf in 1982 and Bohmert in 1988 have advocated this method for high-risk patients (obesity, diabetes, smoking) and also for primary reconstructions. In this technique the medial and lateral fourths of both rectus muscles are left in place, so that only half of each rectus muscle is transposed. Hartrampf, who has experience with more than 500 TRAM flaps, showed that 90% of the perforating arteries emerge in the central portion of the rectus muscles and only 10% in the lateral third. He also showed that innervation of the initially denervated medial fourth occurs very rapidly following its approximation to the lateral fourth. The posterior rectus sheath is reefed to ensure that both portions of the muscle are firmly apposed.

Even when both recti muscles are used, the superior edge of the TRAM flap should be marked 2 fingerwidths above the umbilicus to ensure that the most important perforators are included. Both recti can be divided at the level of the arcuate line and the distal stumps sutured to the posterior rectus sheath to prevent the development of an abdominal hernia.

Besides being more reliable, the double TRAM flap is aesthetically favorable in that the umbilicus remains on the midline and is not drawn toward the ipsilateral side. The physiological umbilical depression can be restored with two nonabsorbable sutures placed between the fascia and dermis above and below the umbilicus.

To guarantee an adequate blood supply for the unilateral TRAM flap, some American authors recommend anastomosing the divided inferior epigastric artery and accompanying vein end-to-end to the thoracodorsal vessels or end-to-side to the axillary artery and vein or to the transposed external jugular vein using *microvascular* technique. While this prolongs the operation by about 2 hours, it provides a level of safety otherwise unobtainable in diabetics, obese patients, and heavy smokers.

Complications

We have not adopted the TRAM flap as a routine method of breast reconstruction because the demand for autogenous tissue is relatively infrequent in Germany, the procedure is complex and time consuming (3 hours), and because absence of the rectus abdominis, especially in younger women, can, in time, produce static changes in the vertebral column predisposing to early spondylosis and associated complaints. To date, several patients have complained of an inability to rise from a squatting position without bracing themselves with their hands and arms.

Five of 53 patients who received a TRAM flap for coverage of radiation ulcers or local recurrences developed an approximately tomato-sized lower abdominal muscle hernia within a few months. So far, however, it has not been necessary to repeat the closure in any of these cases. This could be done by oversewing the hernia with Goretex mesh or repairing it with a trapdoor flap from the contralateral rectus fascia (Mühlbauer and Ramatschi 1988). Eight of the 53 patients developed a partial necrosis or tip necrosis necessitating surgical revision of the flap. When the necrotic areas become demarcated by the 8th–12th day, they are removed; typically this involves the loss of more subcutaneous tissue than corium. The resulting defect is cleansed daily for one week, and granulations are stimulated with sponge cubes. Usually the wound can be closed 1 week later by secondary suture, or if necessary a temporary split-thickness skin graft can be applied.

An important concern in the early postoperative period, especially in older patients, is the intraabdominal pressure elevation that results from closure of the rectus sheath. This can temporarily interfere with respiratory excursions of the diaphragm and may even cause transient congestion in the vena cava. Therefore respiratory and mobilizing exercises are indicated prior to ambulation. We also feel that early ambulation with an abdominal belt will promote wound healing and help the patient to feel better.

Free Gluteal Flap

Very pleasing aesthetic results have also been achieved with a free musculocutaneous gluteus maximus flap (Shaw 1983, Biemer and Steinau 1988). Based either on the superior vascular bundle or preferably (Nahai 1988) on the much longer inferior vascular bundle, the flap can be transferred from the gluteal region with one-fourth of the gluteus maximus muscle. This procedure leaves a relatively long scar but a very inconspicuous defect when subcutaneous fat is simultaneously aspirated from the contralateral side. This freely transplanted superior or inferior gluteal flap may be the breast reconstruction of choice in the hands of a few experienced ones.

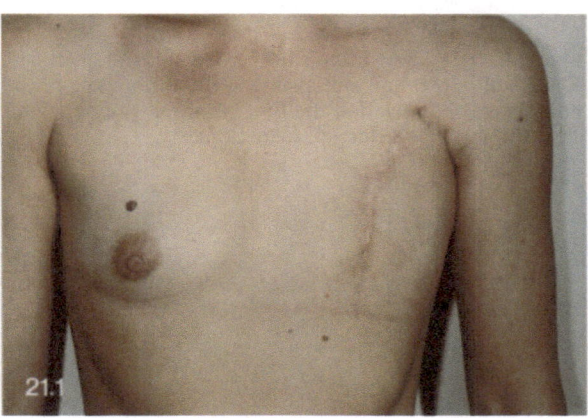

Fig. 21.1. First patient who underwent postmastectomy breast reconstruction at our Frankfurt clinic in 1971

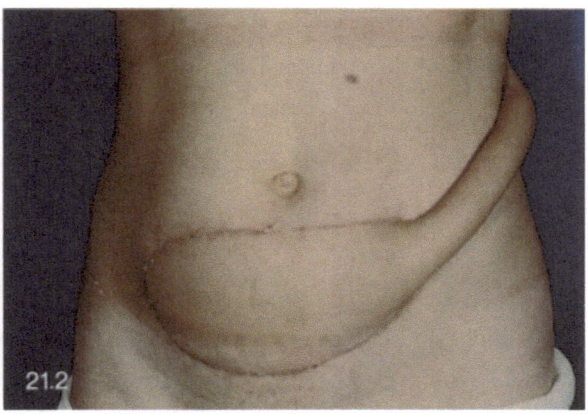

Fig. 21.2. A pedicled lower abdominal flap was established and transposed to the left chest wall in six stages

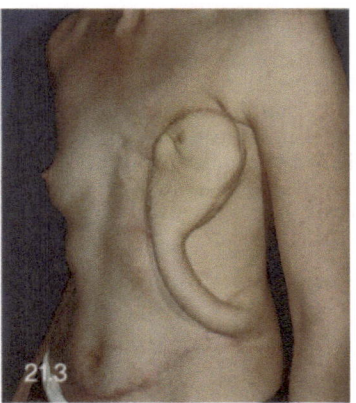

Fig. 21.3. The pedicle provides for inferior volume

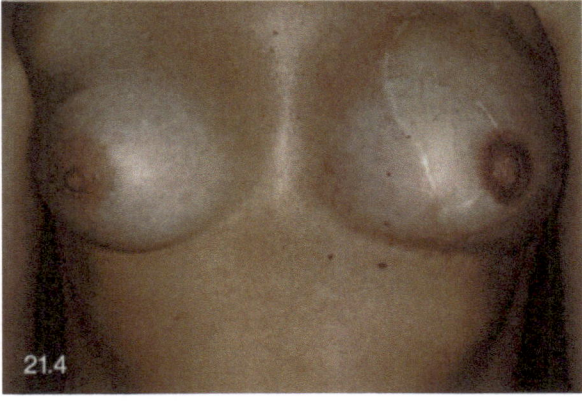

Fig. 21.4. After another six operations the flap was spread out, a silicone implant was inserted beneath it, the nipple was augmented with a free skin graft from the rima ani, and an areola was fabricated by tattooing. The right breast was simultaneously augmented

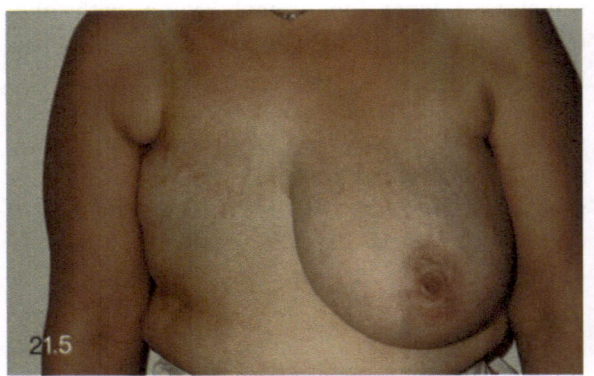

Fig. 21.5. This patient is a poor candidate for superior advancement of the abdominal skin, so the TRAM flap was elected

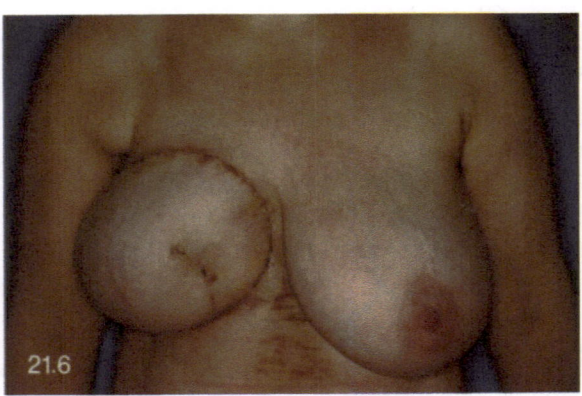

Fig. 21.6. The TRAM flap shows good survival at 8 days. The small depression still visible at the former site of the umbilicus is corrected at the time of nipple-areola reconstruction and left reduction mammoplasty

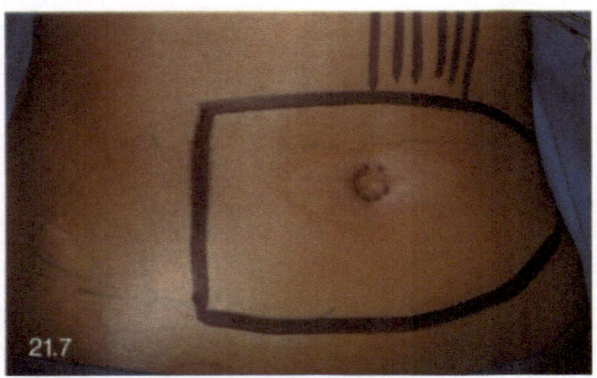

Fig. 21.7. The TRAM flap outlined on the lower abdomen. Most perforators pierce the anterior rectus sheath in the periumbilical area, so the most viable flap can be obtained at that level. The skin on the contralateral side can be taken as far as the lateral border of the rectus

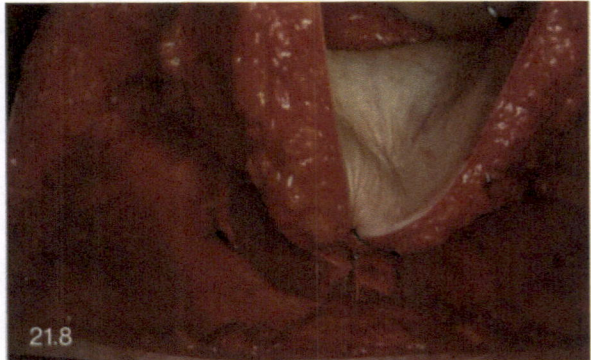

Fig. 21.8. Dissection of the flap proceeds toward the rectus sheath from both sides; the contralateral side that is to be discarded can serve as a control. At the level of the arcuate line, the outer layer of the sheath is divided with a scissors, the muscle is divided with an electrocautery, and the medial and central thirds of the muscle are bluntly separated from the sheath

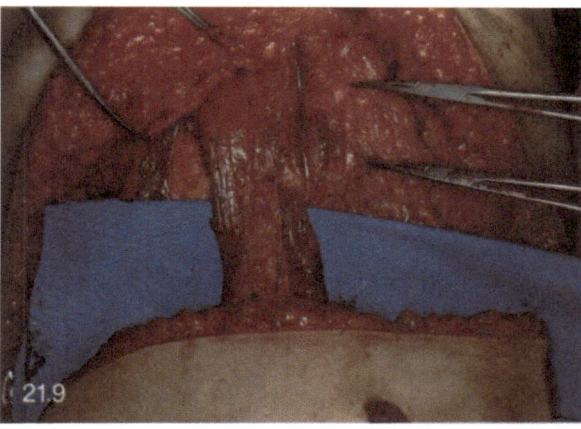

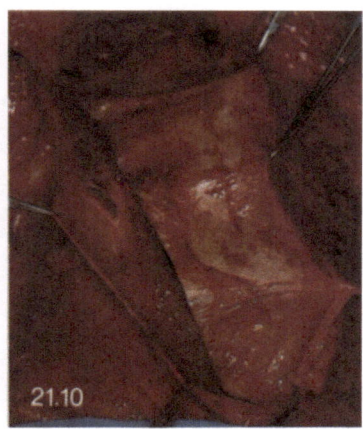

Fig. 21.9. The medial two-thirds of the rectus muscle contain the superior epigastric artery. The intercostal nerves should be divided as far as the sixth intercostal nerve to eliminate contractions in the pedicle

Fig. 21.10. The outer rectus sheath is closed with nonabsorbable interrupted sutures after tacking the caudal portion of the rectus stump with fascia to the arcuate line. This is done to prevent abdominal herniation. The contralateral outer rectus sheath should be imbricated to recenter the umbilicus

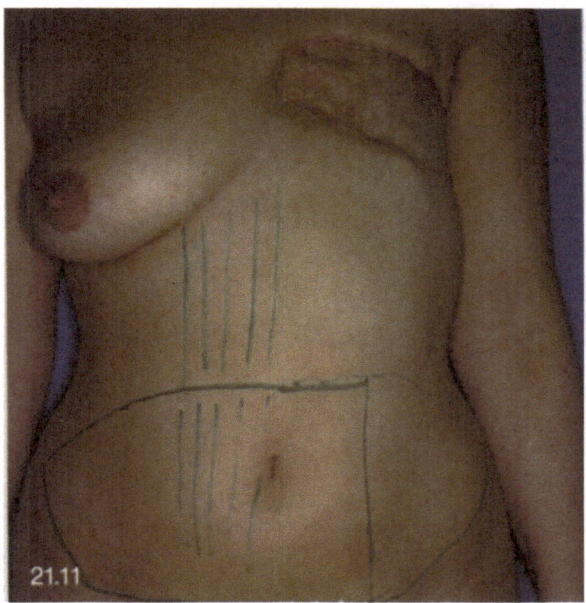

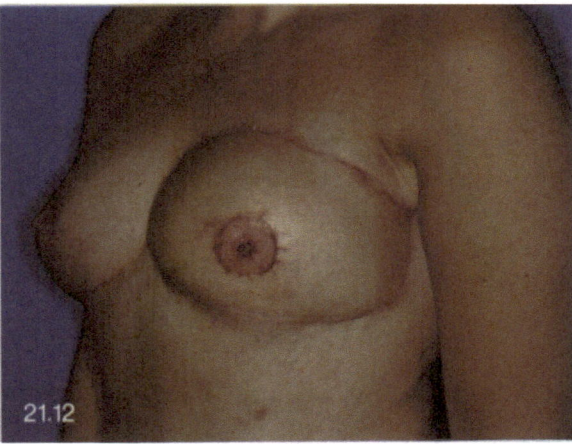

Fig. 21.12. Reconstruction with a TRAM flap and a nipple-areola graft 2 years later

Fig. 21.11. Woman 35 years of age following the excision of local metastases. Premarking should be done in the standing position

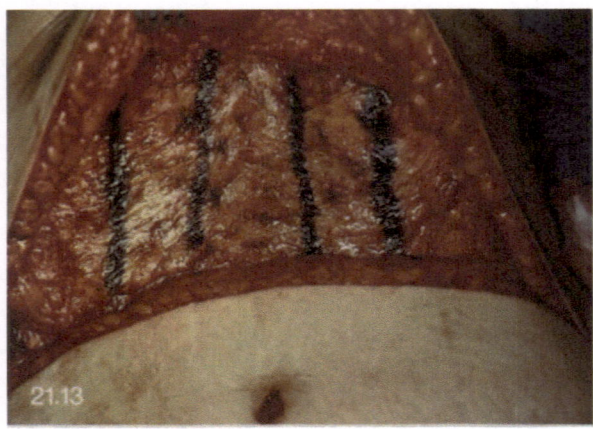

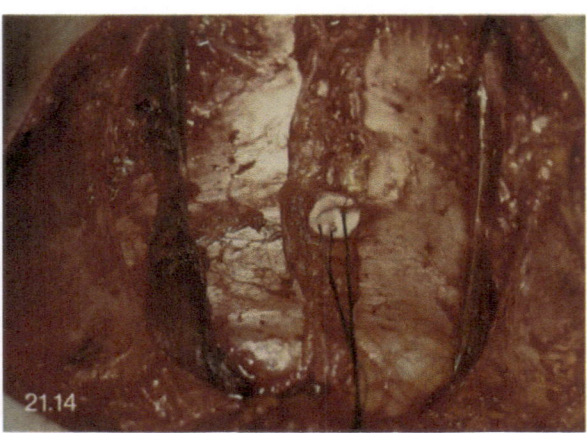

Fig. 21.13. The *bilateral* TRAM flap is larger and more reliable, i.e., less susceptible to distal necrosis. It should be used exclusively in all obese and older patients

Fig. 21.14. Again, the lateral thirds of the rectus muscles should be left on the abdominal wall during the dissection. A strip of rectus fascia should be left on the muscle pedicle to avoid undue stretching of the epigastric artery

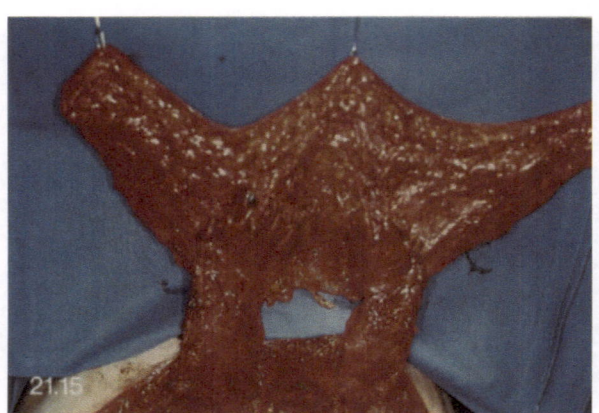

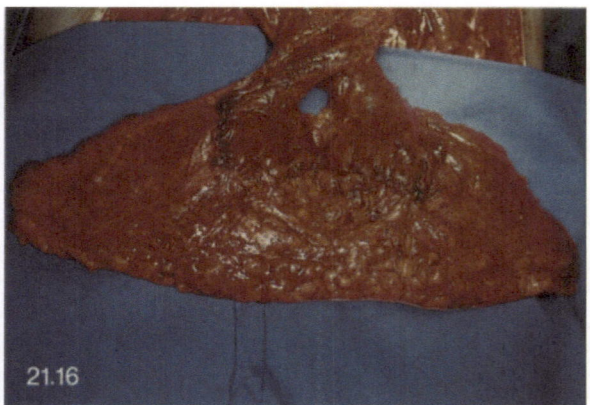

Fig. 21.15. The ends of the muscle are sutured to the fatty tissue to eliminate disruptive shear forces between the muscle, fascial strip, and subcutaneous fat

Fig. 21.16. In the double TRAM flap, the two recti occupy a crossed position in the epigastrium. Adequate mobilization of the skin bridge is essential for unrestricted blood flow

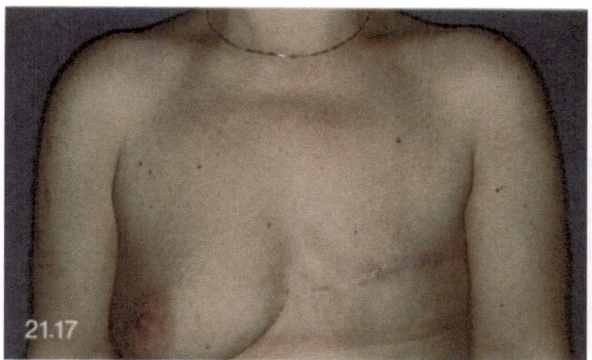

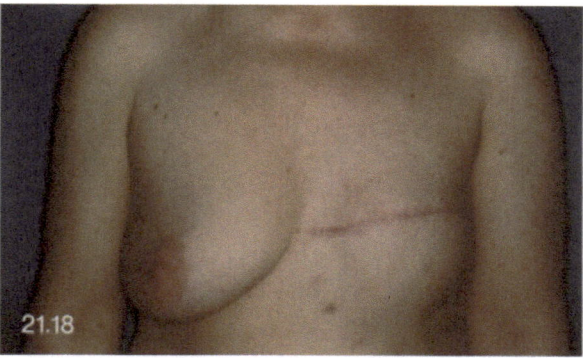

Fig. 21.17. This patient is a good candidate for reconstruction with an upper abdominal advancement flap

Fig. 21.18. Due to "connective tissue weakness," all the silk sutures tore loose on two occasions. This prompted the decision to use a bilateral TRAM flap

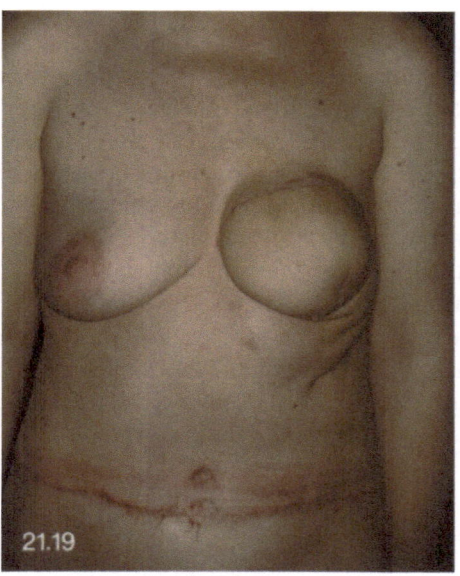

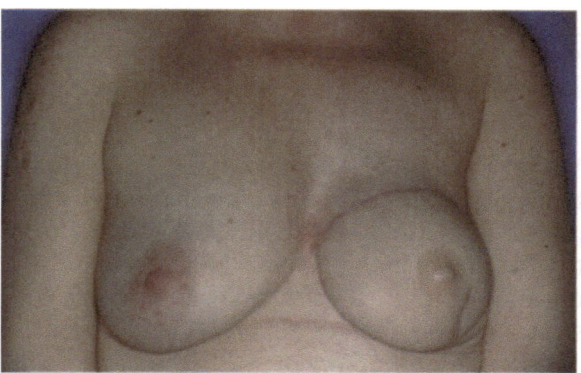

Fig. 21.20. Four months later the breast has assumed its new shape. Note the atrophy of the two rectus pedicles. A "stick on" nipple-areola is shown

Fig. 21.19. At 2 weeks postoperatively the flap is still markedly swollen

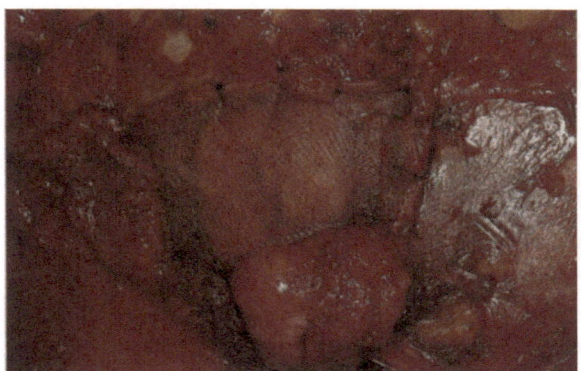

Fig. 21.21. In rare cases a Vicryl (as illustrated here) or, preferably, a nonabsorbable Prolene mesh must be used for closure of the lower rectus sheath

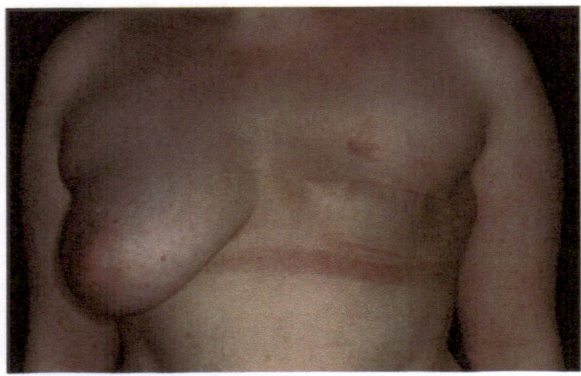

Fig. 21.22. Young obese patients who do not want to alter their [illegible] breast benefit most from a TRAM flap

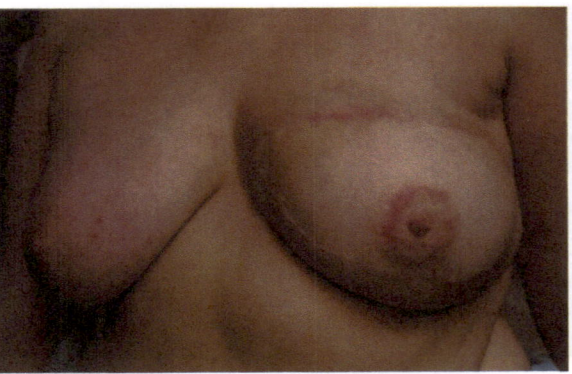

Fig. 21.23. There is no question that the TRAM flap can give the most natural look and feel of any breast reconstruction

22 Contralateral Thoracoepigastric Island Flap

Vasconez in 1982, described the contralateral thoracoepigastric flap based on the superior epigastric artery and vein. This flap is taken from the inframammary region of the normal side and transposed 180° to the side requiring reconstruction (Vasconez et al. 1983). It includes the most superior portion of the rectus abdominis muscle and its anterior fascia, the perforating arteries, and the axial vessels described by Bohmert. The relatively strong traction on the vascular pedicle makes this a risky flap, however. Lejour (1982) reported 10 instances of total necrosis in 33 operations (28%!). For pure breast reconstructions, then, this flap should be considered only as a last resort in patients who refuse a silicone prosthesis, have an irradiated axilla, and have lower abdominal scarring that would preclude the use of a TRAM flap.

If the vascular pedicle appears too short, the xyphoid must be removed and the contralateral costal margin deeply notched to avoid kinking of the pedicle.

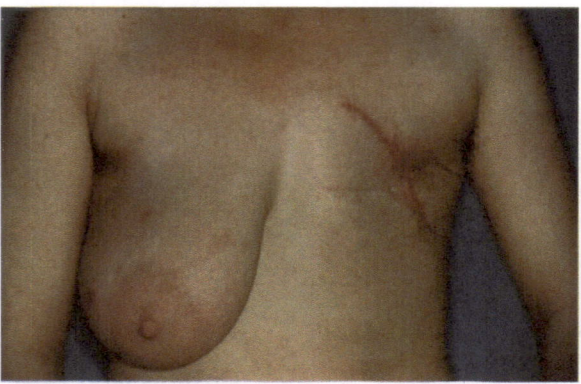

Fig. 22.1. Patient 18 years of age who underwent left mastectomy for chronically recurring abscesses (self-mutilation?)

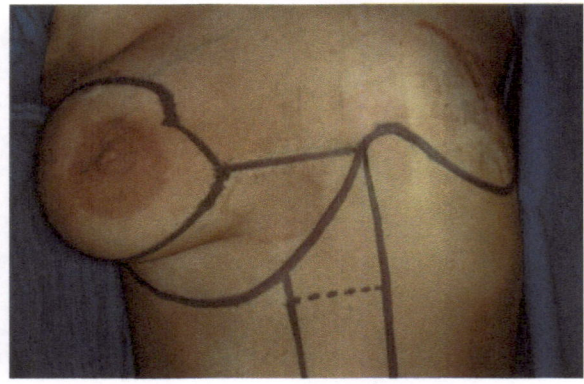

Fig. 22.2. A contralateral thoracoepigastric island flap is outlined below the right breast

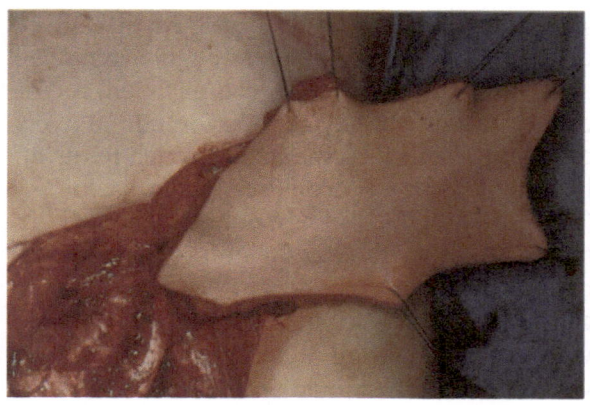

Fig. 22.3. The musculocutaneous island flap is based entirely on the right superior epigastric artery and the posterior insertion of the rectus muscle

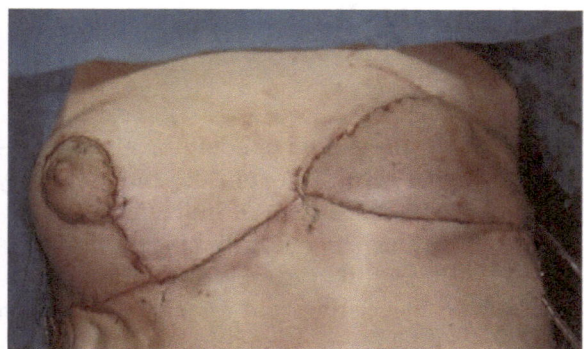

Fig. 22.4. The island flap shows slight venous congestion after it is sutured into place

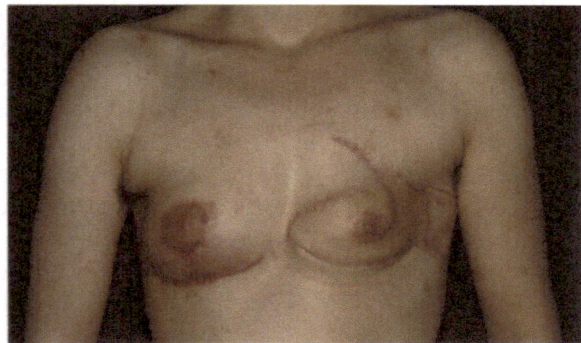

Fig. 22.5. After the island flap has taken, the left nipple-areola is reconstructed. A silicone implant would further improve the result

23 Corrective Procedures

The result of any plastic operation, and especially of a breast reconstruction, depends critically on the strength and extent of individual scar formation. Daily experience with silicone implants has demonstrated that external scar formation – arising from the dermis and often depending on the dermal thickness – has nothing to do with internal scar formation as exemplified by capsular contracture around silicone implants or hypertrophic scarring after intervertebral disc surgery. This is illustrated by the case in Fig. 15.23, where extreme capsular contracture in the breasts coexisted with very heavy internal hypertrophic scarring (and conspicuous external scars) follwing multiple intervertebral disc operations.

If a capsular contracture develops, the path of displacement of the implant is predetermined by the upward taper of the conically shaped thorax. Since the inframammary line is fixed to the chest wall (Fig. 4.3), the rising pressure of the constricting capsule tends to push the prosthesis toward the loose skin of the anterior axilla. In extreme cases this happens as early as the second postoperative week, but usually it develops during the first 6 months. As the degree of constrictive capsule formation cannot be predicted in a given case, the patient should be thoroughly counseled about the possibility of this complication. As the contracture progresses, skin perforation may occur at the site of least resistance, which frequently is the scar. A compression capsulotomy (Figs. 2.14 and 2.15) should not be attempted until at least 6 months after the prosthetic implantation; and, in our experience, a capsulotomy or capsulectomy should not always be combined with the insertion of a double-lumen implant with cortisone (Lemperle and Exner 1990). As a general rule, 6 months should elapse before any corrective procedure is undertaken.

Because the optimum nipple site cannot be determined during the initial reconstruction, we strongly recommend delaying the nipple-areola reconstruction for 2–3 months so that the implant can settle into its definitive position.

Although Z-plasties and W-plasties are the corrective procedures of choice for indrawn scars in the facial region, we do not favor their use on the breast. Angled scars leave a perpetual "signature" from the plastic surgeon, who should leave as few extra scars on the breast as possible. Contracted scars on the body can be managed simply and effectively by the excision of all deep scar tissue and the accurate reapproximation of the fatty tissue.

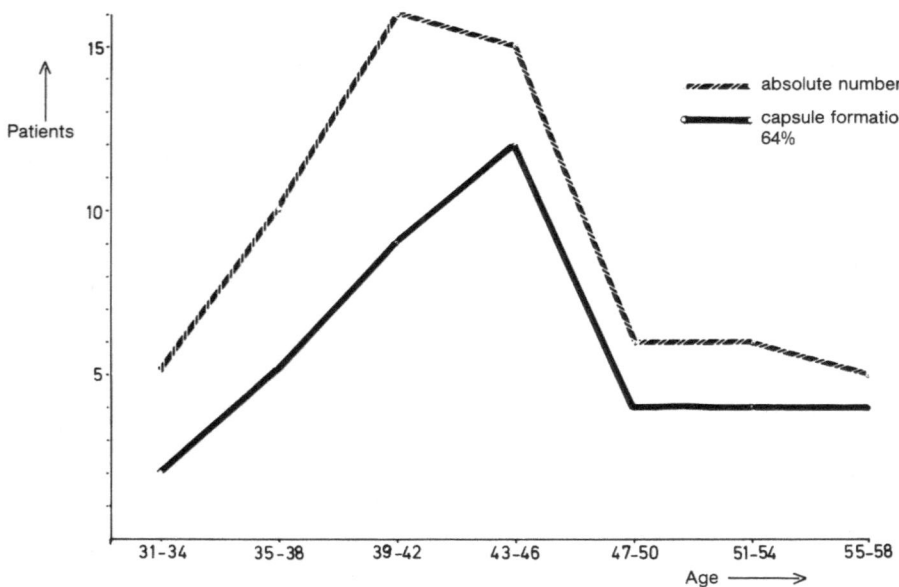

Fig. 23.1. The most frequent complication after breast reconstruction is capsular contracture, which tends to displace the implant laterally and superiorly. As the implant cannot be lowered by closed capsulotomy, it must be operatively repositioned and the cortisone dose increased to 50 or 100 mg

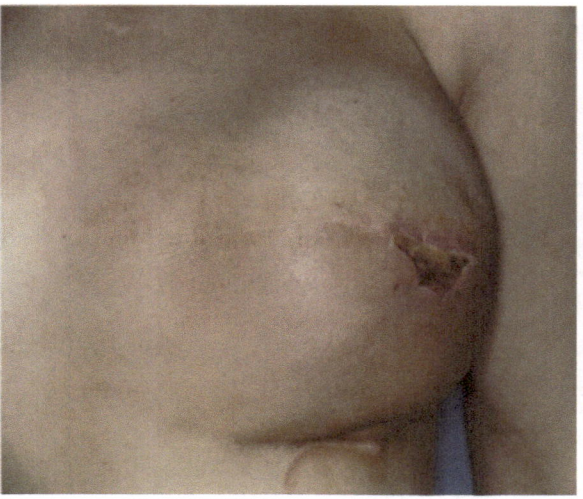

Fig. 23.2. Wound dehiscence can occur after upper abdominal skin advancement if too many sutures were placed on the inframammary crease, restricting blood flow to more cranial tissues. This complication can be managed by secondary excision

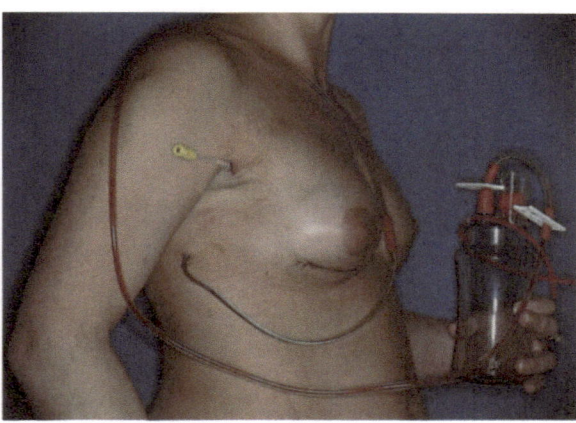

Fig. 23.3. In many cases, infection of the wound cavity can be eradicated with a 6-day regimen of antibiotic irrigations (see Fig. 15.28). Frequently this is followed by constrictive capsule formation, requiring a second operation

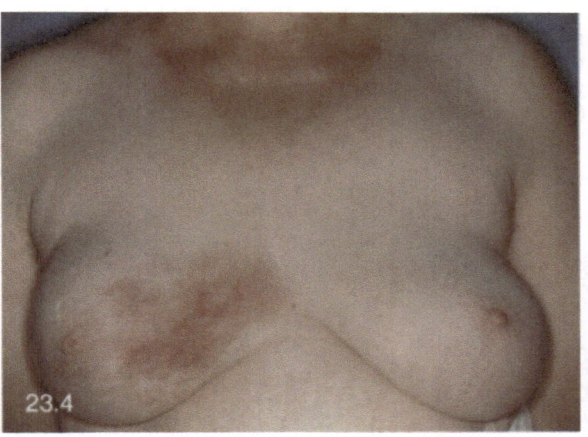

Fig. 23.4. A fulminating infection (e. g., with *Staphylococcus aureus*) necessitates temporary removal of the implant, which is reinserted 2–6 months later

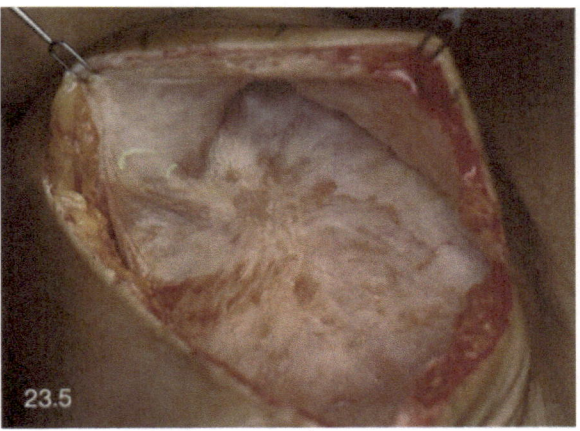

Fig. 23.5. Extremely rare case of a local recurrence behind the implant. This occurred 3 years after a breast reconstruction performed elsewhere

Fig. 23.6. The recurrence was managed by removal of the pectoralis muscle, total capsulectomy, and axillary exploration before reinsertion of the prosthesis. A "second look" at 6 months showed no evidence of disease

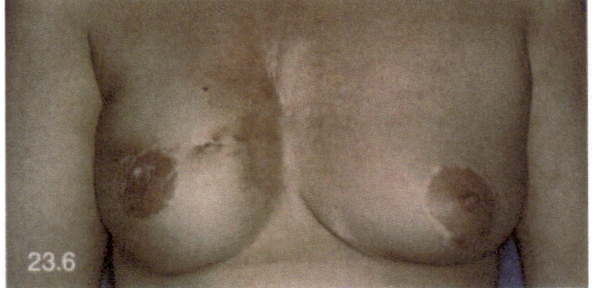

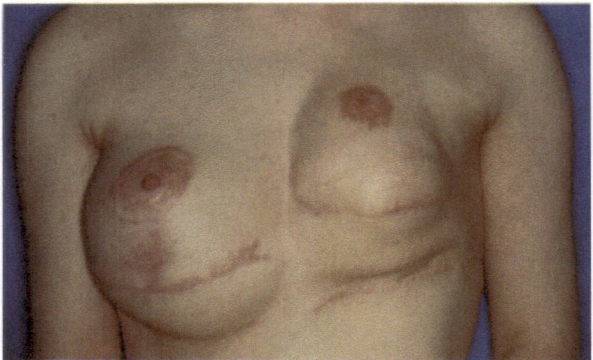

Fig. 23.7. In this young woman with carcinoma of the left breast, almost every mistake was made that a surgeon who "also" does plastic surgery could have made

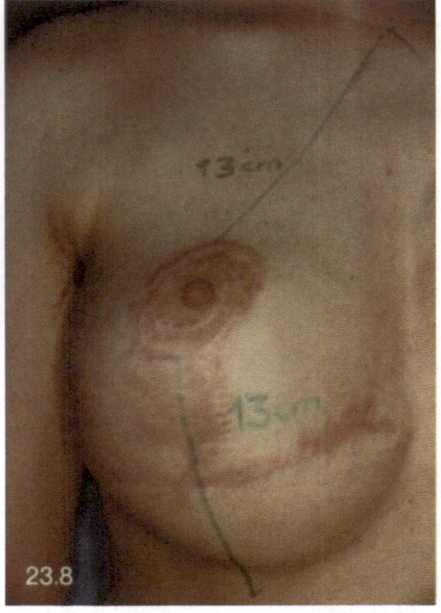

Fig. 23.8. The skin markings for the right reduction mammoplasty were probably drawn with the patient lying down rather than standing. The height of the inframammary line was not considered in determining the level of the nipple-areola but was simply placed 5 cm higher. The glandular tissue inevitably sagged back to its natural level (see Fig. 6.10)

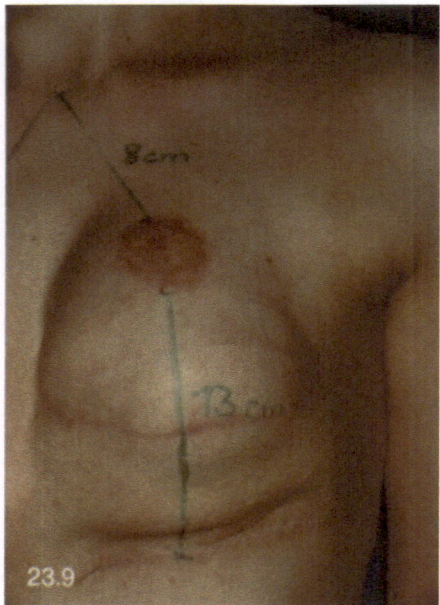

Fig. 23.9. After a silicone implant had been inserted through a separate incision at the level of the original contralateral inframammary line, the nipple height was determined from the opposite nipple, which was displaced superiorly in recumbency. A total of four parallel 10-cm scars (!) are visible over the left breast

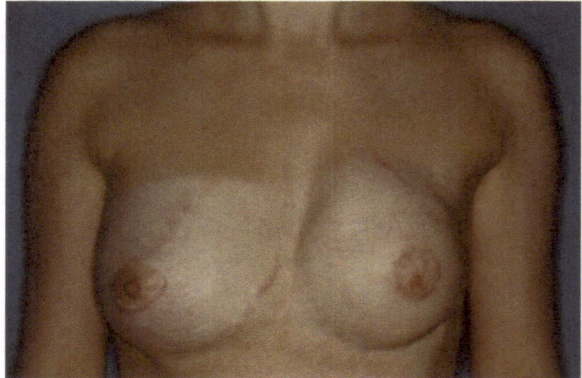

Fig. 23.10. In a first corrective operation, additional glandular tissue was resected from the right breast, and the inframammary crease was restored to its former level while the nipple-areola complex was transposed inferiorly on a glandular pedicle. In addition, the left implant was exchanged for a larger bilumen implant carrying 12 mg of prednisolone. In a second operation the left nipple-areola complex was transplanted and the excisional wound was closed

References

Argenta LC (1984) Reconstruction of the breast by tissue expansion. Clin Plast Surg 11: 257

Berrino P, Campora E, Santi P (1987) Postquadrantectomy breast deformities: Classification and techniques of surgical correction. Plast Reconstr Surg 79: 567–572

Biemer E, Steinau HU (1989) Brustrekonstruktion mit freiem oberen Gluteallappen mit mikrovaskulären Anastomosen. Chirurg 60

Bohmert H (1975) Eine neue Methode zur Rekonstruktion der weiblichen Brust nach radikaler Mastektomie. In: Bohmert H. (Hrsg.) Plastische Chirurgie des Kopf- und Halsbereichs und der weiblichen Brust. Thieme, Stuttgart, S 205–211

Bohmert H (Hrsg) (1982) Brustkrebs und Brustrekonstruktion. Thieme, Stuttgart New York

Bohmert H, Strömbeck JO (1986) Postmastectomy reconstruction. In: Strömbeck JO, Rosato FE (eds) Surgery of the breast. Thieme, Stuttgart New York, pp 243–266

Bostwick J (1983) Aesthetic and reconstructive breast surgery. Mosby, St. Louis

Bostwick J, Vasconez LO, Jurkiewicz MJ (1978) Breast reconstruction after a radical mastectomy. Plast Reconstr Surg 61: 682–693

Brown RG, Vasconez LO, Jurkiewicz MJ (1975) Transverse abdominal flaps and the deep epigastric arcade. Plast Reconstr Surg 55: 416–421

Drever JM (1981) Total breast reconstruction. Ann Plast Surg 7: 54–61

Gillies H (1945) Operative replacement of the mammary prominence. Br J Surg 32: 477–479

Hartrampf CR, Scheflan M, Black PW (1982) Breast reconstruction with a transverse abdominal island flap. Plast Reconstr Surg 69: 216–225

Heidenhain L (1911) Über die Deckung großer Defekte in der Brusthaut. Dtsch Z Chir 108

Höhler H (1977) Reconstruction of the female breast after radical mastectomy. In: Converse JM (ed) Reconstructive plastic surgery. Saunders, Philadelphia, pp 3710–3726

Höhler H, Lemperle G (1975) Der Wiederaufbau der weiblichen Brust nach radikaler Mastektomie. Langenbecks Arch Klin Chir 339: 756 Abstr

Kleinschmidt O (1924) Über Mamma-Plastik. Zentralbl Chir 51: 488–493

Lampe HJ, Lemperle G, Exner K (1985) Der Hautexpander. Technik und Klinik. Chirurg 56: 773–778

Lejour M (1982) Reconstruction of the breast with a contralateral epigastric rectus myocutaneous flap. Chir Plast 6: 181

Lejour M, De Mey A (1983) Experience with 33 epigastric rectus flaps in breast reconstruction. Handchirurgie 15: 257–260

Lemperle G (1982) Verschiedene Schwenk- und Verschiebeplastiken in der rekonstruktiven Brustchirurgie. In: Bohmert H (Hrsg) Brustkrebs und Brustrekonstruktion. Thieme, Stuttgart New York, pp 161–168

Lemperle G, Jäger K (1980) Die Indikation zum Wiederaufbau der weiblichen Brust nach radikaler Mastektomie. Zentralbl Chirurgie 105: 220–226

Lemperle G, Exner K (1989) Der Brustwiederaufbau mithilfe der Oberbauch-Verschiebeplastik. Chirurg 60: 616–617

Lemperle G, Exner K, Nievergelt J (1987) Hauterhaltende Mastektomie beim kleinen Mammacarcinom. Freiburger Chirurgengespräche 19: 42–50

Lemperle G, Exner K, Nievergelt J, Lampe H (1989) Comparison between the abdominal advancement flap and tissue expansion. In: Bohmert H, Leis HP, Jackson IT (eds) Breast cancer – conservative and reconstructive surgery. Thieme, Stuttgart, pp 246–252

Lewis JR (1970) Reconstruction of the breast. Minerva Chir 25: 1223

Lewis JR jun (1971) Reconstruction of the breasts. Surg Clin North Am 51: 429–440

Lewis JR (1979) Use of a sliding flap from the abdomen to provide cover in breast reconstructions. Plast Reconstr Surg 64: 491–497

Maxwell GP, McGibbon BM, Hoopes JE (1979) Vascular considerations in the use of a latissimus dorsi myocutaneous flap after a mastectomy with an axillary dissection. Plast Reconstr Surg 64: 771–780

Mühlbauer W, Ramatschi P (1989) Brustrekonstruktion mit dem vertikalen (VRAM) und transversalen (TRAM) musculocutanen Rectus abdominis-Lappen. Chirurg 60

Mühlbauer W, Olbrisch RR (1977) The latissimus dorsi myocutaneous flap for breast reconstruction. Chir Plast 4: 27

Olbrisch RR, Miericke B, Stolzenberg U von (1989) Brustrekonstruktion mit dem Gewebeexpander. In: Bohmert H (Hrsg) Brustkrebs: Organerhaltung oder Rekonstruktion. Thieme, Stuttgart, S 273

Pennisi VR (1977) Making a definite inframammary fold under a reconstructed breast. Plast Reconstr Surg 60: 523–525

Perrin ER (1976) The use of soluble steroids within inflatable breast prosthesis. Plast Reconstr Surg 57: 163

Radovan C (1982) Breast reconstruction after mastectomy using the temporary expander. Plast Reconstr Surg 69: 195–208

Robbins TH (1979) Rectus abdominis myocutaneous flap for breast reconstruction. Aust N Z J Surg 49: 527–530

Ryan JJ (1982) A lower thoracic advancement flap in breast reconstruction after mastectomy. Plast Reconstr Surg 70: 153–158

Schneider WJ, Hill HL, Brown RG (1977) Latissimus dorsi myocutaneous flap for breast reconstruction. Br J Plast Surg 30: 277–281

Shaw WW (1983) Breast reconstruction by superior gluteal microvascular free flaps without silicone implants. Plast Reconstr Surg 72: 490

Snyderman RK, Guthrie RH (1971) Reconstruction of the female breast following radical mastectomy. Plast Reconstr Surg 47: 565–567

Spahn I (1987) Brustrekonstruktion nach Ablatio mammae – eine Nachuntersuchung an 416 Patientinnen. Dissertation, Frankfurt

Spitalny HH, Lemperle G, Radu D (1981) Reconstruction of the breast by advancement of abdominal skin. Chir Plastica 6: 87–93

Spitalny HH, Lemperle G (1978) Brustwiederaufbau mit der Oberbauch-Verschiebeplastik. Videothek der Dt. Gesellschaft für Chirurgie, Braun-Dexon, Spangenberg

Tansini I (1906) Sopra il mio nuovo processo di amputazione della mammella. Gaz Med Itali 57: 141

Vasconez LO, Psillakis J, Johnson-Giebeik R (1983) Breast reconstruction with contralateral rectus abdominis myocutaneous flap. Plast Reconstr Surg 71: 668–675

Woods JE (1986) Breast reconstruction: Current state of art. Mayo Clin Proc 61: 579–585

Part F

Nipple-Areola Reconstruction

Like reconstruction of the breast mound itself, reconstruction of the nipple-areola complex has made significant strides in the last 10 years. While women were content with a "brassiere" breast in the early phase of breast reconstruction (1971 to 1976), today it would be impossible to judge the result of a breast and nipple-areola reconstruction in the clothed condition. Although many women claim that they can do without a nipple-areola complex prior to reconstruction, we find that 86% of our patients ultimately want to have a "complete" breast.

Nearly all techniques of nipple-areola reconstruction will give a satisfactory though less-than-optimum result. Four basic methods are employed:

1. Banking the patient's own nipple-areola in the groin for later replantation.
2. Tattooing of the nipple and areola.
3. Free grafts from the contralateral nipple and areola.
4. Construction of a nipple with local rotating flaps, and construction of an areola from the skin of the inner thigh or upper eyelids.

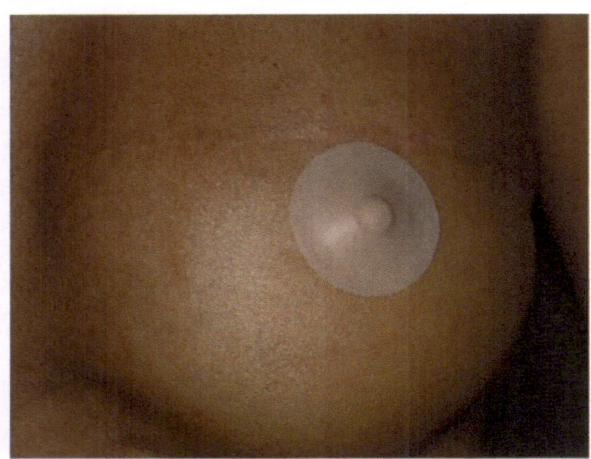

Fig. 24.1. The correct nipple site should not be determined with a measuring tape but by visual estimation. As this may differ from the patient's own concept, we recommend using a "stick-on" nipple-areola that the patient herself can apply before a mirror preoperatively

24 Banking of the Nipple-Areola

To a woman suddenly faced with the amputation of a breast, it can be a great comfort to know that it may be possible to preserve her own nipple and areola ("... then there's still hope!").

Although banking of the nipple-areola was practiced in the early years of breast reconstruction (Millard 1971; Höhler 1977), it has been largely abandoned because three authors (Bouvier 1977; Allison and Howorth 1978; Rose 1980) described the simultaneous transplantation of cancer cells to the groin with subsequent involvement of local lymph nodes. In all cases the base of the graft had been checked only by frozen section before the transfer.

There is still much discrepancy in published reports on the frequency of nipple involvement in breast carcinoma (Anderson et al. 1981; Quinn and Barlow 1980). In our series of patients with primary breast carcinoma, the total incidence of nipple involvement was 8.6% (Walther 1986). In 121 banked nipple-areolas, we did not find a single instance of metastasis in the groin region. On the other hand, the 67% incidence of pigmentation loss after replantation (Fig. 24.5) and the 32% incidence of partial nipple slough suggest that this method should be applied selectively.

Banking the nipple-areola in the lower abdomen (Fig. 24.3) is appropriate only if:

1. the opposite nipple-areola complex is small,
2. the tumor size is no greater than T1,
3. the nipple-areola complex is clinically uninvolved and at least 4 cm from the tumor margin, and
4. the carcinoma is solid but shows no intraductal growth.

Transfer of the graft to the groin should be delayed 2 days until it has been confirmed by examination of paraffin-block sections that the nipple-areola complex is free of tumor involvement (Fig. 24.4).

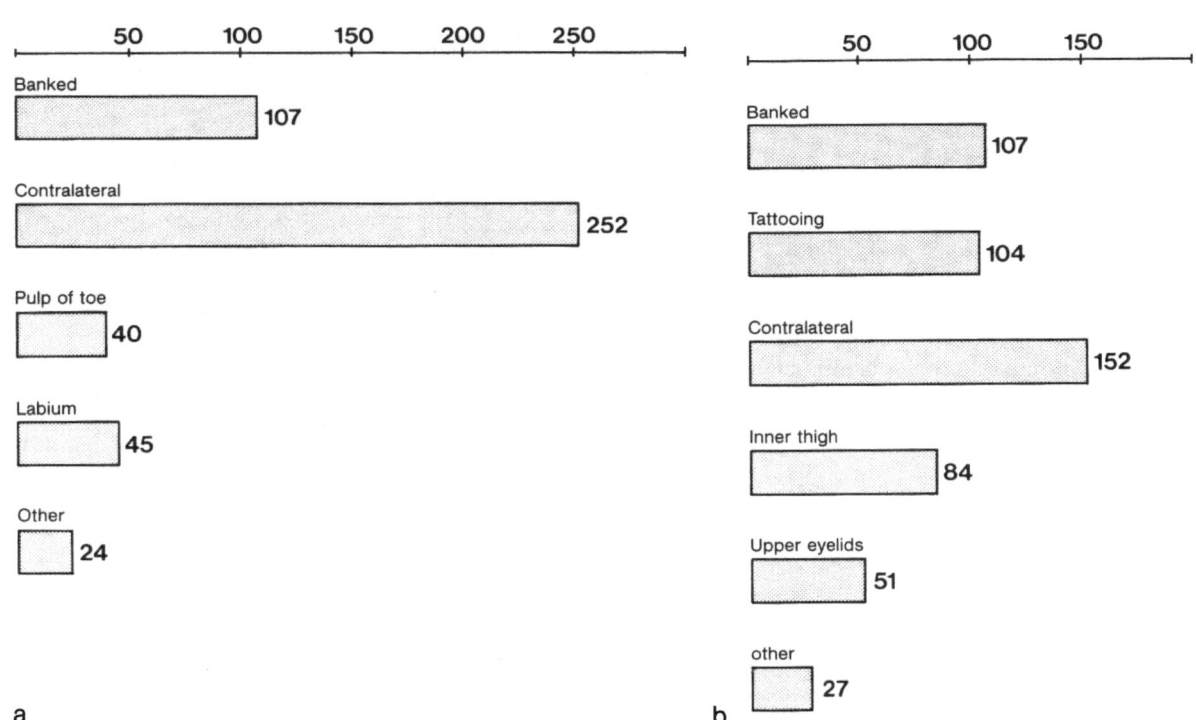

a

b

Fig. 24.2. a Nipple reconstructions performed at St. Markus Hospital, Frankfurt, from 1971 to 1985 ($n = 468$). **b** Areolar reconstructions during the same period ($n = 525$)

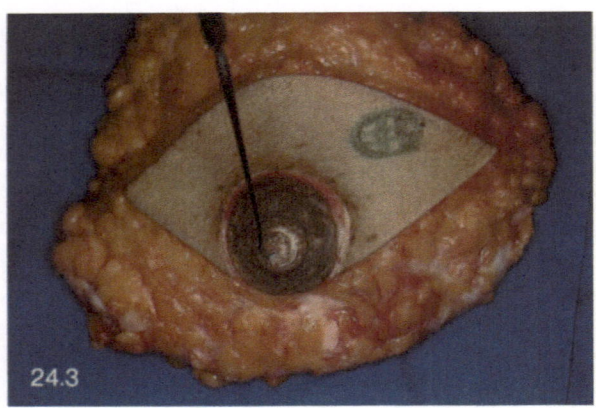

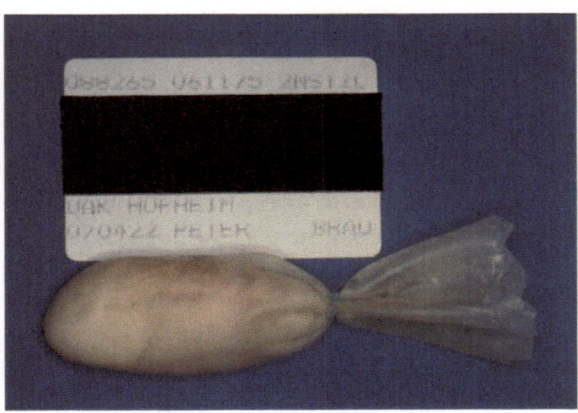

Fig. 24.3. If the tumor is more than 4 cm from the nipple-areola complex, the latter can be banked in the lower abdomen for reuse after histologic examination has confirmed the absence of cancer cells

Fig. 24.4. Pending receipt of the pathology report, the nipple-areola complex, with its raw wound surfaces apposed, is wrapped in a moist compress in a glove finger and stored in a refrigerator. We have successfully stored grafts for up to 12 days using this method

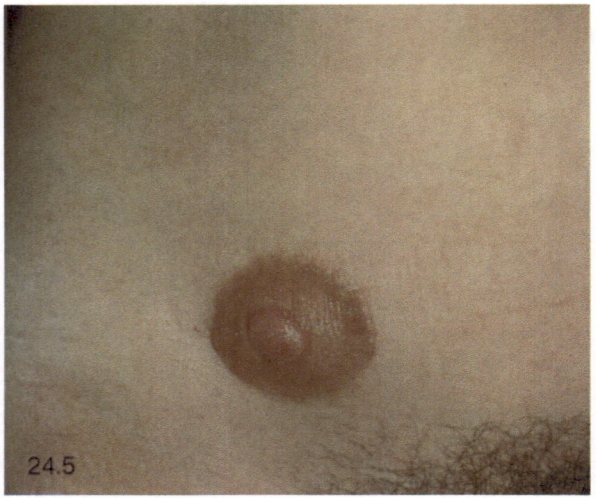

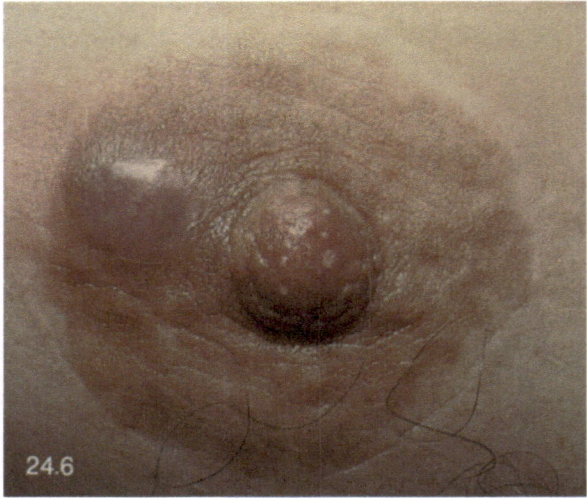

Fig. 24.5. Nipple-areola complex banked in the right lower abdomen

Fig. 24.6. Here an epithelial cyst has developed from the Montgomery glands on an areola still banked in the waiting position. The cyst is treated by incision and drainage. We have found no local recurrences in any of our 121 banked nipple-areola grafts, which in any case would have been detected promptly by the patient herself

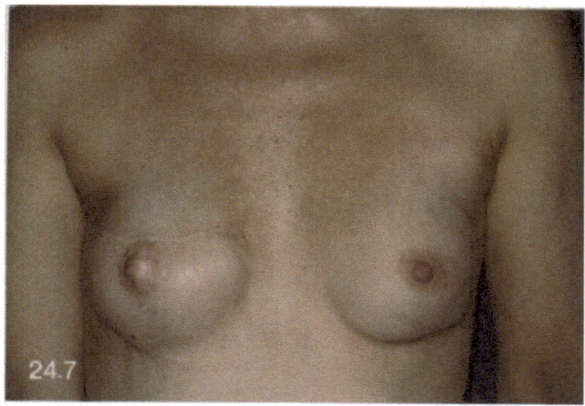

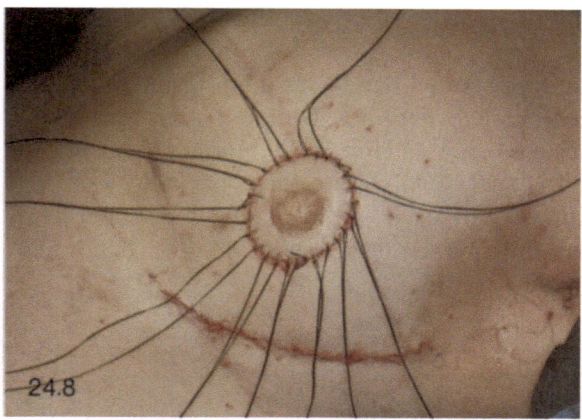

Fig. 24.7. Typical depigmentation of a replanted nipple-areola. The complex is usually healthy, however, and its color is easily restored by tattooing

Fig. 24.8. The nipple-areola complex is removed from the lower abdomen by an elliptical excision and replanted at the most prominent site on the reconstructed breast. The graft, though relatively thick, is devoid of scar tissue

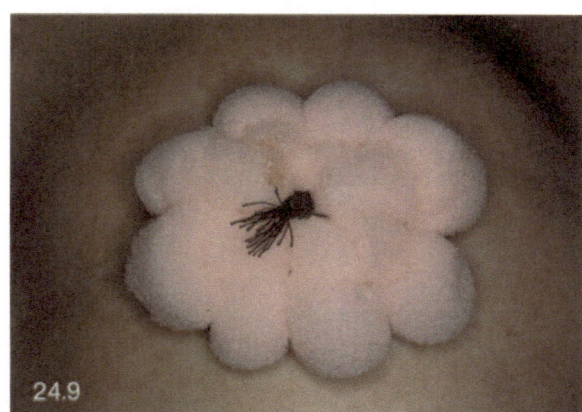

Fig. 24.9. The interrupted sutures are tied over a foam bolus dressing, which covers the replanted complex for 8 days

25 Tattooing of the Areola

In experienced hands, tattooing offers a simple, economical, low-risk method for producing an attractive areola (Fig. 25.7) (Höhler 1977; Becker 1987; Little 1988). Since the color intensity of the tattooed areola needs to be "overcorrected" and can fade markedly over time, the procedure may eventually have to be repeated. Areolar tattooing is a rational alternative to the full-thickness skin graft from the inner thigh, especially when high color intensity is desired. Due to the danger of AIDS transmission, we caution against using a professional tattooer and recommend the use of sterile, disposable heads with a sealed pigment reservoir (Fig. 25.3).

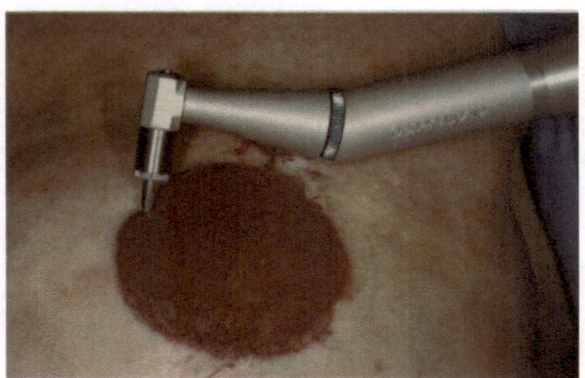

Fig. 25.1. Tattooing of the nipple and areola is a simple and effective procedure but requires some experience due to the need for overcorrection

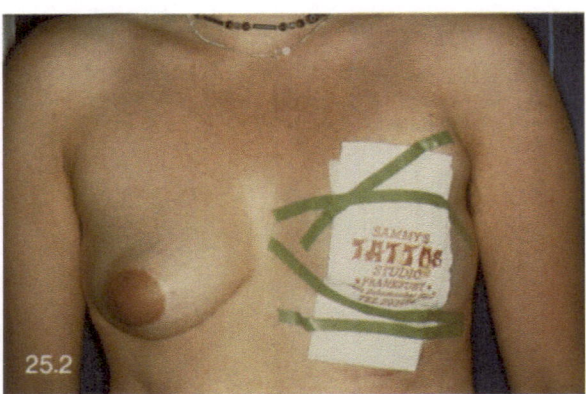

Fig. 25.2. The ointment dressing remains on the breast for 6 days, until the superficial crust has separated

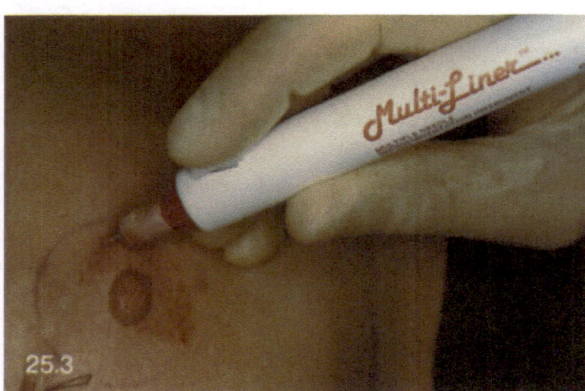

Fig. 25.3. Today, single-use tattooing pencils and motorized tattooing instruments are available which eliminate the risk of AIDS transmission

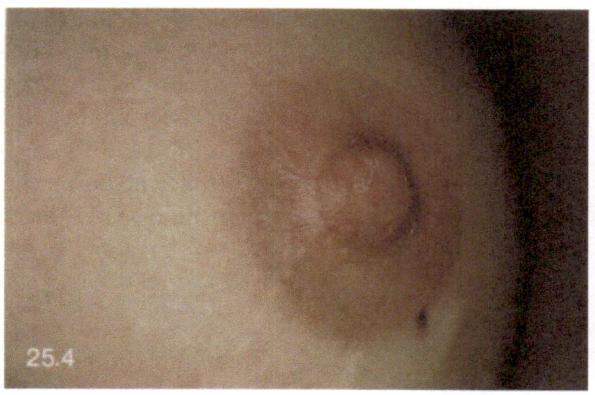

Fig. 25.4. Appearance of the tattooed areola 5 months later

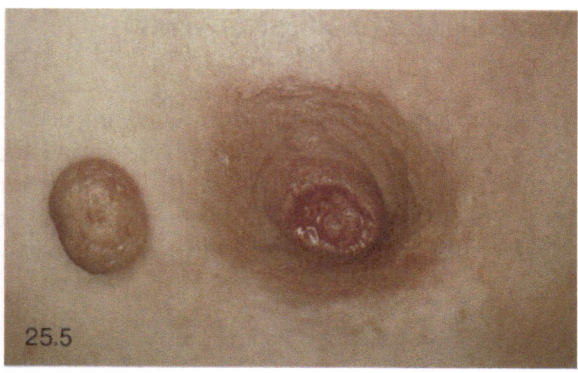

Fig. 25.5. The nipple itself was taken from the contralateral side

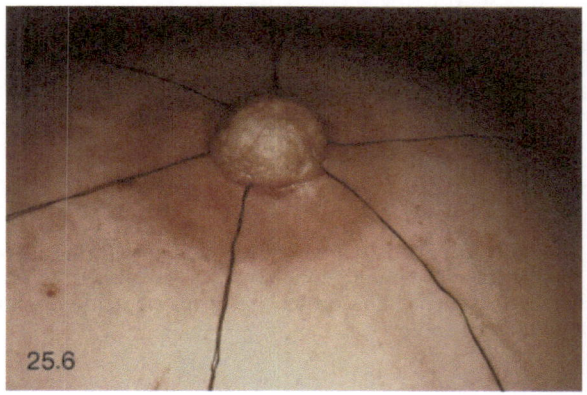

Fig. 25.6. The nipple is held in place with a bolus pressure dressing for 8 days. The areola has been tattooed

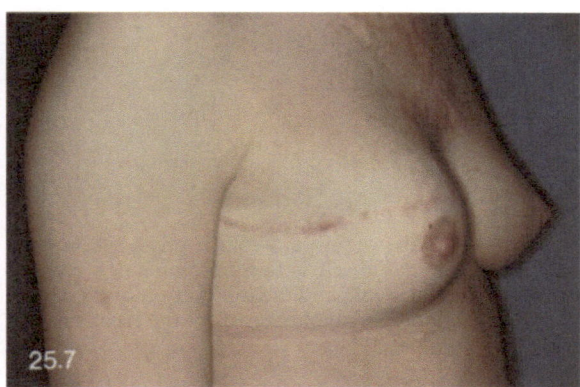

Fig. 25.7. Final result 5 months later

26 Full-Thickness Skin Grafts

1. Areolar graft. The best aesthetic result is provided by skin taken from the opposite nipple and areola. If the areolar diameter is greater than 5 cm and mastopexy is also required, at least a 1.5-cm wide circumferential strip will be available for harvesting when the areola is transposed (Fig. 26.1). The tissue is harvested as a full-thickness graft in one or perhaps two concentric strips (never as a spiral!) and is pressed against the deepithelized bed for 1 week with a bolus dressing. In hundreds of areolas reconstructed by this method, we have seen no instances of partial graft loss.

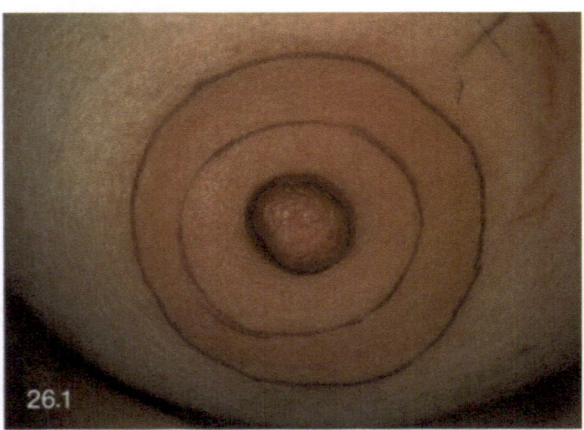

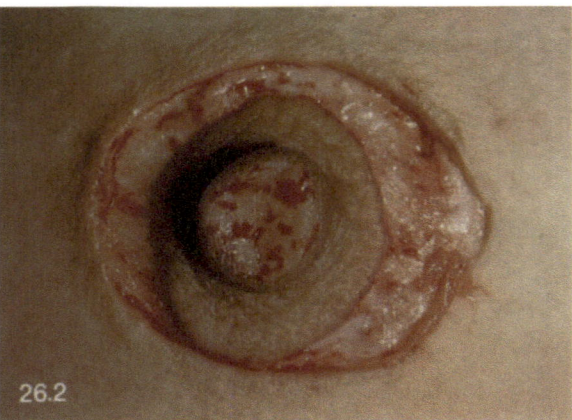

Fig. 26.1. When the opposite areola is greater than 4 cm in diameter and the nipple is fairly prominent, a concentric strip from the areola and the top portion of the nipple can be used to make a nipple-areola for the reconstructed side

Fig. 26.2. The areolar donor site is closed with intradermal sutures. The nipple donor site may be allowed to epithelize, or, depending on its size, it may be closed with two crossed sutures

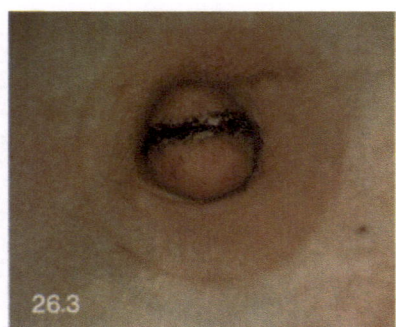

Fig. 26.3. If the nipple is very broad and flat, the lower half can be harvested as a wedge-shaped graft. The inferior edge of the remaining half is turned down and sutured

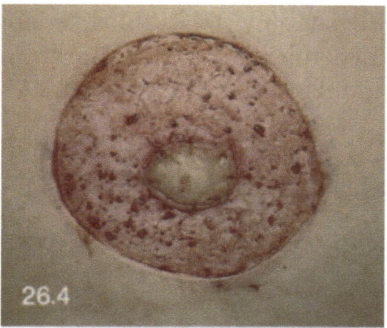

Fig. 26.4. The nipple is sutured to the deepithelized bed

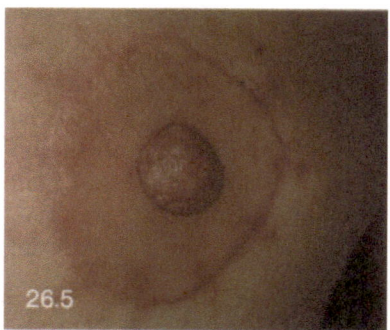

Fig. 26.5. Appearance after healing of the concentric areolar graft and shared nipple

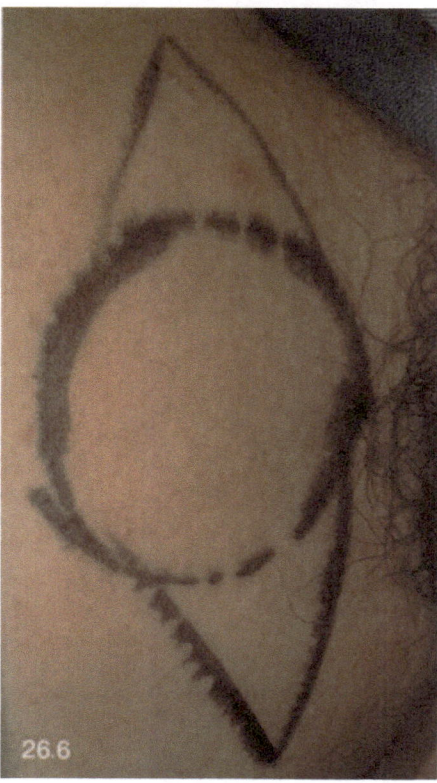

2. From the inner thigh. If the opposite areola is small, the donor site of second choice is the upper inner thigh (Fig. 26.6). This area near the vulva has a naturally heavy pigmentation and, like all free skin grafts, will increase its pigmentation several-fold when transplanted.

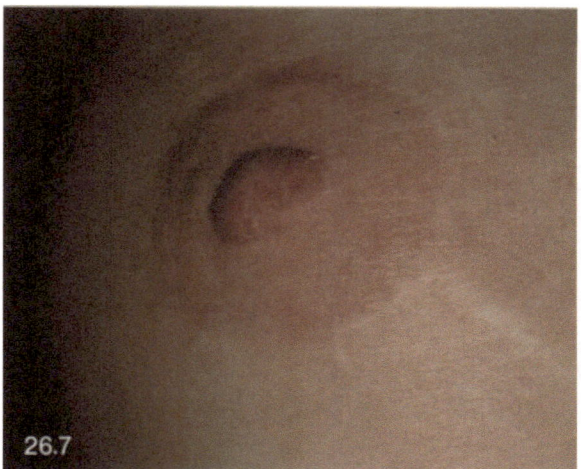

Fig. 26.6. The donor site of second choice is the hairless inner surface of the upper thigh, which often is naturally hyperpigmented. This pigmentation increases further when the skin is transplanted as a full-thickness graft

Fig. 26.7. This areola reconstructed from the upper inner thigh has healed well, as has the nipple, which was constructed from the top of the opposite nipple

3. From the upper eyelids. In patients over 40 years of age who have generally little pigment and correspondingly light-colored areolae, skin can be harvested from the upper eyelids instead of the thigh (Juri et al. 1984) for areolar reconstruction (Fig. 26.8). These grafts are easier to obtain than thigh grafts, leave unobtrusive scars, and can even widen the visual field without additional cost (Fig. 26.8). Remarkably, this skin does not show the usual hyperpigmentation response to transplantation, and its texture closely resembles that of the areolar skin (Fig. 26.10).

If the eyelids are unsuitable as donor sites, pink skin also may be harvested from the postauricular area.

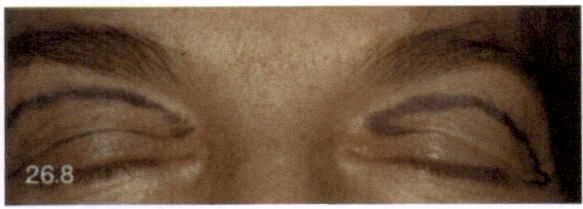

Fig. 26.8. In women over 40 years of age, 1.5-cm strips of skin can be taken from the upper eyelids in the form of a blepharoplasty

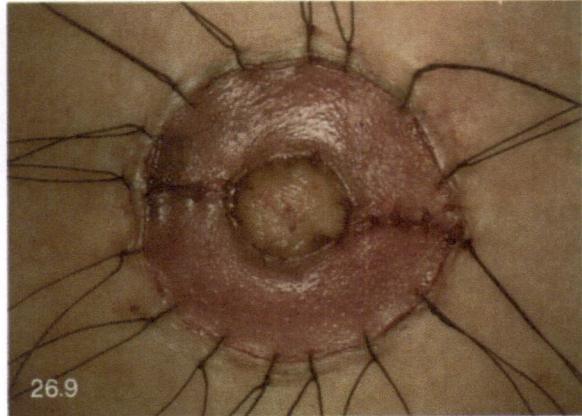

Fig. 26.9. The full-thickness skin grafts are attached and secured with a bolus pressure dressing for 8 days

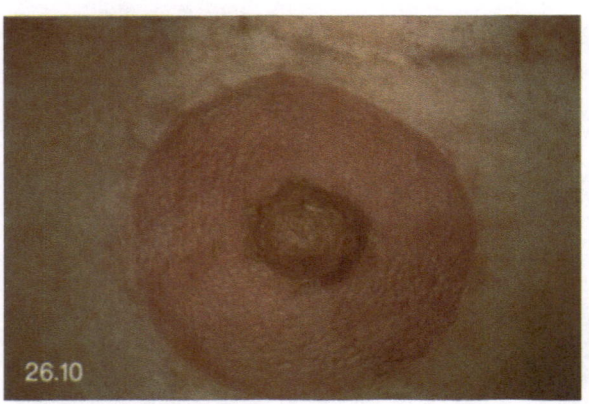

Fig. 26.10. Appearance 4 months later. The palpebral skin provides an especially good areolar replacement in light-skinned individuals with little nipple-areola pigmentation

4. Contralateral nipple. A nipple can be constructed from the upper 5 mm of the opposite nipple, or, if the latter is broad and flat, the lower half may be excised (Fig. 26.3). In the latter method the donor site is closed with simple interrupted sutures, while the truncated nipple may be allowed to epithelize from the milk ducts.

In patients with a dark nipple-areola, a wedge from the labium minus may occasionally be used for nipple reconstruction (Fig. 26.11). Wedges from the earlobe (Fig. 26.12), toe pulp (Fig. 26.13), or tongue have not proven satisfactory.

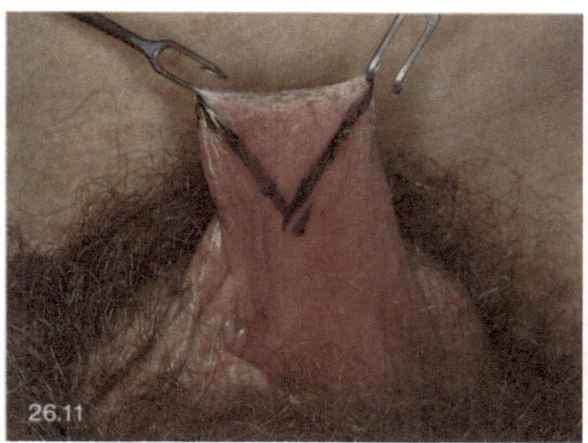

Fig. 26.11. If the opposite nipple is too flat, other donor sites must be considered. In patients with heavy pigmentation, the nipple-areola complex can be reconstructed with a full-thickness graft from the labia minora, although this tissue has a much softer consistency than a normal nipple

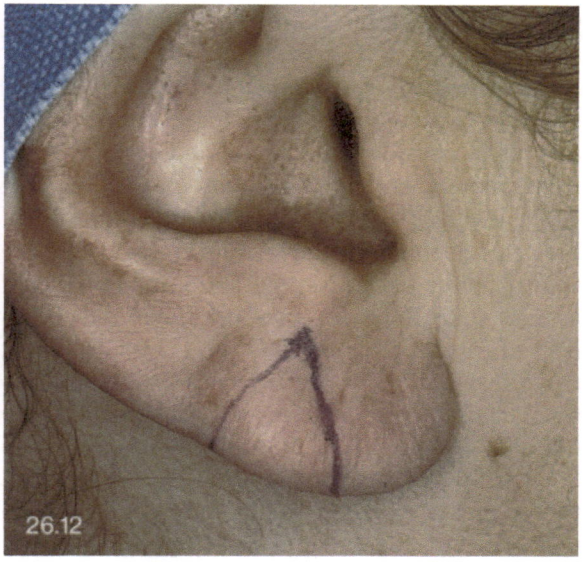

Fig. 26.12. If the opposite nipple-areola is very light, a wedge of earlobe can be used for nipple reconstruction. However, this wedge will remain as pale as the auricular skin for the patient's lifetime and therefore is not recommended

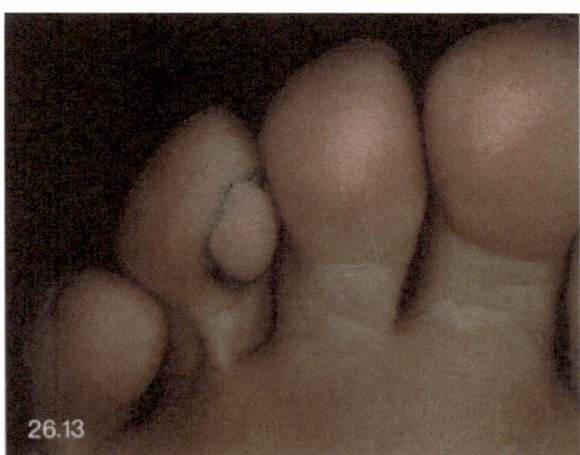

Fig. 26.13. The same applies to a wedge from the pulp of the toe. While this graft offers favorable projection, it remains pale and may require tattooing

5. Secondary nipple augmentation. If the subcutaneous tissue was too thin for the primary construction of a projecting nipple with local flaps, a deepithelized full-thickness dermal graft from the rima ani can be interposed between the full-thickness skin graft and dermis at a later time, making sure that the undermined area is no larger than 5 mm in diameter.

In addition, the new generation of microspheres for soft-tissue augmentation (Bioplastique, Arteplast) may offer a new alternative for nipple augmentation (Lemperle 1990).

6. Increasing the nipple-areola projection. The normal nipple-areola has a thin, loose dermis which affords a physiological protuberance in the upright posture and in the lateral projection. But when the nipple-areola area of a reconstructed breast is deepithelized, the thicker dermis of the skin from the back or upper abdomen remains in a tense state. Therefore, we incise the deepithelized area circumferentially and radially in a cloverleaf pattern if the thickness of the subcutaneous tissue permits. This incision creates three dermal islands (Fig. 27.5) and loosens the whole area, so that part of the full-thickness skin graft now apposes to the dermal islands and part directly to the subcutaneous fat. Depending on individual scar formation, this provides a good loosening effect that gives an adequate nipple projection in some patients (Fig. 27.8); in others no discernable improvement is achieved. In patients with thin subcutaneous tissue, this projection can be augmented at a later stage by dividing the dermis circumferentially and inserting a small, 1.5-ml silicone prosthesis (the type used in mice to study fibrous contracture) between the capsule and subcutaneous tissue.

7. Positioning of the nipple-areola complex. It is best to determine the prospective nipple site not with a measuring tape or ruler but by *visual estimation* while viewing the standing patient from a distance of 2 m. For a given fixation of the silicone prosthesis, there will be only one optimum nipple site, i. e., on the greatest projection of the breast mound. Only after the new nipple site has been established should one determine the nipple position on the opposite breast that will require mastopexy. During selection of the nipple sites, the patient must know that the reduced breast will sag again over time while the reconstructed breast will not. Even after a period of years, the healthy nipple-areola can be raised to the level of the reconstructed nipple-areola by means of a supraareolar skin excision (see Fig. 3.12).

27 Local Rotating Flaps

Many procedures have been devised for nipple reconstruction (Little 1984) that have not proven successful in our hands and therefore are not included in this text. Methods that involve pulling the nipple forward do not afford a permanent projection because of the high skin tension that exists over the most prominent portion of the breast.

On the other hand, the local flap procedure described by Hartrampf and Culbertson in 1984 is more effective when a deepithelized rotating flap is used and the donor site is closed with permanent intradermal sutures. As this closure distorts the outer border of the areola, that area must be deepithelized!

We have developed another technique using a Maltese cross (Figs. 27.1–27.3) or "Mercedes star" (Figs. 27.4–27.6) in which 3 or 4 deepithelized flaps are swung toward the center and fixed with simple interrupted sutures. It is our experience that a primary full-thickness skin graft survives poorly over these rotated flaps. Therefore this graft should not be applied until granulation has commenced, i. e., after 6–8 days. Until then the graft (e. g., from the inner thigh) can be stored in a refrigerator at 4° C.

In 1988, Little introduced his "skate" technique; a very reliable, constant flap for nipple reconstruction. He also recommended tattooing of the areola and new nipple.

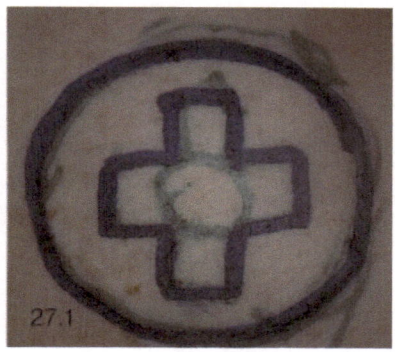

Fig. 27.1. A relatively small nipple can be constructed with four flaps cut in a Maltese cross pattern

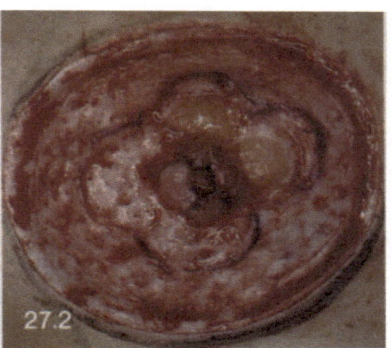

Fig. 27.2. After deepithelization of the recipient area, the flaps are cut from the dermis and sutured together at the center

Fig. 27.3. The nipple constructed from local flaps is often underperfused and makes a precarious substrate for full-thickness skin grafts. But even if superficial sloughing occurs, an adequate prominence usually remains. Alternatively, application of the skin graft may be delayed for 7 days to allow the nipple to recover

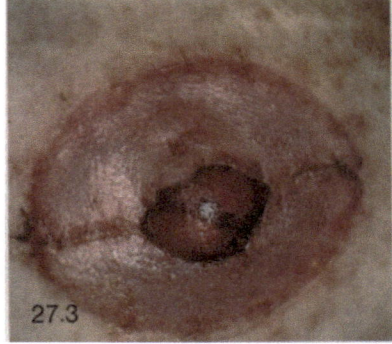

The most simple and reliable way of creating a new nipple – even from scar tissue – is the methode of Anton and Hartrampf (1990) who developed the scale-flap of Little (1988) into a star-flap.

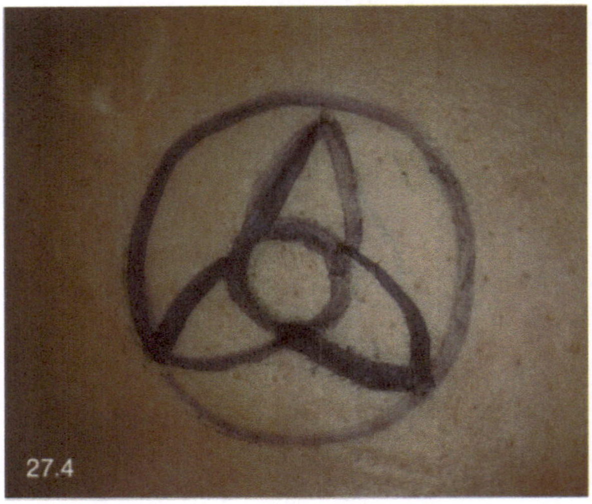

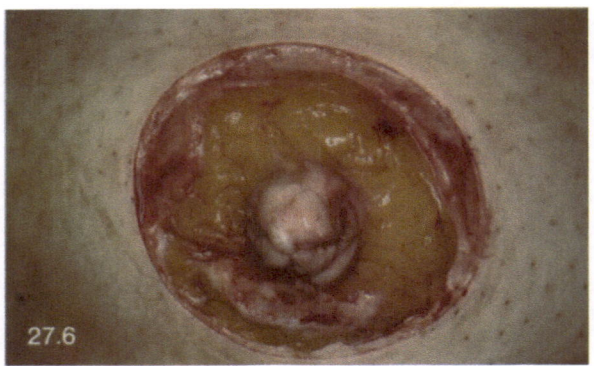

Fig. 27.4. If there is sufficient subcutaneous fat to provide blood flow to the new nipple-areola (e. g., over a latissimus island flap), the nipple can be constructed from flaps cut in a three-pointed "Mercedes star" pattern

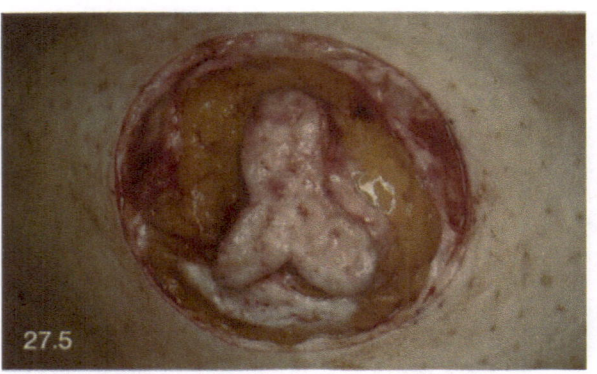

Fig. 27.5. The star is surrounded by a deepithelized dermal bed

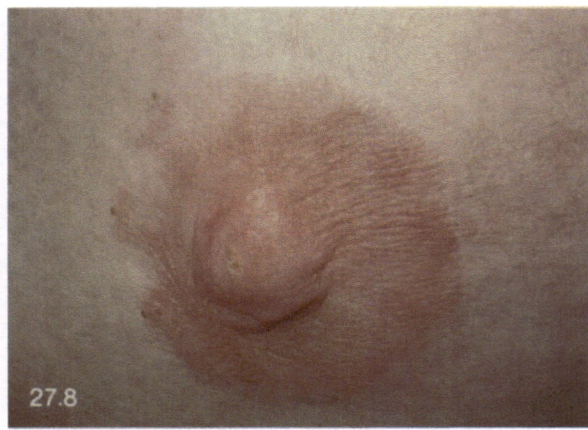

Fig. 27.6. The three arms of the star are elevated toward the center. This simultaneously loosens the subcutaneous fat, causing some protuberance of the areola

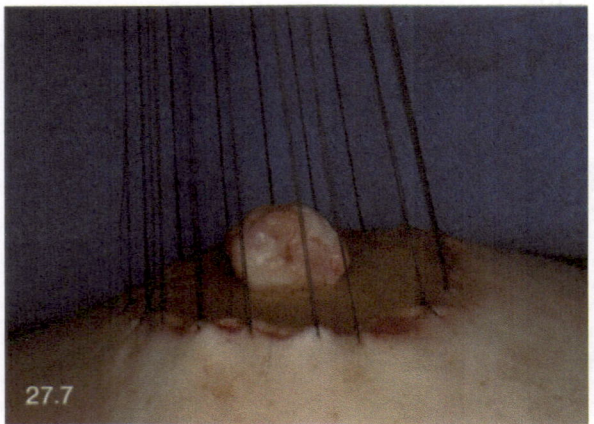

Fig. 27.7. The subcutaneous tissue is covered, and a separate graft is used for coverage of the nipple

Fig. 27.8. Final result 3 months later

References

Adams WM (1949) Labial transplant for correction of loss of the nipple. Plast Reconstr Surg 4: 295–298

Allison AB, Howorth MG (1978) Carcinoma in a nipple preserved for heterotropic auto-implantation. N Engl J Med 298: 1132

Andersen JA, Gram JB, Pallesen RM (1981) Involvement of the nipple and areola in breast cancer, value of clinical findings. Scand J Plast Reconstr Surg 15: 39–42

Anton MA, Hartrampf CR (1990) Nipple reconstruction with the star flap. Plast, Surg. Forum 13: 100–103

Becker H (1986) The use of intradermal tattoo to enhance the final result of nipple-areola reconstruction. Plast Reconstr Surg 77: 673–675

Brent B, Bostwick J (1977) Nipple-areola reconstruction with auricular tissues. Plast Reconstr Surg 60: 353–361

Broadbent TR, Woolf RM, Metz PS (1977) Restoring the mammary areola by a skin graft from the upper inner thigh. Br J Plast Surg 30: 220–222

Bouvier B (1977) Problems in breast reconstruction. Med J Aust 1: 937

Gruber RP (1979) Nipple-areola reconstruction: a review of techniques. Clin Plast Surg 6: 71–83

Hartrampf CR, Culbertson JH (1984) A dermal-fat flap for nipple reconstruction. Plast Reconstr Surg 73: 982–986

Höhler H (1977) Reconstruction of the female breast after radical mastectomy. In: Converse JM (ed) Reconstructive Plastic Surgery Saunders, Philadelphia pp 3710–3726

Juri J et al. (1984) Mammary reconstruction. Rev Argent Cir 46: 6

Kroll SS (1987) Nipple reconstruction with a double opposite tab flap. Plast Surg Forum 10: 219–220

Lemperle G, Exner K (1989) Verschiedene Möglichkeiten der Mamillenrekonstruktion. Chirurg 60: 627–630

Lemperle G, Ott H, Charrier U et al (1991) PMMA-microspheres for intradermal implantation. Ann Plast Surg 26: 57–63

Lemperle G, Spitalny HH (1980) Reconstruction of the nipple and areola after radical mastectomy. Acta Chir Belg 79: 155–157

Little JW (1984) Nipple-areola reconstruction. Clin Plast Surg 11: 351–364

Little JW (1988) Nipple-areola reconstruction. In: Bostwick J (Ed) Perspectives in Plastic Surgery. Quality Medical Publishing, St. Louis

Millard DR, Devine J Jun, Warren WD (1971) Breast reconstruction: A plea for saving the uninvolved nipple. Am J Surg 122: 763

Muruci D, Jose J, Nogueira LR (1978) Reconstruction of the nipple-areola complex. Plast Reconstr Surg 61: 558

Quinn RH, Barlow JF (1981) Involvement of the nipple and areola by carcinoma of the breast. Arch Surg 116: 1139–1140

Rose JH (1980) Carcinoma in a transplantated nipple. Arch Surg 116: 1131

Spilker G, Oeking G, Biemer E (1986) Eine neue Technik der Mamillenrekonstruktion. Handchirurgie 18: 19

Spitalny HH, Lemperle G (1982) Techniken zur Wiederherstellung der Brustwarze. In: Bohmert H (Hrsg) Brustkrebs und Brustrekonstruktion. Thieme, Stuttgart New York, S 190

Part G

Radiotherapy

28 Radiation Damage

An effective course of radiotherapy will inevitably cause injury to the skin, subcutaneous tissue, periosteum, and perhaps even the lung. The tragedy of chronic radiation injuries is that they are progressive throughout the patient's lifetime, i.e., ulcerations and radiocarcinomas can develop even several decades following the exposure. The typical picture of radiodermatitis with vascular congestion, fibrosis, and superficial ulceration was most commonly seen in the era of X-irradiation. While gamma radiation (e.g., cobalt-60) is less damaging to the skin, it can sometimes lead to severe induration and fibrosis of the subcutaneous tissue and muscle, while the fast electrons emitted by high-voltage sources (betatron, linear accelerators) often incite fibrosis at deeper levels such as the lung or mediastinum.

Unfortunately, radiation damage cannot be predicted in a given case, because the radiologist cannot yet take into account all individual parameters such as the responses of the immune

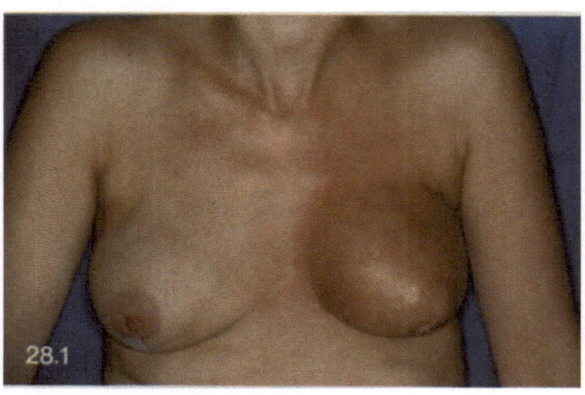

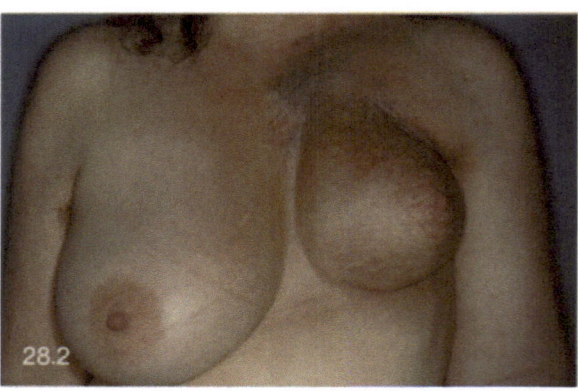

Fig. 28.1. Appearance 2 years after tumorectomy and subsequent irradiation. The left breast is hot, hard, and without sensation. Adjuvant postoperative radiotherapy is controversial and will remain so until the biologic factors that determine individual radiosensitivity can be taken into account when calculating the dose. These patients were all irradiated between 1982 and 1987!

Fig. 28.2. This patient underwent left quadrantectomy and subsequent irradiation. The breast is very hard but is not painful. The patient presented with a suspected tumor recurrence, but this was not confirmed histologically

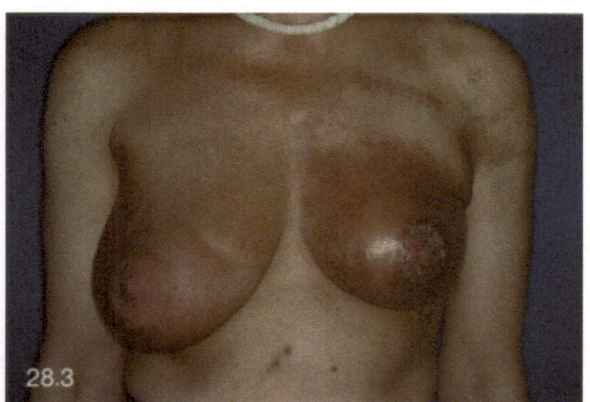

Fig. 28.3. Woman 44 years of age with a small carcinoma in the lower outer quadrant of the left breast, treated by breast-conserving surgery and postoperative radiation. Now the entire breast is involved by recurrent disease

system, skin, and autonomic nervous system, eating and smoking habits, and local factors such as the thickness of the dermis and subcutaneous tissue, local blood flow, darkness or lightness of the complexion, and so forth when calculating the radiation dose.

Patients with severe, chronic radiation injuries commonly report that skin maceration and severe inflammatory skin changes were already apparent during the course of the radiotherapy, but that they "went through it" anyway. Because most patients who require plastic surgery for radiation damage have received prophylactic irradiation, the plastic surgeon tends to take a critical view of adjuvant radiotherapy. Yet there is no question that therapeutic irradiation has an established place in the management of breast carcinoma (e. g., in lymphangiosis and hemangiosis) and in cases where surgical treatment options have been exhausted.

Since radiation damage may be the price to pay for the destruction of a malignant tumor, the plastic surgeon has, in the last decade, developed a musculocutaneous flap – either pedicled or

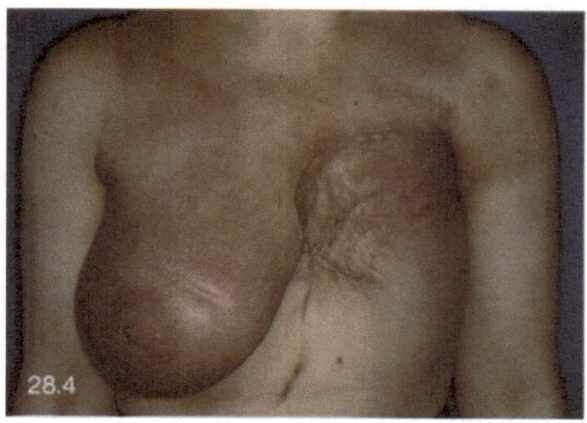

Fig. 28.4. Simple split-thickness skin grafting is advised initially after mastectomy to facilitate evaluation for further local recurrence

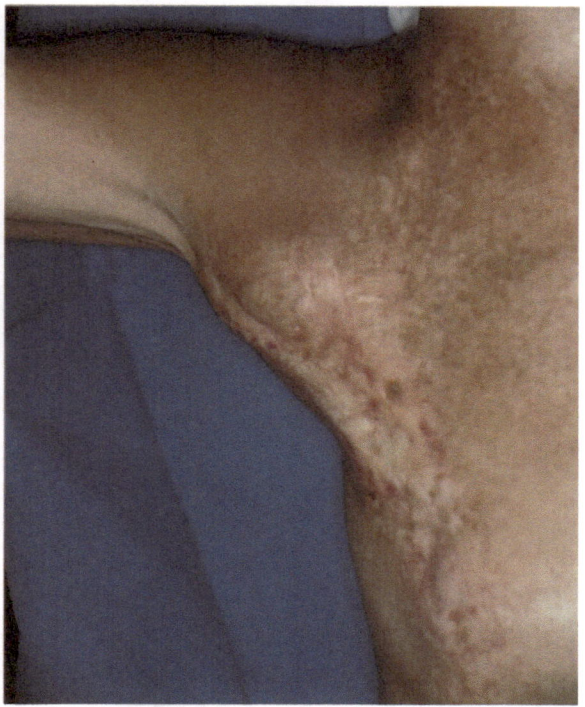

Fig. 28.5. Subcutaneous fibrosis following cobalt irradiation of the axilla. Fortunately this condition did not represent a recurrence of carcinoma

freely transferred using microanastomotic technique – for almost every area of the body. Today there is no longer any basis for the therapeutic nihilism that has persisted among radiologists and surgeons due to previous bad experiences in the treatment of irradiated tissues. To be sure, wound healing is delayed in the irradiated area, which is why free split-thickness and full-thickness skin grafts are very slow to "take" and often leave residual defects. Local rotating flaps are likewise associated with a high complication rate because the skin adjacent to the irradiated area is itself usually damaged, perhaps imperceptibly, by scattered rays. The treatment of choice for all radiation ulcers, therefore, is deep excision followed by reconstruction of the defect with a musculocutaneous flap.

Massive radiation-induced pleural thickening will benefit the patient with a longstanding radiation ulcer on the chest wall by stabilizing the chest in cases where it was necessary to perform a rib resection in that area.

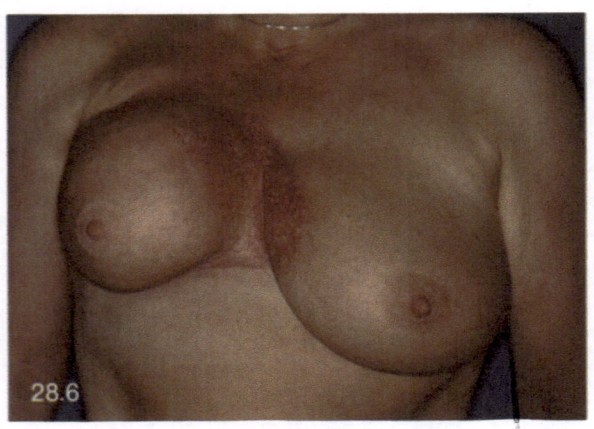

Fig. 28.6. Painful, stony hard breast following tumorectomy and postoperative irradiation

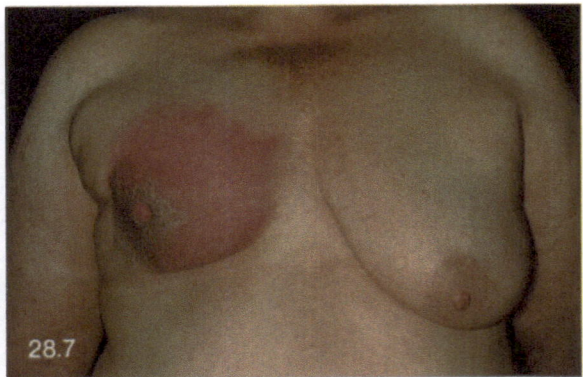

Fig. 28.7. Inflammatory recurrence of carcinoma in an irradiated breast. Two years previously a stage 1 tumor was removed from the right lower quadrant

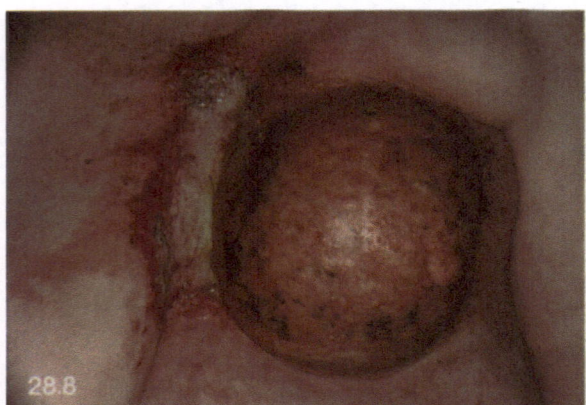

Fig. 28.8. Ulceration in the sternal field and maximum contraction of the left breast 3 years following tumorectomy and irradiation

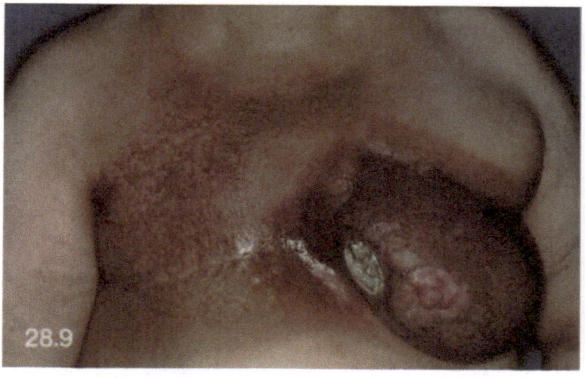

Fig. 28.9. Foul-smelling ulceration 2 years following radiotherapy for recurrent breast carcinoma

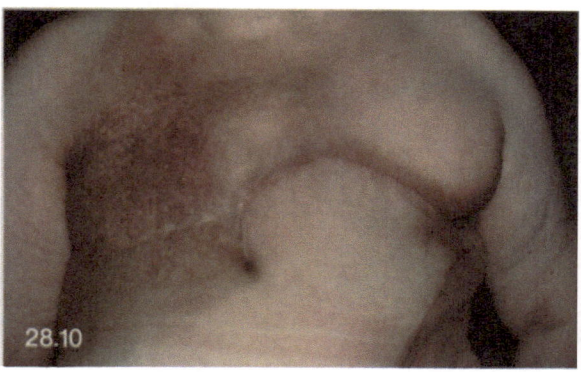

Fig. 28.10. The tumor was widely excised and the defect reconstructed with a broad thoracoepigastric flap

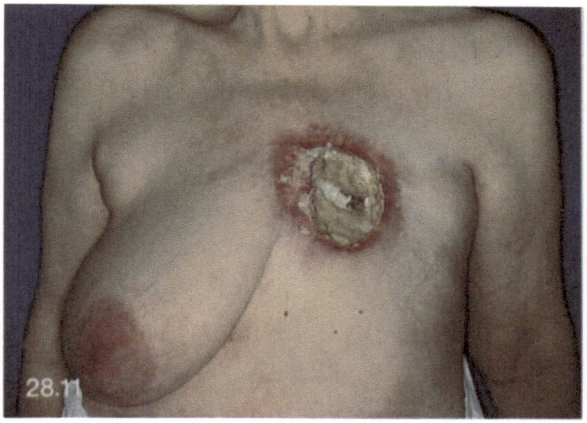

Fig. 28.11. Extremely foul-smelling radiation ulcer of the left chest wall with exposure of the sternum and ribs. The lesion had been treated conservatively for 8 years

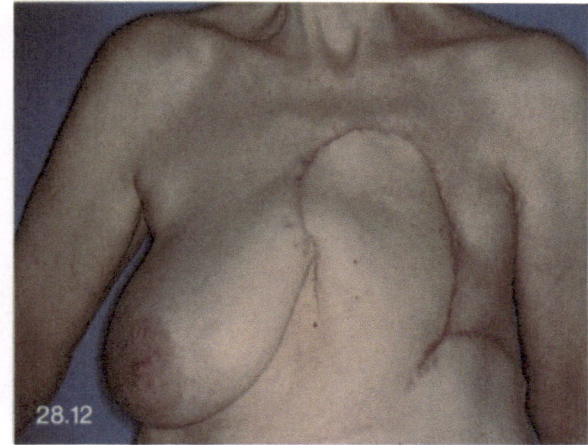

Fig. 28.12. The lesion was widely excised down to the characteristically indurated pleura, and primary reconstruction with a thoracoepigastric flap was performed. We prefer specific antibiotic therapy

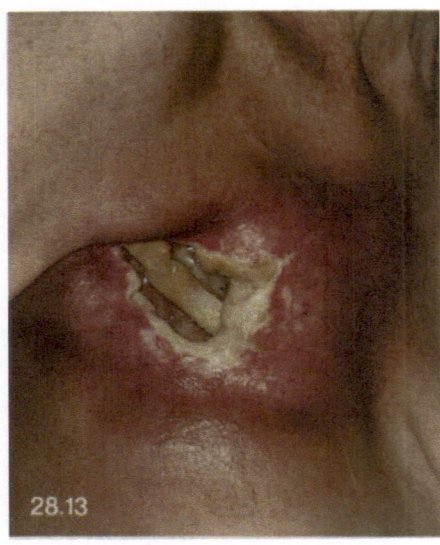

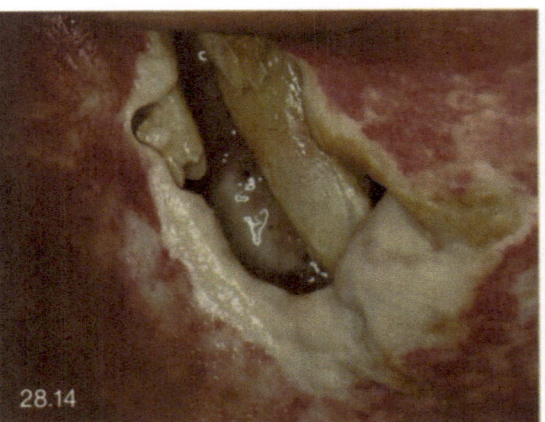

Fig. 28.14. One cup of pus daily had to be drained from the pleural cavity. A TRAM flap is well suited for this type of reconstruction (see Fig. 34.2)

Fig. 28.13. Severe radionecrosis of the right chest wall with massive pleural empyema and induration

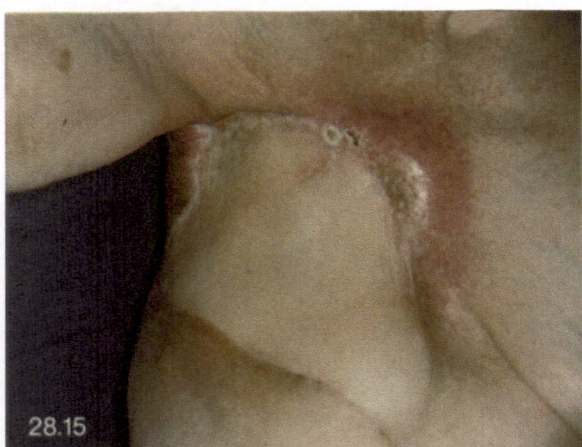

Fig. 28.15. Appearance following the resection of three ribs, suction-irrigation of the pleural cavity, and transposition and healing of a contralateral TRAM flap

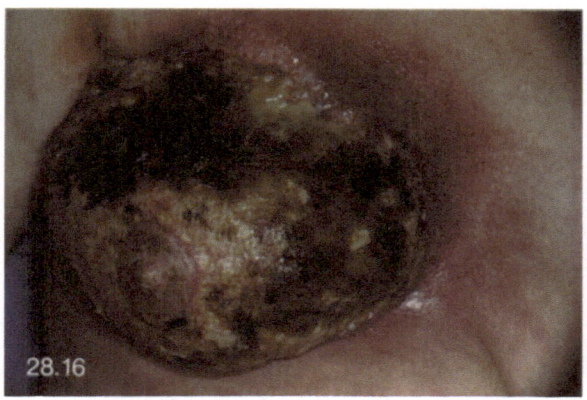

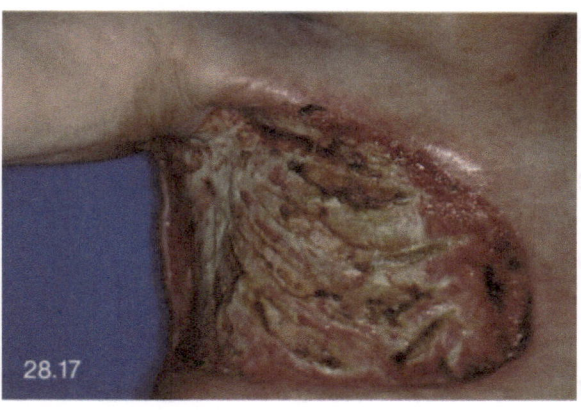

Fig. 28.16. Acute radiation necrosis of the right breast skin with an intact nipple-areola. A fulminating infection developed after a small scar excision, 4 months following prophylactic irradiation of the breast

Fig. 28.17. After mastectomy, reconstruction is delayed for 1 week due to the danger of infection

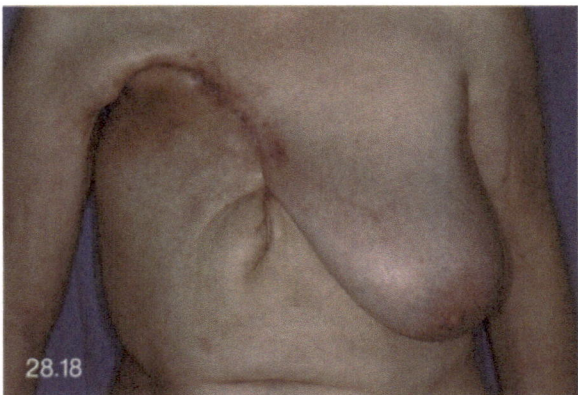

Fig. 28.18. Appearance 3 weeks after reconstruction with a large thoracoepigastric flap moved in two stages

References

Berrino P, Campora E, Santi P (1987) Postquadrantectomy breast deformities: Classification and techniques of surgical correction. Plast Reconstr Surg 79: 567-572

Krebs H (1984) Mammatransposition und Omentumtransposition bei Strahlenfolgen im Thoraxbereich. In: Lemperle G, Koslowski L (Hrsg) Chirurgie der Strahlenfolgen. Urban & Schwarzenberg, München, S 114-118

Lemperle G, Koslowski L (1984) Chirurgie der Strahlenfolgen. Urban & Schwarzenberg, München

Lemperle G, Radu D (1981) Die plastisch-chirurgische Deckung von Strahlenulcera im Thorax- und Beckenbereich. Langenbecks Arch Chir 355: 187-192

Mühlbauer W, Olbrisch RR (1977) The latissimus dorsi myocutaneous flap for breast reconstruction. Chir Plastica 4: 27-34

Olivari N (1984) Deckung von Thoraxwanddefekten mit dem latissimus-dorsi-Lappen. In: Lemperle G, Koslowski L (Hrsg) Chirurgie der Strahlenfolgen. Urban & Schwarzenberg, München, S 91-101

Petit IY (1987) Reconstruction problems in the postradiation contracted breast after conservative treatment. In: Bohmert H (Hrsg) Brustkrebs: Organerhaltung oder Rekonstruktion. Thieme, Stuttgart

Przybilski R, Lemperle G (1984) Verschiedene Schwenklappenplastiken zur Deckung von Strahlenulcera. In: Lemperle G, Koslowski L (Hrsg) Chirurgie der Strahlenfolgen. Urban & Schwarzenberg, München, S 80-90

Radu D, Lemperle G (1984) Der musculocutane Rectuslappen für Strahlenulcera der Brustwand und der Leiste. In: Lemperle G, Koslowski L (Hrsg) Chirurgie der Strahlenfolgen. Urban & Schwarzenberg, München, S 124-130

Scherer E, Busch M, Müller RD (1984) Heilungschancen und Schädigungsmöglichkeiten bei der radiologischen Tumortherapie. In: Lemperle G, Koslowski L (Hrsg) Chirurgie der Strahlenfolgen. Urban & Schwarzenberg, München, S 14-30

Trott KR (1984) Strahlenbiologische Faktoren bei der Entstehung von Strahlenfolgen an der Haut. In: Lemperle G, Koslowski L (Hrsg) Chirurgie der Strahlenfolgen. Urban & Schwarzenberg, München, S 31-35

Part H

Local Recurrence

Indications

In the United States it is widely held that local recurrence is always a manifestation of systemic disease (Willis 1973; Deutsch et al. 1986; Bostwick et al. 1986). As a result, surgery is often withheld for local recurrences, and patients generally are referred to an oncologist.

In Europe, however, it is believed that some local recurrences arise from cells that were implanted into lymph channels before or during mastectomy and for some reason remained there. A retrospective analysis of 80 patients with local recurrence who were referred to us for operative treatment (Enke 1984) showed that systemic spread developed in only 17.5% of the women within 6 years after excision of the local recurrence. Thirty-one percent developed further local disease, giving a figure of 48.5% for the total mortality in all patients with local recurrence, i. e., no higher than the prognosis for the corresponding tumor stages would imply. It is our practice, therefore, to excise a local recurrence if it is at all resectable and then reconstruct the defect using plastic surgical techniques. We also recognize a psychological indication for resection and reconstruction in patients whose tumors have already metastasized to the lung, liver, or bone. Our rationale is that the latter foci are not perceived as such by the patient, whereas a local recurrence persistently reminds the patient of her disease and its grim prognosis.

Of course, all available options in oncology and radiology are applied as an adjunct to the surgical treatment of a local recurrence. Even so, it is common to see a severe local recurrence develop during chemotherapy or 6–12 months after its discontinuation, implying that the chemotherapy often does not kill the cells but merely inhibits or delays their replication.

We see similar effects after prophylactic radiation to the chest wall: Of the 80 patients reviewed, 35 (44%) had received postoperative irradiation. Recurrent tumors seemed to grow faster and more aggressively in the irradiated skin than in nonirradiated areas, which remained free of metastases until the terminal stage. This is why adjuvant radiation was abandoned as a routine therapy in the mid-1970s.

Technique

If a recurrent tumor develops in the skin of a reconstructed breast or following subcutaneous mastectomy, large elliptical skin areas will have to be excised with adequate margins, and the prosthesis may have to be removed. In these cases it is difficult to decide whether to start postoperative radiotherapy or resume chemotherapy.

Because the "radical" removal of a local recurrence often involves the resection of one or more ribs, experience in thoracic surgery is a prerequisite for operations of this kind. However, many patients present with lentil-sized cutaneous or subcutaneous nodules that can be removed together with the underlying muscle and possibly the rib periosteum a 1-cm safety margin. The surgical defect is closed by undermining and mobilizing the wound margins (this can lead to wound-edge necrosis in irradiated tissues!) or by elevating and rotating a local flap.

If the intercostal muscle is involved by tumor, the pleura must be resected along with the adjacent ribs. This offers a good opportunity to palpate the chest wall from the pulmonary side and, if necessary, excise a pleural specimen for histologic study. In many cases, the fluid aspirated from a pleural effusion will not contain demonstrable cancer cells, and the diagnosis must rely on pleural biopsy! Rib and pleural defects are best reconstructed with musculocutaneous flaps, most notably the latissimus dorsi flap, pectoralis island flap, or the vertical or transverse rectus abdominis flap. It is unnecessary to replace the missing pleura, as the muscles will become firmly adherent to the visceral pleura and produce an airtight closure of the chest. It is amazing how many ribs can be removed - even the entire sternum - without provoking clinically apparent or subjective respiratory complaints. Since Freilinger (1983, personal communication) described two adolescents who underwent surgical repair of pectus excavatum and experienced no respiratory problems following total removal of the infected sternum, we have been very liberal in our surgical attack on sternal metastases and try to encompass them broadly (Fig. 32.15) with a resection that may include the heads of the clavicles and cartilaginous portions of the ribs. We found that even hand-sized defects with five missing ribs could be securely closed, primarily with a latissimus dorsi flap (Fig. 32.21), although these patients later demonstrated paradoxical chest motion with no clinical complaints.

Complications

The complications are like those that invariably arise in a certain percentage of patients who un-

dergo a major flap reconstruction. Smokers are at much greater risk than nonsmokers for "tip necrosis" and wound dehiscence and should discontinue their habit as soon as possible once the recommendation for surgery has been made. We demand 4 weeks of strict abstinence preoperatively!

When complications arise it is much better to undertake a prompt second operation than try to achieve second-intention healing. Secondary healing, especially in cancer patients, belongs to the surgery of the nineteenth century.

29 Skin Grafts

In patients with skin metastases, temporary coverage of the excisional defect with a split-thickness skin graft offers the safest approach. Even tiny recurrent growths on the split-thickness graft can be promptly detected and removed. On the other hand, the survival of this graft depends on a good substrate that must not consist of exposed ribs, a poorly perfused indu-

rated pleura, or radiation fibrosis. In borderline cases a meshed skin graft may be tried, or the wound may first be covered with a synthetic material (Epigard) for 8–10 days until initial, deep granulations appear.

If the grafted skin heals well under the pressure of a bolus dressing for 8 days and remains free of recurrent disease for 1 year, the split-thickness graft, often contracted and unsightly, may be excised and the defect resurfaced with a rotating flap.

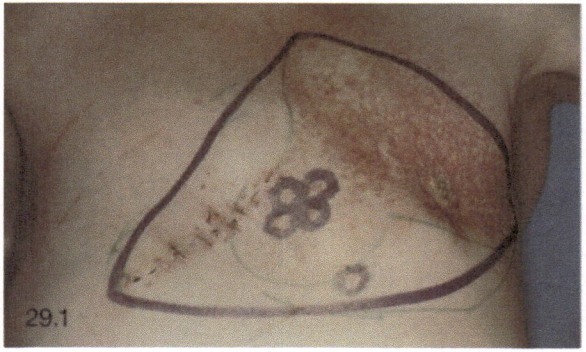

Fig. 29.1. In a patient with multiple skin recurrences – these developed 7 and 9 months after bilateral mastectomy – a large skin area should be excised down to the fascia and grafted with split-thickness skin so that any further recurrence or local metastases can be promptly detected

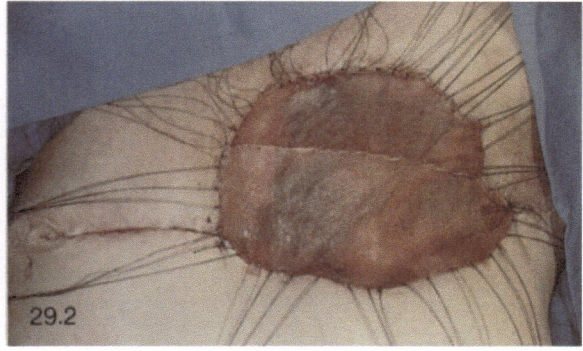

Fig. 29.2. These very aggressive skin recurrences are often associated with a lymphangiosis calling for postoperative radiation 3 weeks after the graft procedure. The reluctance of many radiologists to irradiate split-thickness skin grafts is unfounded. They are no more sensitive than normally perfused skin

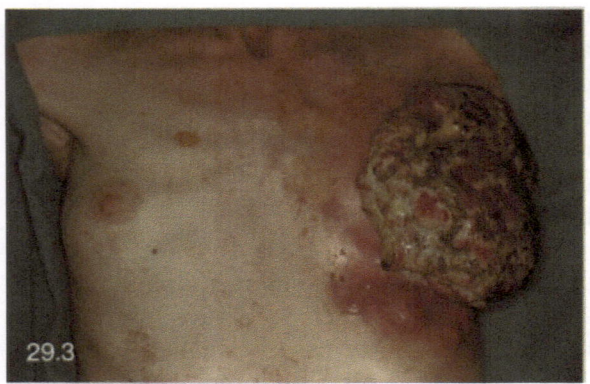

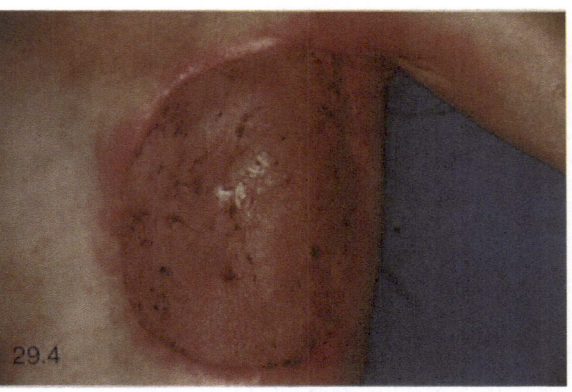

Fig. 29.3. Even with a large ulcerating tumor that can be separated from the ribs, primary split-thickness skin grafting is indicated

Fig. 29.4. The split-thickness skin heals very well over the rib periosteum, provided the latter has not been irradiated

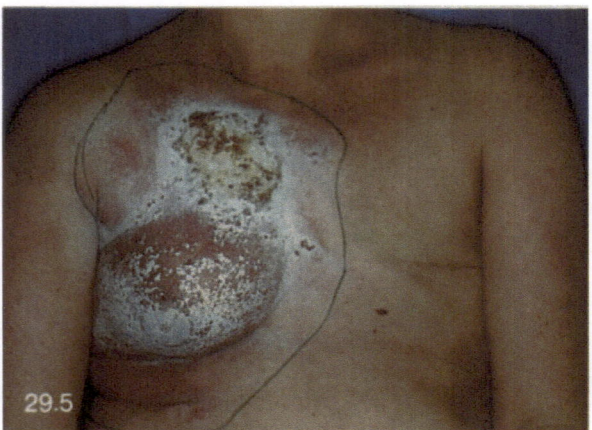

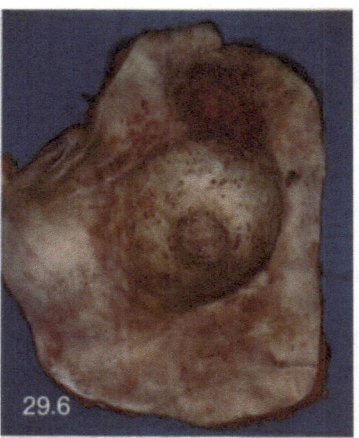

Fig. 29.5. Even on a chest wall that has been irradiated twice, initial split-thickness skin grafting may be attempted

Fig. 29.6. The surgical specimen is easily separated from the chest wall

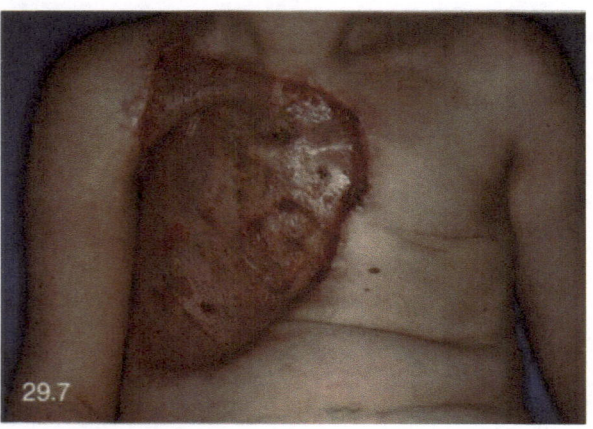

Fig. 29.7. Five weeks later the irradiated area is covered with split-thickness skin

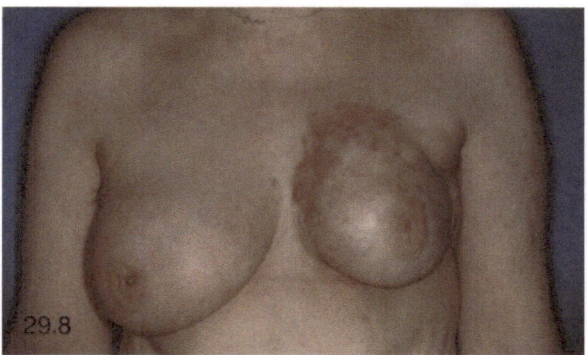

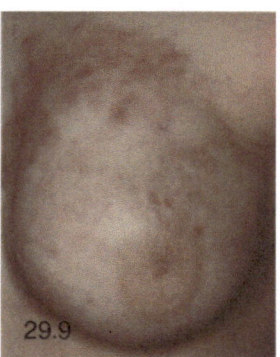

Fig. 29.8. Skin recurrences 2 years after subcutaneous mastectomy and reconstruction with a silicone implant

Fig. 29.9. Considerable local spread developed within 4 months

30 Local Rotating Flaps

A defect that includes exposed ribs, exposed pleural peel, or even an open portion of the chest cavity following the radical excision of a metastatic or recurrent tumor may be covered by transferring a musculocutaneous flap or by rotating a local fasciocutaneous flap. The former method is more complex and should be reserved for deeper defects, while the latter provides a relatively simple, effective solution even in elderly and infirm patients (Figs. 30.9–30.12). Local flap procedures can sometimes be done under local anesthesia.

We routinely use specific, local antibiotic therapy, combined if necessary with suction-irrigation drainage, in all patients with infected defects.

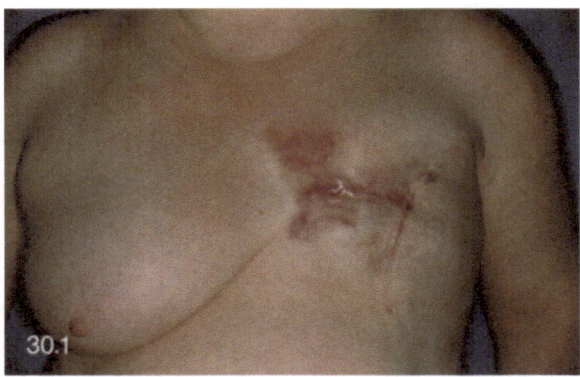

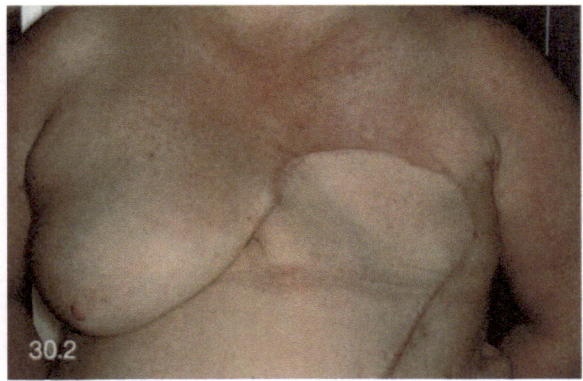

Fig. 30.1. Fulminating local recurrence of breast carcinoma

Fig. 30.2. After wide excision of the tumor and partial resection of the fourth and fifth ribs, the defect is reconstructed with a broad thoracoepigastric flap. The fascial component of the flap is placed directly over the visceral pleura, by which it is "pleuralized," or covered with pleural epithelium

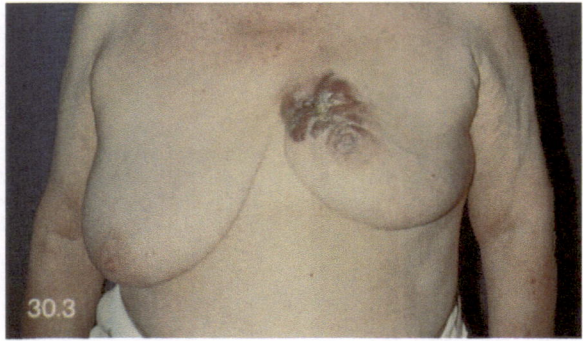

Fig. 30.3. Large breast carcinoma, still quite mobile, which the patient had "successfully" concealed from her family doctor for 8 years

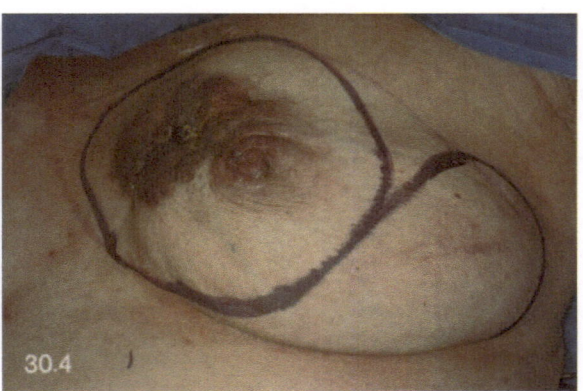

Fig. 30.4. The lateral portion of the breast is used to create a flap that will be rotated into the surgical defect

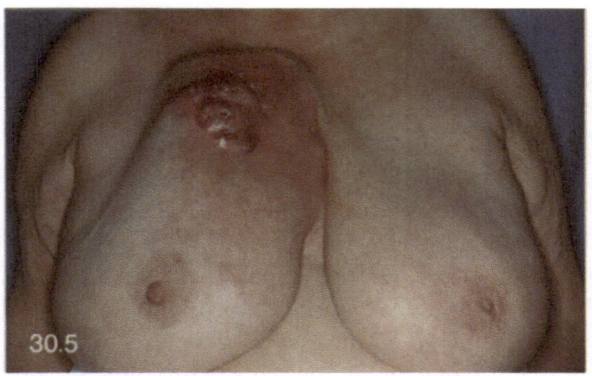

Fig. 30.5. Woman 75 years of age, known to have breast carcinoma for 10 years

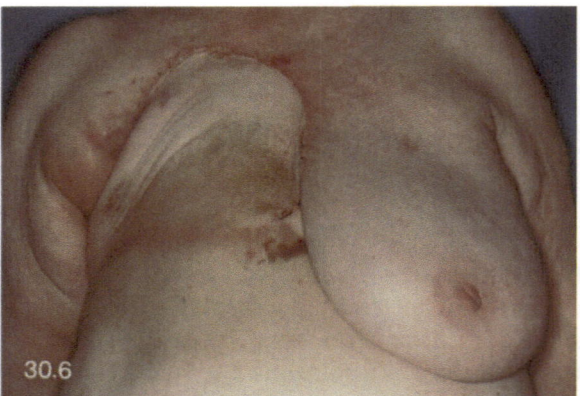

Fig. 30.6. The tumor was widely excised and the defect covered with skin from both lower breast quadrants. There was no demonstrable lymph node involvement

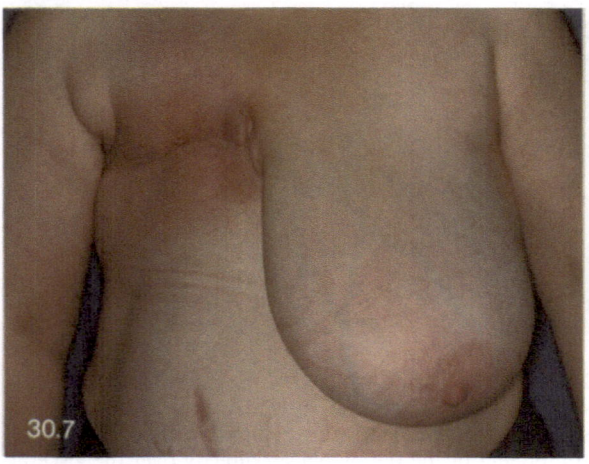

Fig. 30.7. Radiation ulcer with a local recurrence

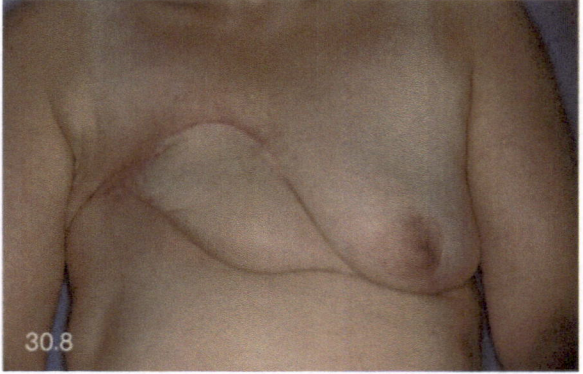

Fig. 30.8. At reduction mammoplasty of the left breast for symmetry, the local recurrence was excised and the defect covered with a skin flap from the breast undersurface based on the inframammary line

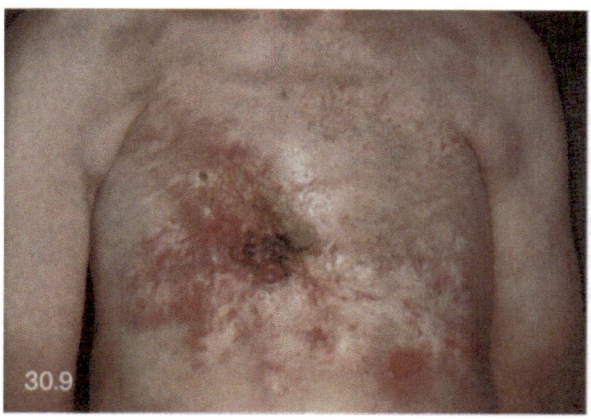

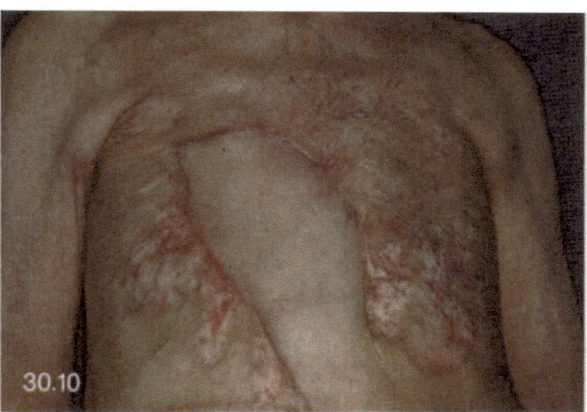

Fig. 30.9. Locally recurrent adenocarcinoma 40 years (!) after bilateral mastectomy and subsequent irradiation of the chest wall

Fig. 30.10. The extirpative defect was covered with a thoracoepigastric flap

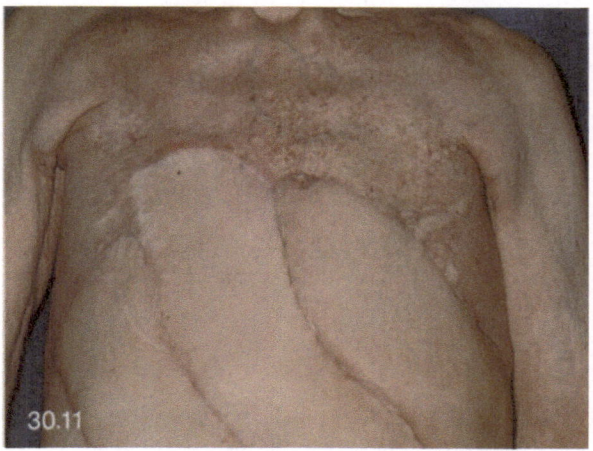

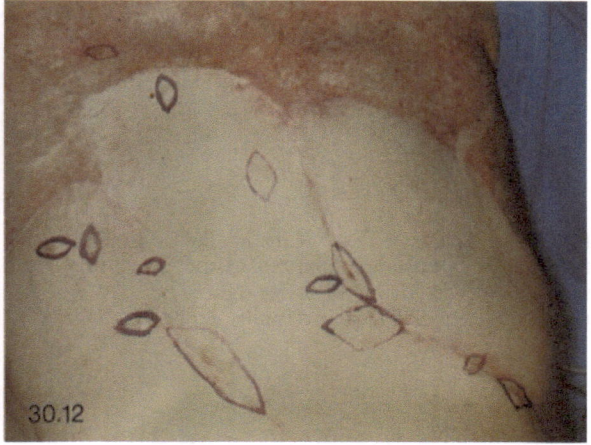

Fig. 30.11. Additional local recurrences at adjacent sites were removed and reconstructed with two local flaps, which could be safely taken from the loose skin of this 82-year-old patient

Fig. 30.12. Additional skin metastases in the abdominal skin used for the reconstruction are individually excised. There is no evidence of distant metastasis

31 Pectoralis Island Flap

The contralateral pectoralis island flap is available for the reconstruction of large sternal defects. To obtain good flap mobility, the muscle must be completely released from its thoracic origins and humeral insertion.

With its excellent vascularity, the pectoralis island flap can reliably cover a palm-sized skin area located half above and half below the inframammary line (Fig. 31.1). Small sternal defects can also be covered with vascularized segments of the pectoralis major that are swung into the cavity in trapdoor fashion. These segments are supplied by perforators from the internal mammary artery.

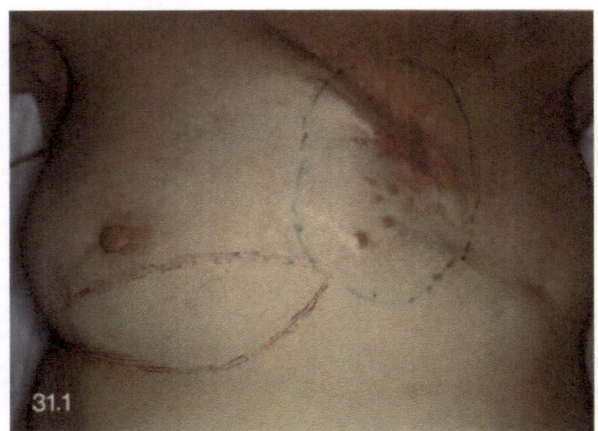

Fig. 31.1. Local recurrence in the medial portion of the irradiated field. Postexcisional reconstruction can be done with a skin ellipse from the lower right breast that receives its blood supply from the pectoralis major muscle

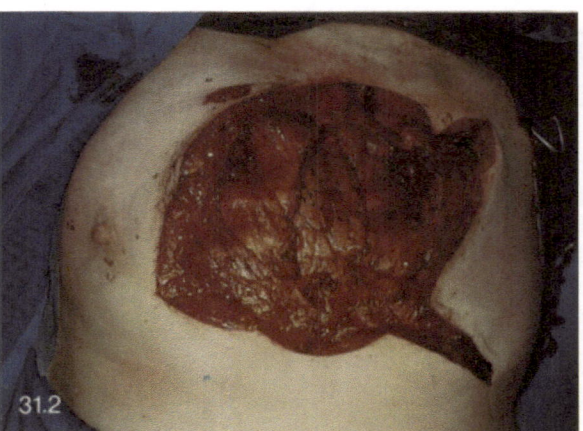

Fig. 31.2. The sternum and portions of adjacent ribs have been resected. Exposed lung tissue is covered directly with the pectoralis major muscle

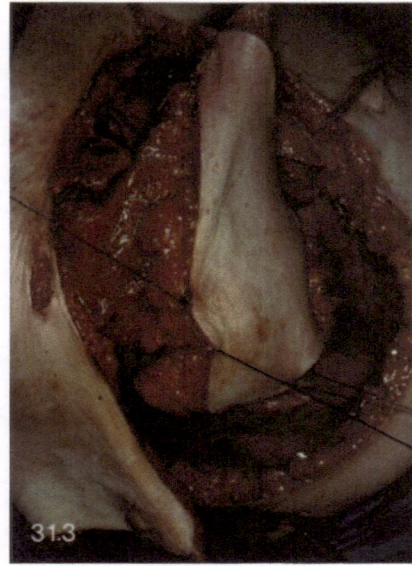

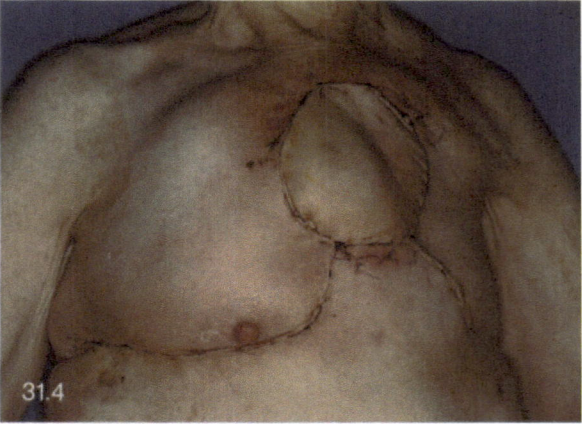

Fig. 31.4. Postoperative result

Fig. 31.3. The pectoralis muscle is completely released from its origins on the ribs and from its humeral insertion

32 Latissimus Island Flap

The latissimus dorsi island flap offers the greatest transfer radius of all the musculocutaneous flaps. Even when its humeral insertion is left intact, the muscle can reach well past the thoracic midline and will cover any sternal defect (Figs. 32.10–32.12). In a patient with cancer en cuirasse, Baudet (1987, personal communication) mobilized all of the dorsal skin on both latissimus dorsi muscles and transposed it anteriorly, achieving good primary flap healing. Olivari (1976) used pedicled latissimus island flaps almost exclusively for the primary repair of very large radiation ulcers and defects following the resection of metastases on the chest. With its excellent blood supply and correspondingly high bacteriostatic potential, the latissimus dorsi is the flap of choice for infected wounds as well. This presumes, of course, that the thoracodorsal artery has not been damaged during the initial operation or by subsequent irradiation!

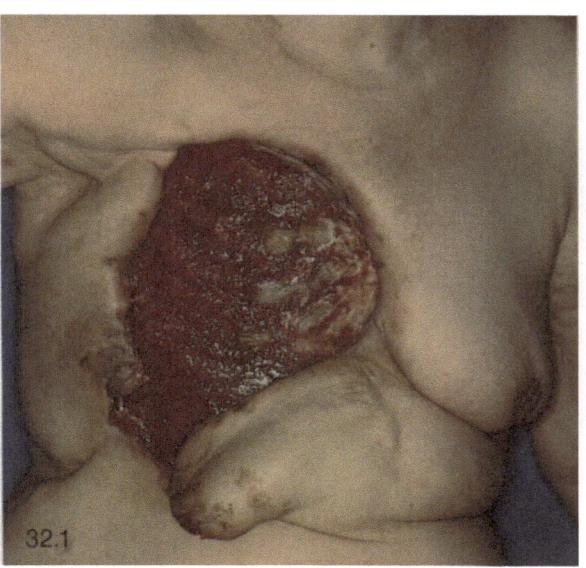

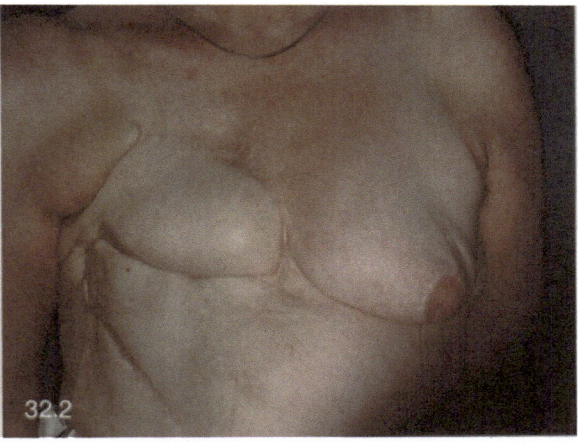

Fig. 32.2. Stable coverage at 6 years

Fig. 32.1. A fulminant periprosthetic infection developed following attempted breast reconstruction with a thoracoepigastric flap. After resection of the partially necrotic ribs, the thoracoepigastric flap was reflected and the defect reconstructed with a latissimus island flap

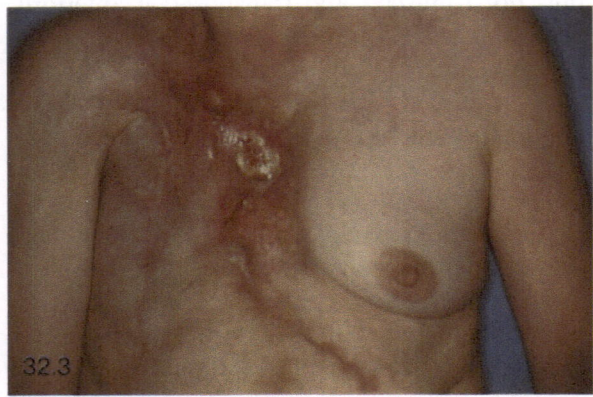

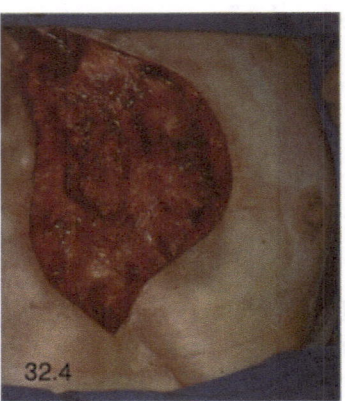

Fig. 32.3. Local recurrence and chronic radiation ulcer previously resurfaced with an omental flap

Fig. 32.4. The entire sternum is excised

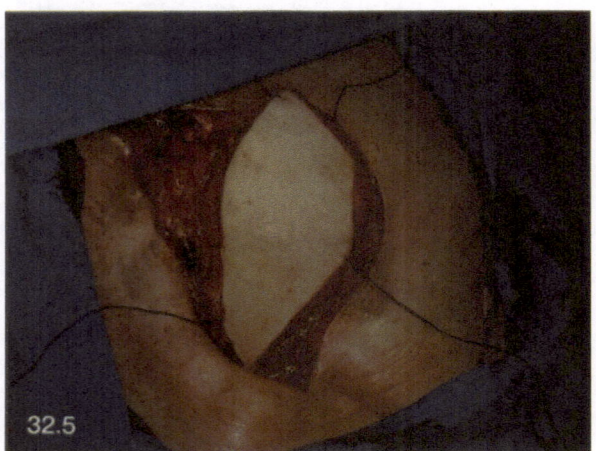

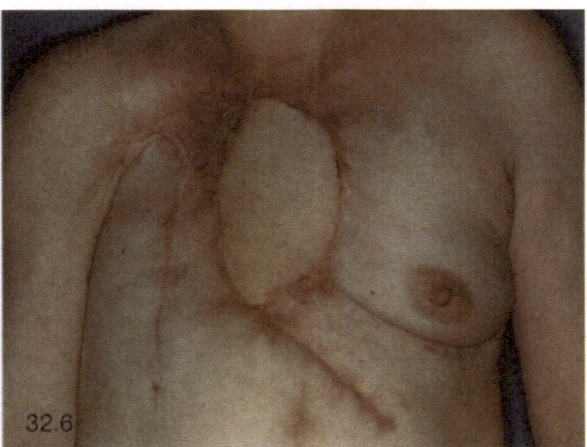

Fig. 32.5. Because there is radiation damage to the right lateral chest wall with inevitable compromise of blood flow to the ipsilateral latissimus dorsi muscle, a latissimus dorsi island flap is mobilized from the healthy left side

Fig. 32.6. The copious blood supply of the latissimus dorsi ensures primary healing with good defect coverage

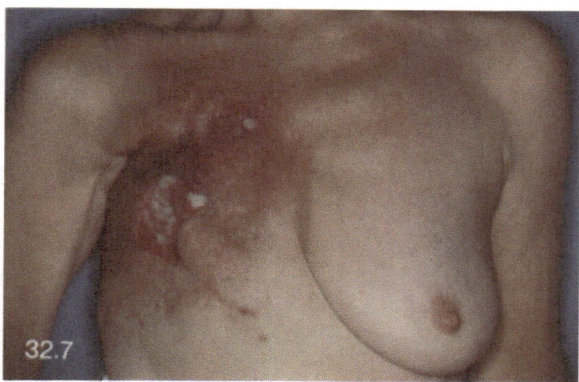

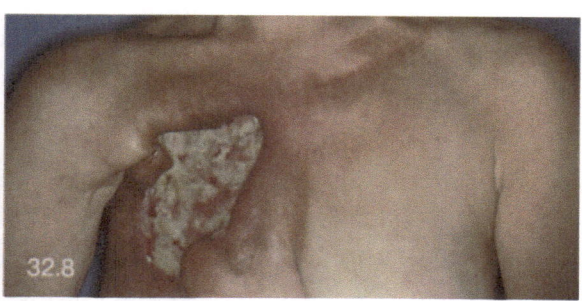

Fig. 32.8. By 6 weeks there was rapidly spreading infection with a palm-sized ulceration. Again, latissimus dorsi circulation was compromised on the right side, so the defect was reconstructed with a *free* latissimus flap using microvascular technique

Fig. 32.7. Radiation-damaged chest wall 4 years after mastectomy and postoperative irradiation. Reconstruction was attempted by the rotation of a thoracoepigastric flap. Because the flap was taken from the irradiated area, partial flap loss ensued

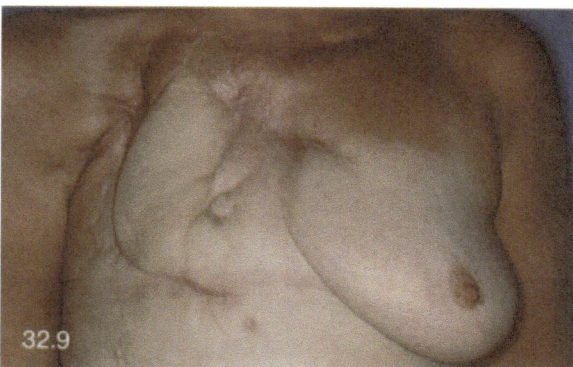

Fig. 32.9. The healed flap has also led to improved circulation in the surrounding radiation-damaged skin

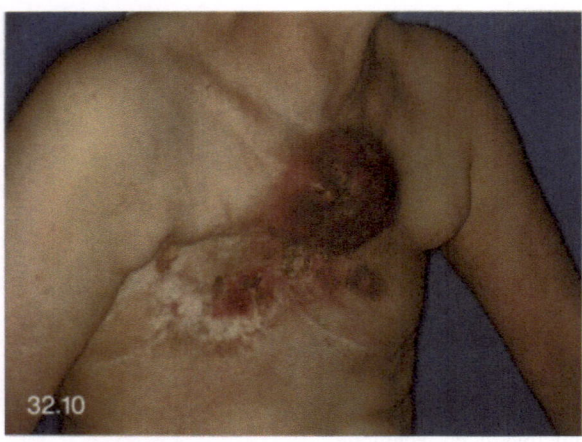

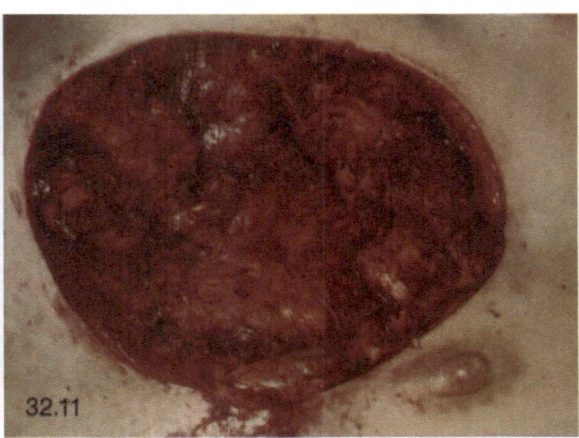

Fig. 32.10. Recurrence of breast cancer with involvement of the manubrium sterni

Fig. 32.11. A wide excision was performed that included partial resection of the right clavicle

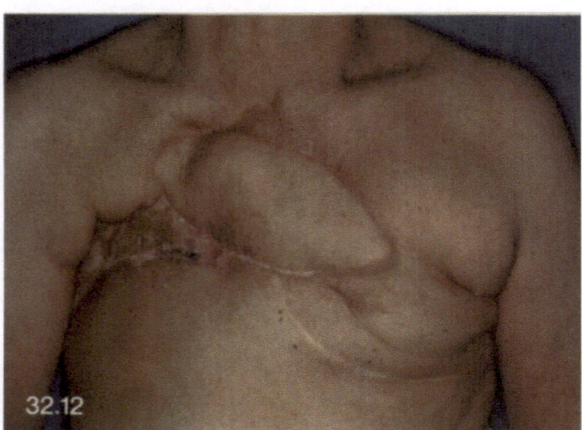

Fig. 32.12. The defect was reconstructed with a latissimus dorsi flap from the left side. Due to the length of the transfer, the skin paddle had to be placed far medially and inferiorly on the latissimus muscle

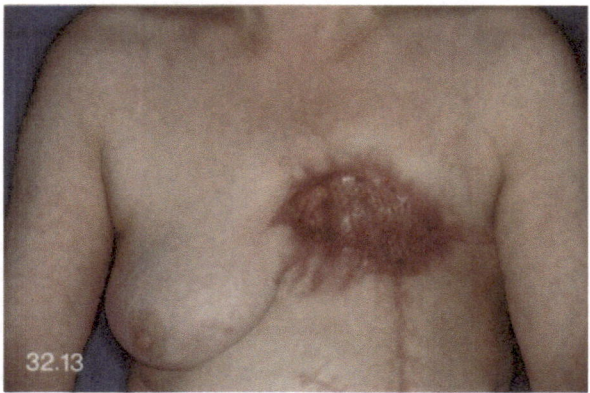

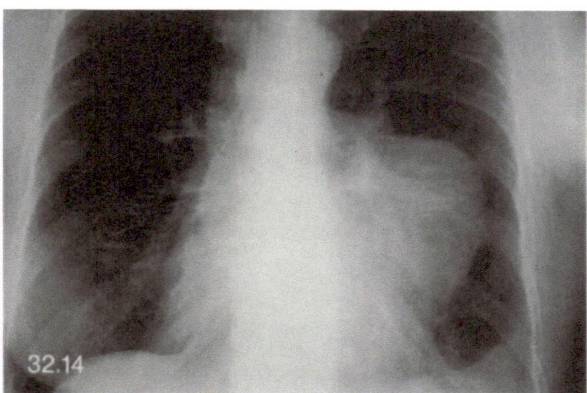

Fig. 32.13. Appearance 12 years after the resection of a cystadenoma phyllodes. The patient had had six recurrences of a fibrosarcoma, and reconstruction with an omental flap had been attempted elsewhere

Fig. 32.14. The preoperative chest radiograph demonstrates the extent of the tumor

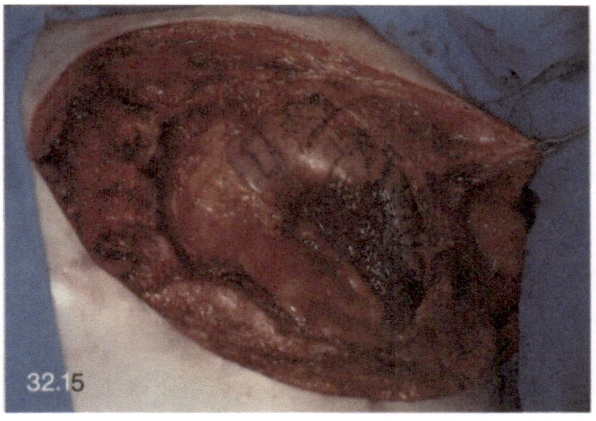

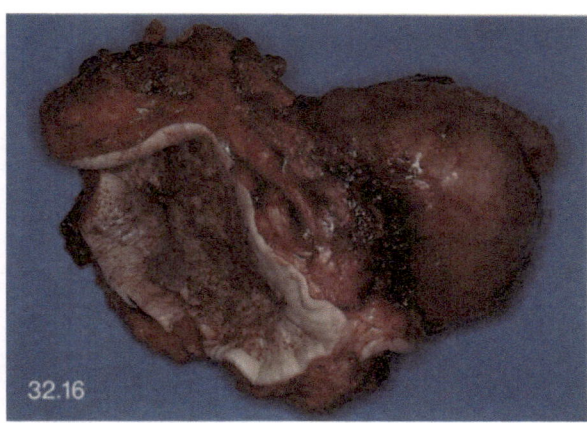

Fig. 32.15. The latest recurrence, which was mainly intrathoracic, was separated from the mediastinum, and the entire sternum was removed

Fig. 32.16. Surgical specimen

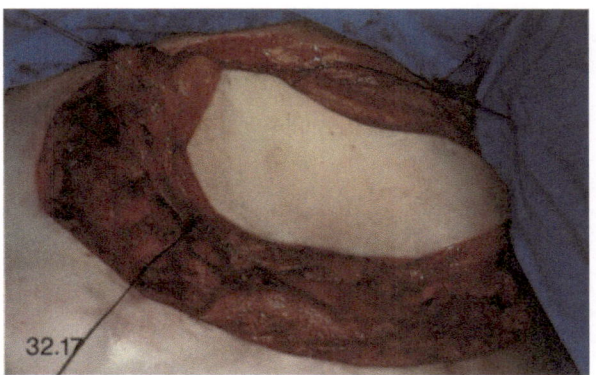

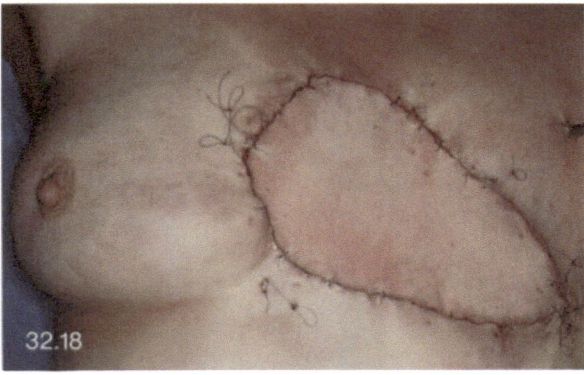

Fig. 32.17. Inset of a latissimus dorsi flap with a large skin island, transposed from the left side

Fig. 32.18. Perfect flap healing

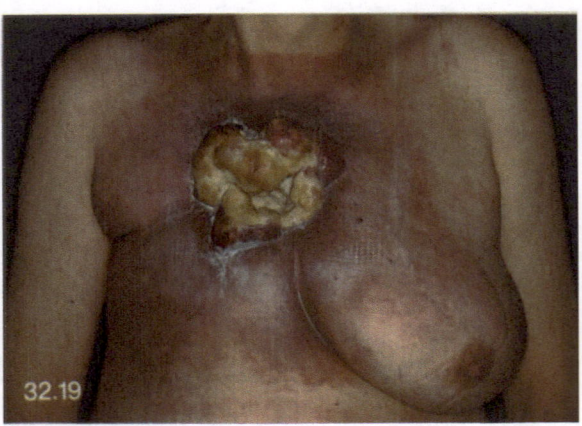

Fig. 32.19. Fist-sized, ulcerating, locally recurrent breast cancer after right mastectomy with subsequent radiation to the sternum

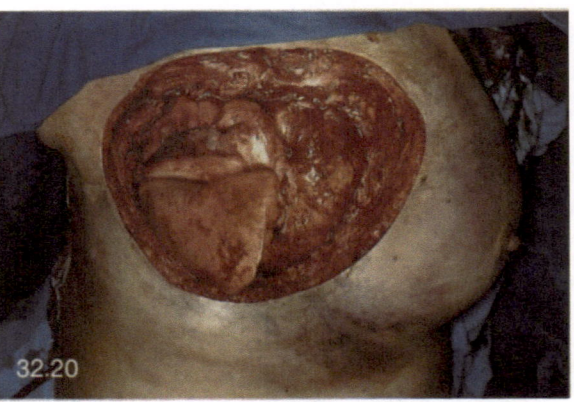

Fig. 32.20. Resection of the entire sternum and the second through sixth ribs on the right side

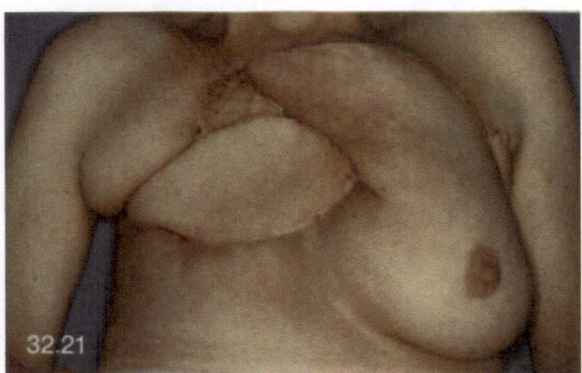

Fig. 32.21. The large defect is covered with a latissimus dorsi flap from the right side, an advancement flap from the left side, and a triangular split-thickness skin graft

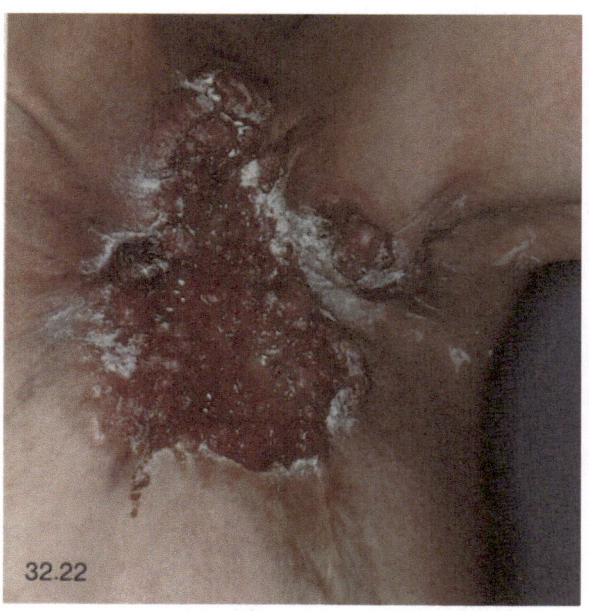

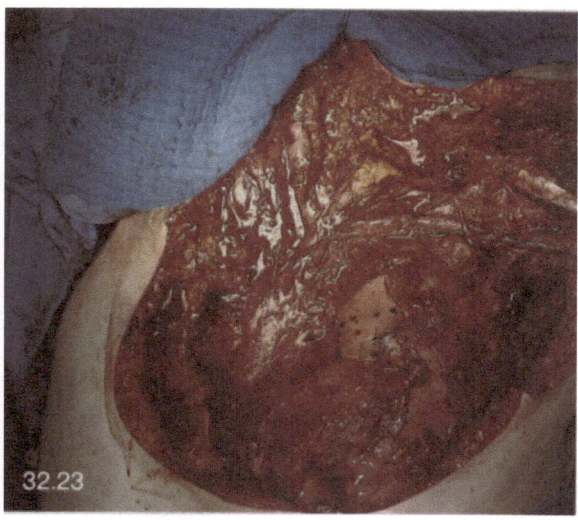

Fig. 32.23. The excision includes resection of the clavicle and the first through fourth ribs

Fig. 32.22. Local recurrence in irradiated skin

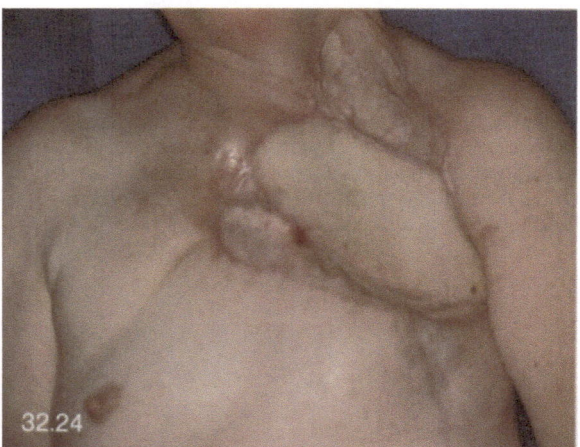

Fig. 32.24. Six months after reconstruction with a latissimus island flap and two mesh grafts

33 Vertical Rectus Abdominis Flap

The vertical rectus flap is as reliable as the latissimus flap but may be easier to elevate since the patient does not have to be repositioned (Robbins 1976). For a large thoracic defect, an L-shaped flap combining the patterns of the VRAM and TRAM flaps can also be designed (Fig. 28.14). During planning of the flap, it must

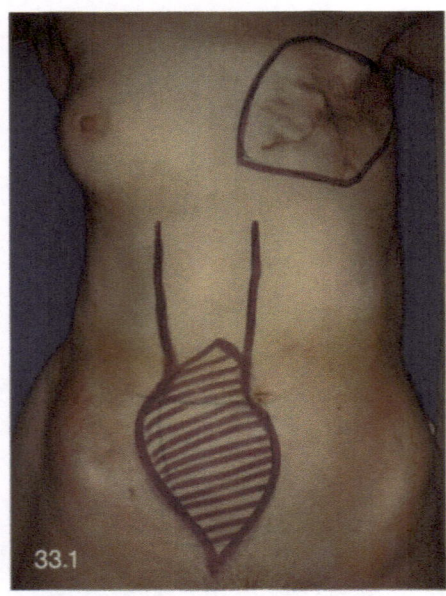

Fig. 33.1. Fifteen years after mastectomy. For the past 6 years the patient had repeated local recurrences that were excised as outpatient procedures. The latest recurrences developed at weekly intervals under chemotherapy despite two irradiations of the chest wall. The proposed excision and vertical rectus flap are outlined

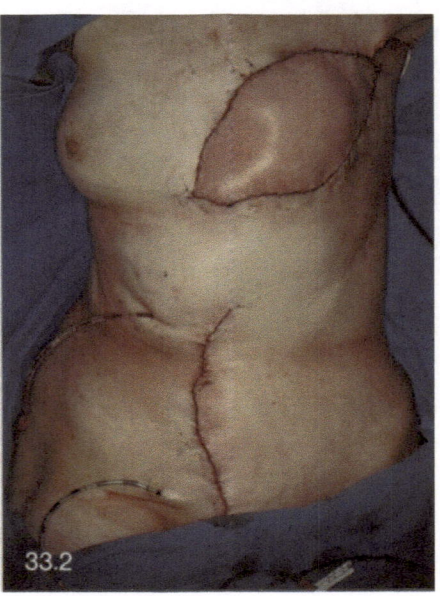

Fig. 33.2. The well-perfused rectus flap is inset into the excisional defect

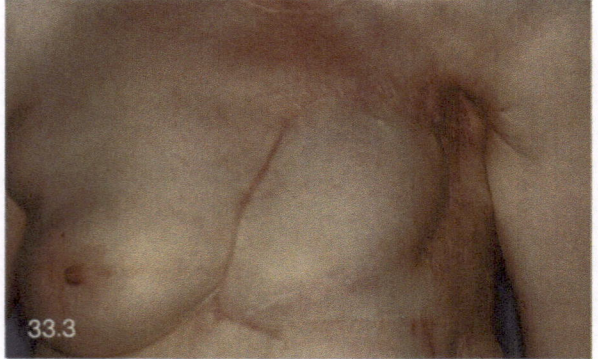

Fig. 33.3. No additional recurrences develop below the musculocutaneous flap, but skin metastases developed in the region of the occiput, left neck, left back, left chest wall, and umbilicus

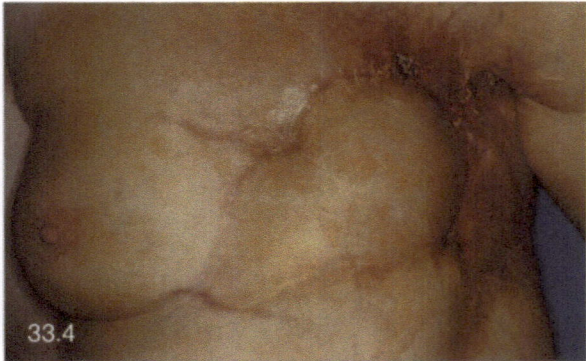

Fig. 33.4. Over a 6-month period the patient underwent 116 outpatient surgical procedures, each involving the removal of 2–5 skin metastases. There is advanced radiofibrosis of the left shoulder with paralysis of the left arm and severe scoliosis

be considered whether the contralateral internal mammary artery is fibrosed due, say, to previous irradiation. While Doppler scanning is an effective tool in the axilla, scans of the superior epigastric artery are less rewarding due to the depth of the vessel.

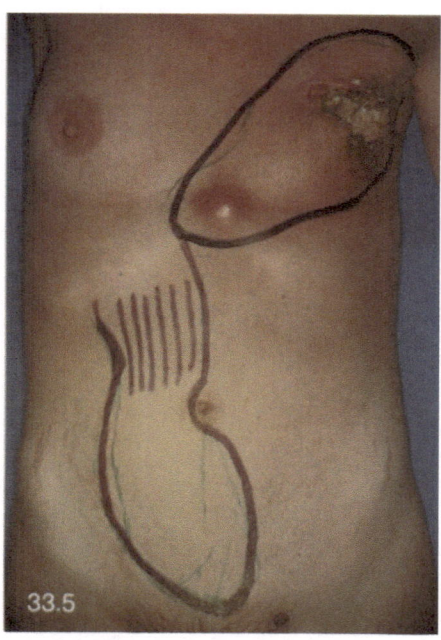

Fig. 33.5. Ulcerating local recurrence in the left anterior axillary line and another local recurrence in the xiphoid region

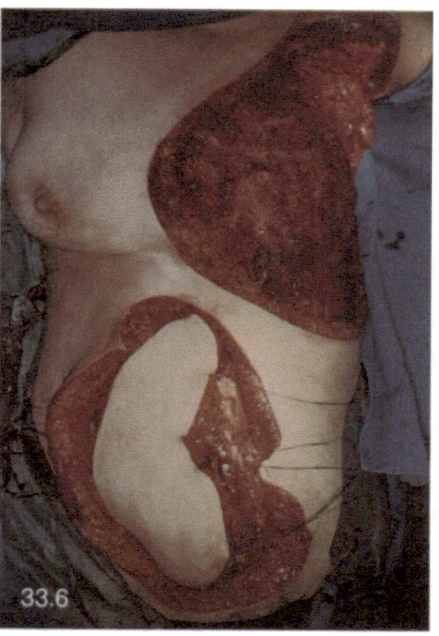

Fig. 33.6. After wide resection of the inferior sternum and partial resection of the third and fourth ribs, the defect is covered with a vertical rectus flap

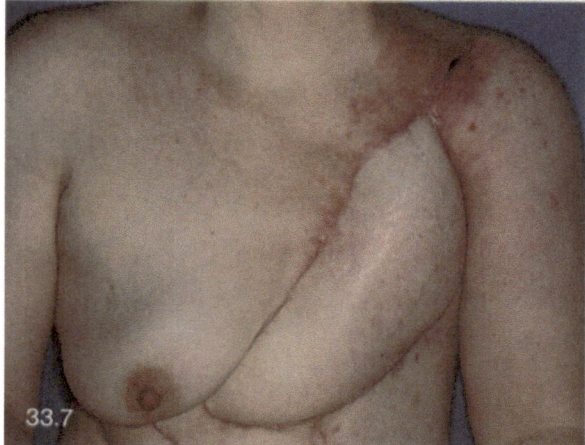

Fig. 33.7. This reliable, well-perfused flap has healed optimally

34 Transverse Rectus Abdominis Flap

The unilateral TRAM flap (Hartrampf and Scheflan 1981) is at much greater risk for tip necrosis than the VRAM flap. Therefore, it should be reserved for breast reconstructions in women who are slender and have not been irradiated. At the same time, the lower abdomen of older, slender patients offers a particularly abundant supply of excess skin. It is a basic rule that the more corpulent a patient is, the poorer the perfusion of the subcutaneous fatty tissue and the greater the

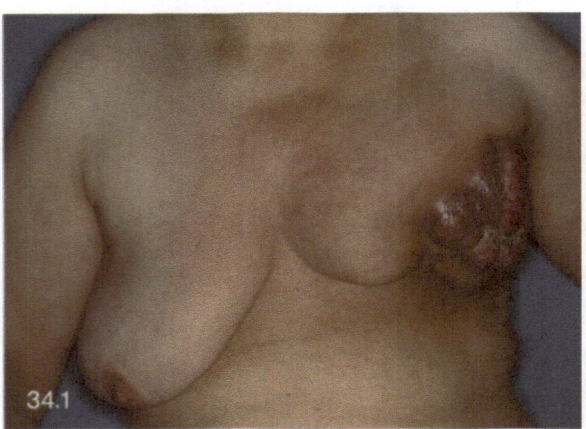

Fig. 34.1. Ulcerating recurrence of breast carcinoma in the irradiated area

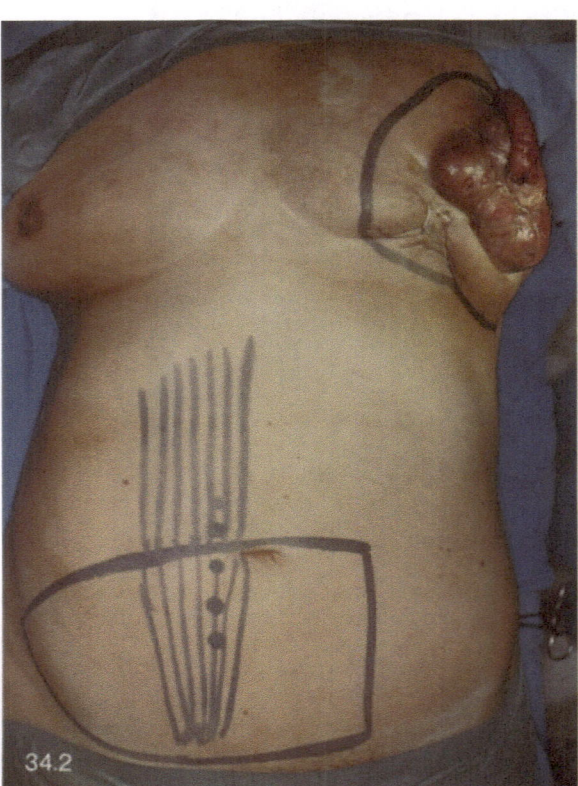

Fig. 34.2. Outline of a transverse rectus flap on the contralateral side

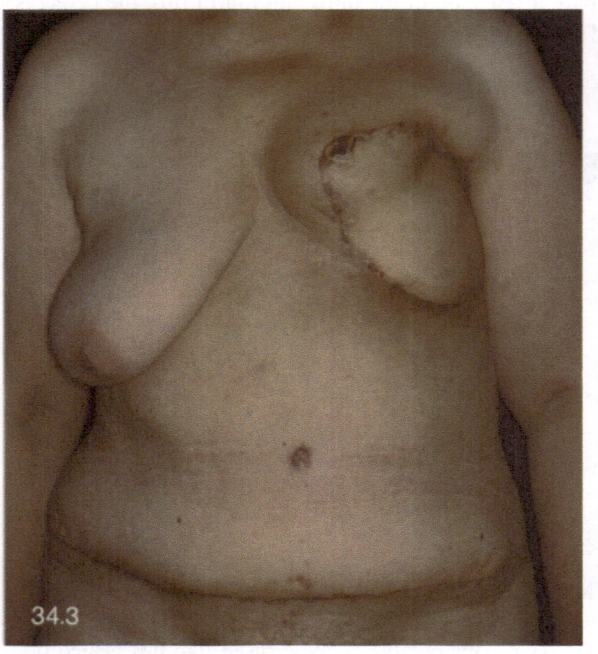

Fig. 34.3. Despite the resection of two ribs, tumor-involved brachial plexus had to be left behind at operation. The defect was easily covered with the rectus abdominis flap. One year later two skin metastases were excised in the cranial portion of the flap

risk of extensive fat necrosis. If the patient also happens to be a heavy smoker, the failure of a rotating flap or island flap is all but inevitable.

With the TRAM flap, this risk can be minimized by using a bipedicled flap if at all possible (Fig. 21.14). This permits the transfer of a relatively large tissue volume from the lower abdomen to the chest wall, and the spine is not subjected to an unbalanced load upon standing. On the other hand, some older patients who have had this procedure complain that they are unable to rise from a squatting position without assistance.

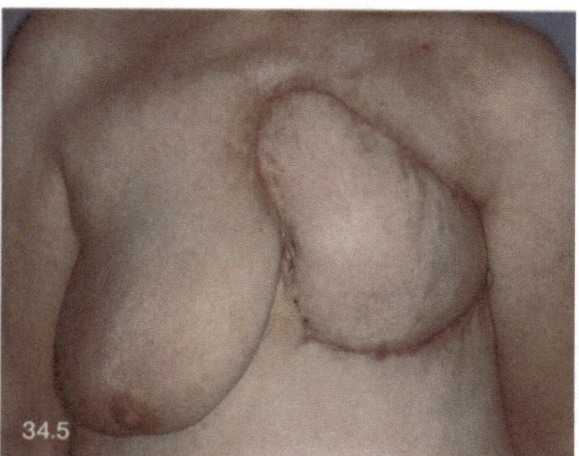

Fig. 34.5. Perfectly healed flap

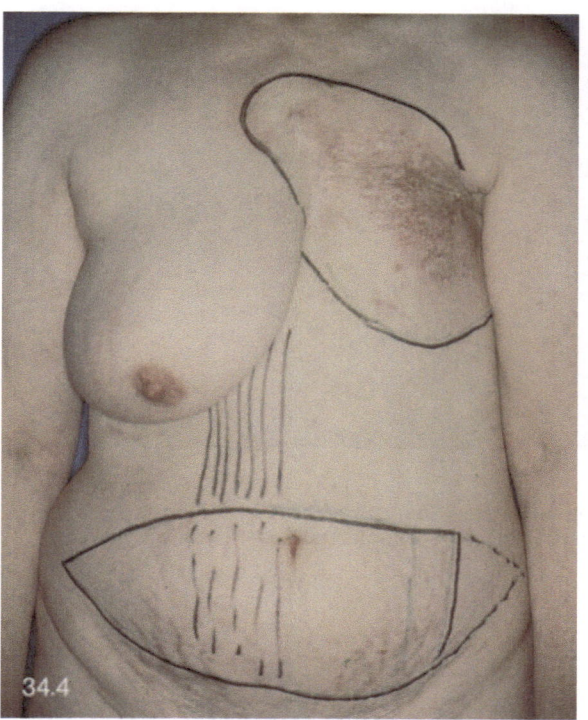

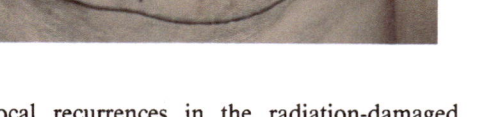

Fig. 34.4. Local recurrences in the radiation-damaged area. The proposed excision and contralateral TRAM flap are outlined

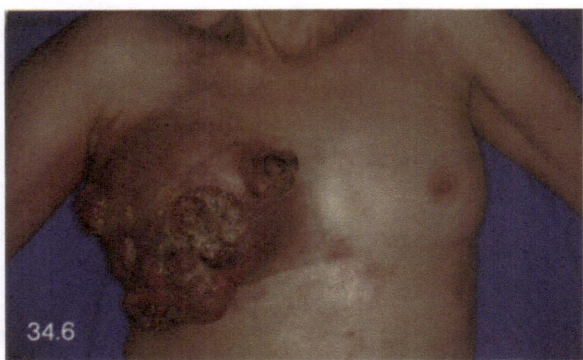

Fig. 34.6. Primary breast carcinoma in a patient who was "reassured" for 4 years and treated "biologically"

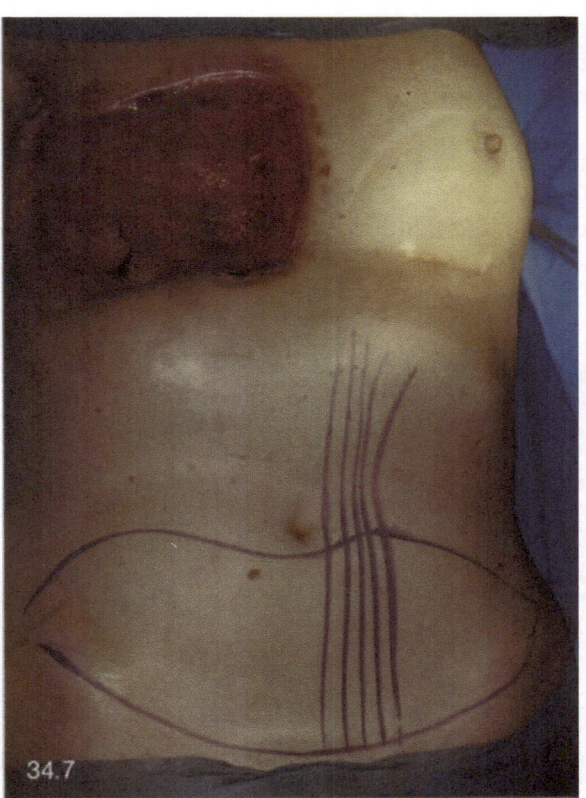

Fig. 34.7. The tumor was heavily infected, so 8 days elapsed before a contralateral TRAM flap was elevated

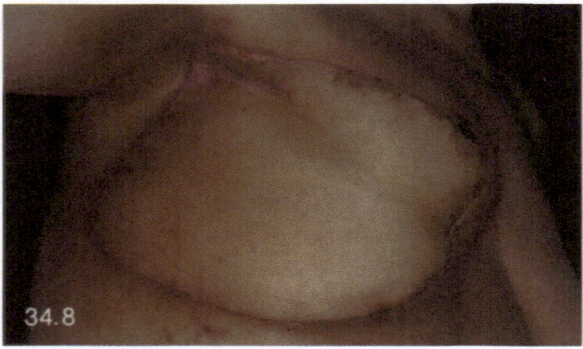

Fig. 34.8. The healed flap 2 weeks later. The patient died 5 months later from distant metastases

35 Upper and Lower Arm Flap

In some breast cancer patients, the arm on the irradiated side is paralyzed due to radiation fibrosis of the brachial plexus or its metastatic encasement. In a number of cases where the paralyzed arm seriously interfered with dressing, turning in bed, and many other activities, we have amputated the arm and afterward seen remarkable improvements in the patient's outlook on life.

In patients with massive metastatic disease of the axilla and also of the chest wall, the skin over part or all of the upper arm can be used to cover the surgical defect. In many cases the humeral head can be exarticulated at the shoulder and shelled from its muscular envelope while pre-

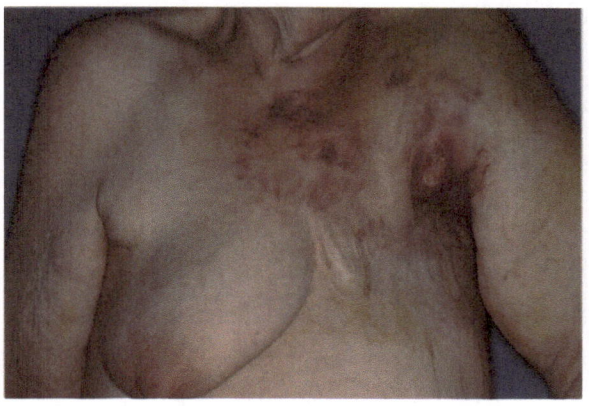

Fig. 35.1. Patient 68 years of age with excruciating pain and paralysis of the left arm due to encasement of the brachial plexus by carcinoma

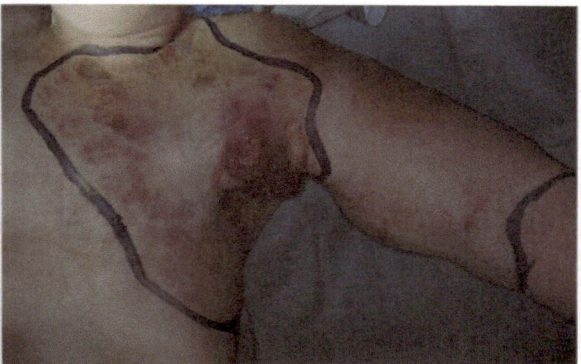

Fig. 35.2. The skin of the paralyzed upper arm is available for reconstruction of the defect

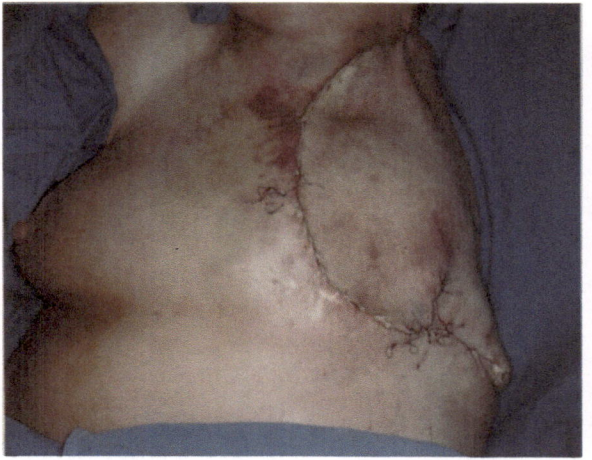

Fig. 35.3. Adequate perfusion of the expanded upper arm flap following removal of the humerus and shoulder joint, scapula, plexus, and clavicle. The prognosis is grave, but the patient's quality of life is substantially improved

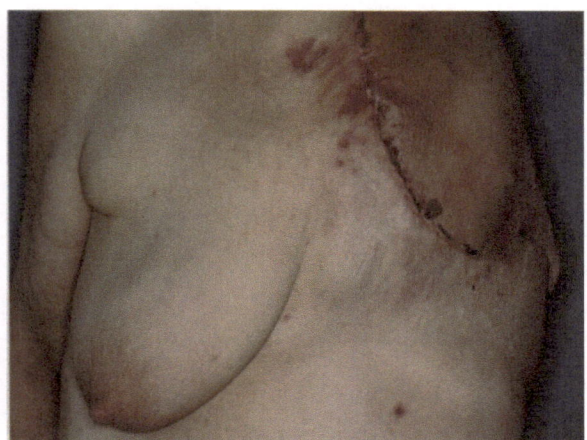

Fig. 35.4. Appearance at discharge. Suddenly relieved of her pain, the patient blossomed psychologically, but she died 2 months later from a pathologic fracture of the cervical spine

serving the axillary artery. In advanced cases, however, it may be necessary to extend the resection to include the clavicle, the entire plexus with the lateral vertebral processes, the scapula, and possibly the thoracic inlet. The trapezius and deltoid muscles should be spared, if possible, to maintain blood supply to the outside of the upper arm, but as much subcutaneous tissue as possible can be removed along the flap margins.

Of course, we recognize that this mutilating operation is palliative in nature, but no other means are available for relieving pain and improving the quality of life in advanced cases of this kind.

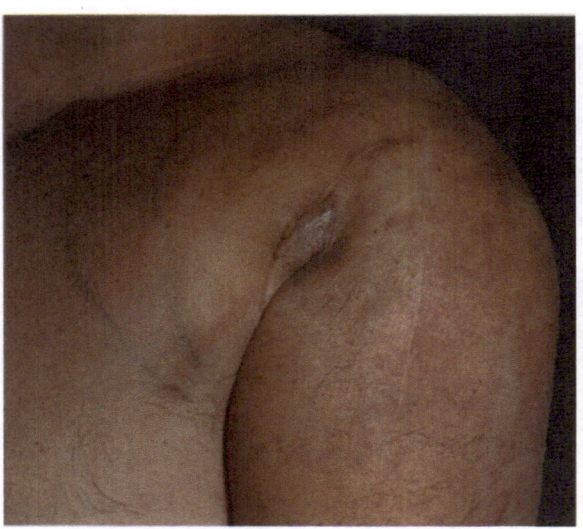

Fig. 35.5. Patient with recurrent sarcoma of the axilla unresponsive to radiotherapy. Radical removal of the whole arm appears to be the only recourse

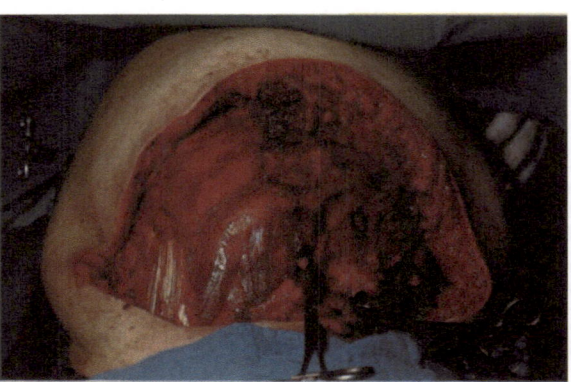

Fig. 35.6. High amputation of the arm including the clavicle, scapula, and plexus. Frozen sections confirm that the thoracic inlet and surrounding skin are free of tumor

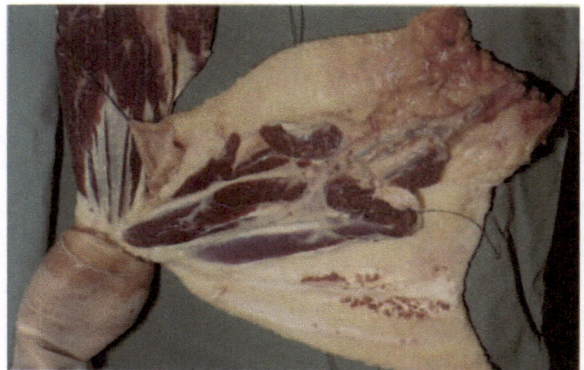

Fig. 35.7. A free lower arm flap that includes all of the skin and some flexor muscles is excellently suited for coverage of the defect. The brachial vessels above the elbow are anastomosed to the stumps of the subclavian vessels

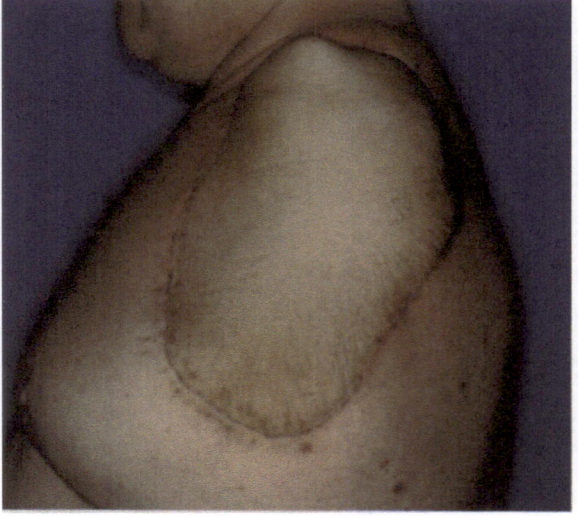

Fig. 35.8. Perfect healing of the lower arm flap to the chest wall (courtesy of Dr. Exner)

References

Arnold PG, Pairolero PC (1979) Use of pectoralis major muscle flap to repair defects of anterior chest wall. Plast Reconstr Surg 63: 205-212

Berrino P, Campora E, Santi P (1987) Postquadrantectomy breast deformities: Classification and techniques of surgical correction. Plast Reconstr Surg 79: 567-572

Bostwick J, Paletta C, Hartrampf CR (1986) Conservative treatment for breast cancer: Complications requiring reconstructive surgery. Ann Surg 203: 481-490

Deutsch M, Parsons JA, Mittal BB (1986) Radiation therapy for local-regional recurrent breast carcinoma. Int J Radiat Oncol Biol Phys 12: 2061-2065

Enke U (1984) Zur Pathogenese der Lokalmetastasierung des Mammacarcinoms. Dissertation, Frankfurt

Exner K, Nievergelt J, Lemperle G (1989) Surgical treatment of local recurrence on the thoracic wall. In: Bohmert H, Leis HP, Jackson IT (eds): Breast cancer - conservative and reconstructive surgery. Thieme, Stuttgart, pp 441-448

Fisher ER, Sass R, Fisher B, Gregorio R, Brown R, Wickerham L (1986) Pathologic findings from the National Surgical Breast Project (Protocol 6). II: Relation of local breast recurrence to multicentricity.Cancer 57: 1717-1724

Herzog P, Exner K, Wollbruck W, Lemperle G, Holtermüller KH (1989) Sonographie in der Diagnostik des lokalen Rezidivs und der Lymphknotenmetastasierung nach Mammakarcinom. Ultraschall Klin Prax 4: 95-98

Koch HI, Voss AC, Ahlemann LP (1980) Die Prognose des Rezidivs beim operierten und nachbestrahlten Mammacarcinom. Strahlentherapie 156: 705-753

Larson DL, Mc Murtrey MJ (1984) Musculocutaneous flap reconstruction of chest wall defects. An experience with 50 patients. Plast Reconstr Surg 73: 734-740

Lejour M, de Mey A, Mattheien W (1983) Local recurrences and metastases of breast cancer after 194 reconstructions. Chir Plast 7: 131-134

Mc Craw JB, Penix JO, Baker JW (1978) Repair of major defects of chest wall and spine with the latissimus dorsi myocutaneous flap. Plast Reconstr Surg 62: 197-206

Olivari N (1976) The latissimus dorsi flap. Br J Plast Surg 29: 126

Tai Y, Hasegawa H (1974) A transverse abdominal flap for reconstruction after radical operations for recurrent breast cancer. Plast Reconstr Surg 53: 52-54

Tansini I (1896) Nuovo processo per l'amputazione della mammaella per cancre. La Reforma Medica 12: 3

Willis RA (1973) The spread of tumors in the human body, 3rd edn. Butterworths, London

Further Reading

Bohmert H, Leis HP, Jackson IT (eds) (1989) Breast cancer – conservative and reconstructive surgery. Thieme, Stuttgart New York

Bostwick J (1989) Plastic and reconstructive breast surgery. Quality Medical Publishing, St. Louis

Lalardrie JP, Jouglard JP (1974) Chirurgie plastique du sein. Masson, Paris

Lejour M (1988) Third International Course on Plastic and Reconstructive Surgery of the Breast. Brussels Congress Centre Publishers, Brussels

Lemperle G, Koslowski L (Hrsg) (1984) Chirurgie der Strahlenfolgen. Urban & Schwarzenberg, München Wien Baltimore

Maillard GF, Montandon D, Goin JL (1983) Plastic reconstructive breast surgery. Médecine et Hygiène, Genève

Mathes SJ, Nahai F, (1989) Reconstructive surgery. Quality Medical Publishing, St. Louis

Maxwell GP (ed.) (1988) Plastic and reconstructive breast surgery. Clin Plast Surg [Suppl]

Mc Craw JB, Arnold PG (1986) Mc Craw and Arnold's atlas of muscle and musculocutaneous flaps. Hampton, Norfolk

Millard DR (1987) Principlization of plastic surgery. Little, Brown, Boston

Strömbeck JO, Rosato FE (1986) Surgery of the breast. Thieme, Stuttgart New York

Subject Index

As of 1991 Organ of the European Association of Plastic Surgeons

Editor-in-Chief:
I. T. Jackson, Southfield, MI

European Co-editor:
D. E. Tolhurst, Rotterdam

Editorial Board Members:
L. Argenta, Winston-Salem, NC
A. Berger, Hannover
W. Boeckx, Leuven
A. Brčić, Ljubljana
L. Clodius, Zurich
    (Book reviews)
M. Costagliola, Toulouse
R. Daoud, Paris
A. De Mey, Brussels
P. Eckert, Würzburg
J. M. Fernandez-Villoria, Madrid
J. Fisher, Nashville, TN
T. Fujino, Tokyo
D. Hauben, Petah Tiqva
J. Holle, Vienna
N. J. Lüscher, Basel
G. Maillard, Lausanne
J. van der Meulen, Rotterdam
T. Milward, Leicester
J.-P. A. Nicolai, Arnhem
B. Palmer, Malmö
Ch. Papp, Innsbruck
G. Pohl, Magdeburg
J. L. del Rio Legarreta, Madrid
D. Soutar, Glasgow
F. Vandenbussche, Lille
D.-M. Wang, Beijing
M. Westreich, Tzrifin
E. Yormuk, Ankara

Members of the societies supporting the journal are entitled to a special reduced subscription rate. Please contact the secretary of your society.

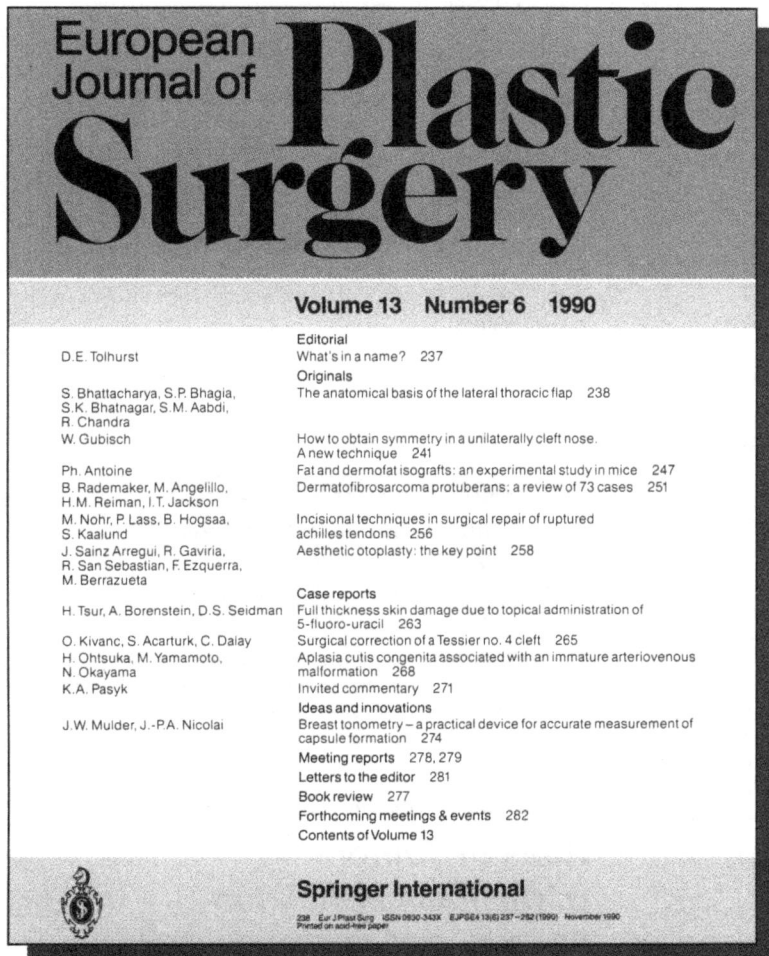

**Official Journal of the Association of German Plastic Surgeons,
Austrian Society for Plastic and Reconstructive Surgery,
Belgian Society for Plastic Surgery,
Dutch Society for Plastic and Reconstructive Surgery,
Turkish Society of Plastic Surgeons**

Send now for your free sample copy or subscription!

Subscription Information:

ISSN 0930-343X   Title No. 238
1991, Volume 14 (6 issues): DM 338,– (suggested list price)
plus carriage charges:
FRG DM 12,20; other countries DM 17,40.

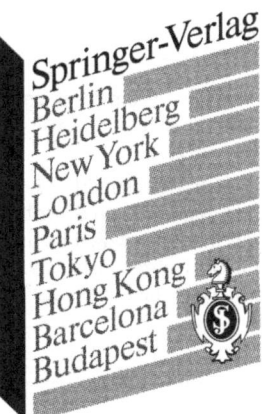

Springer-Verlag
Berlin
Heidelberg
New York
London
Paris
Tokyo
Hong Kong
Barcelona
Budapest

D. Marchac, Paris

Surgery of Basal Cell Carcinoma of the Face

1988. VIII, 115 pp. 80 figs. and 2 color plates.
Hardcover DM 170,- ISBN 3-540-18034-6

The main purpose of this atlas is to show how basal cell carcinomas can be treated in a simple, safe, and effective manner by surgery. The importance of histological confirmation of complete excision is discussed at length. Careful repair according to the principles of plastic surgery can produce excellent aesthetic results.

D. Marchac, Paris (Ed.)

Craniofacial Surgery

Proceedings of the First Congress of the International Society of Cranio-Maxillo-Facial Surgery

1987. XXXVI, 495 pp. 603 figs. in 956 separate illustrations.
Hardcover DM 398,- ISBN 3-540-16924-5

J. Glicenstein, J. Ohana, C. Leclercq, Paris

Tumours of the Hand

1988. XIII, 229 pp. 130 figs., mostly in colour.
Hardcover DM 198,- ISBN 3-540-17439-7

This book deals with both benign and malignant tumours of the hand classified under the following headings: skin tumours, soft tissue tumours, bone tumours and tumours of the nail. It analyzes the different aspects of each of these tumours on a clinical, radiologic, pathologic, histologic and therapeutic level.

"A unique book..."

Annals of the Royal College of Surgeons of England

R. T. Manktelow, Toronto

Microvascular Reconstruction

Anatomy, Applications and Surgical Technique

1986. XIII, 221 pp. 288 figs. Hardcover DM 390,-
ISBN 3-540-15271-7

This book is aimed at experienced surgeons and trainees as a "when, what, and how to" guide to microvascular reconstruction surgery.

"The book is superb. The author does not try to cover every flap that has been described, instead he covers 10 different types of flaps which he uses frequently and with which the majority of reconstructive problems can be solved. The book is cleverly laid out to facilitate its use as a reference source."

The Medical Journal of Australia

R. Loeb, University of São Paulo, Brazil

Aesthetic Surgery of the Eyelids

Translated from the Portuguese by S. Braley

1989. XI, 155 pp. 167 figs. in 474 parts, incl. 260 in color.
Hardcover DM 360,- ISBN 3-540-96912-8

Contents: Anatomical Considerations. - Scleral Show. - Bulges of the Skin, Fat, Muscle and Bone Tissue. - Depressions of the Eyelids. - Complementary Surgeries. - Ectropions, Hematomas, and Other Complications. - Index.

This unique volume distills the proven techniques of an internationally respected plastic surgeon.
The "Scleral Show" chapter is the most complete treatment on this topic and the section on surgical correction of depression deformities masterfully demonstrates the author's original techniques.

D. J. David, North Adelaide, South Australia; **D. C. Hemmy,** Milwaukee, WI; **R. D. Cooter,** North Adelaide, South Australia

Craniofacial Deformities

Atlas of Three-Dimensional Reconstruction from Computed Tomography

1990. X, 147 pp. 106 figs. in 461 parts. Hardcover DM 236,-
ISBN 3-540-96969-1

The authors have assembled a comprehensive atlas which analyzes the three-dimensional reconstruction techniques and compares and contrasts computed tomography images with standard X-ray images of various craniofacial disorders.

J. Prein, Basel; **W. Remagen, B. Spiessl, E. Uehlinger,** Zürich

Atlas of Tumors of the Facial Skeleton

Odontogenic and Nonodontogenic Tumors

Central Registry of DÖSAK (German-Austrian-Swiss Association for the Study of Tumors of the Face and Jaws)

1986. X, 162 pp. 264 figs. mostly in color.
Hardcover DM 368,- ISBN 3-540-16167-8

"This volume is an essential addition to the library of head and neck surgeons from whatever discipline. It will be continually referred to by the 'physician' presented with a rare facial bony tumor."

British Journal of Plastic Surgery

Prices are subject to change without notice.

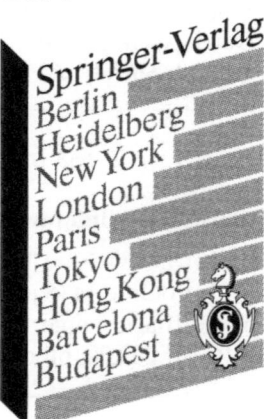

Springer-Verlag
Berlin
Heidelberg
New York
London
Paris
Tokyo
Hong Kong
Barcelona
Budapest